Lymphoma

METHODS IN MOLECULAR MEDICINE™

John M. Walker, Series Editor

123. **Marijuana and Cannabinoid Research:** *Methods and Protocols,* edited by *Emmanuel S. Onaivi, 2006*
122. **Placenta Research Methods and Protocols:** *Volume 2,* edited by *Michael J. Soares and Joan S. Hunt, 2006*
121. **Placenta Research Methods and Protocols:** *Volume 1,* edited by *Michael J. Soares and Joan S. Hunt, 2006*
120. **Breast Cancer Research Protocols,** edited by *Susan A. Brooks and Adrian Harris, 2005*
119. **Human Papilloma Viruses:** *Methods and Protocols,* edited by *Clare Davy and John Doorbar, 2005*
118. **Antifungal Agents:** *Methods and Protocols,* edited by *Erika J. Ernst and P. David Rogers, 2005*
117. **Fibrosis Research:** *Methods and Protocols,* edited by *John Varga, David A. Brenner, and Sem H. Phan, 2005*
116. **Inteferon Methods and Protocols,** edited by *Daniel J. J. Carr, 2005*
115. **Lymphoma:** *Methods and Protocols,* edited by *Timothy Illidge and Peter W. M. Johnson, 2005*
114. **Microarrays in Clinical Diagnostics,** edited by *Thomas O. Joos and Paolo Fortina, 2005*
113. **Multiple Myeloma:** *Methods and Protocols,* edited by *Ross D. Brown and P. Joy Ho, 2005*
112. **Molecular Cardiology:** *Methods and Protocols,* edited by *Zhongjie Sun, 2005*
111. **Chemosensitivity:** *Volume 2, In Vivo Models, Imaging, and Molecular Regulators,* edited by *Rosalyn D. Blumethal, 2005*
110. **Chemosensitivity:** *Volume 1, In Vitro Assays,* edited by *Rosalyn D. Blumethal, 2005*
109. **Adoptive Immunotherapy:** *Methods and Protocols,* edited by *Burkhard Ludewig and Matthias W. Hoffman, 2005*
108. **Hypertension:** *Methods and Protocols,* edited by *Jérôme P. Fennell and Andrew H. Baker, 2005*
107. **Human Cell Culture Protocols,** *Second Edition,* edited by *Joanna Picot, 2005*
106. **Antisense Therapeutics,** *Second Edition,* edited by *M. Ian Phillips, 2005*
105. **Developmental Hematopoiesis:** *Methods and Protocols,* edited by *Margaret H. Baron, 2005*
104. **Stroke Genomics:** *Methods and Reviews,* edited by *Simon J. Read and David Virley, 2004*
103. **Pancreatic Cancer:** *Methods and Protocols,* edited by *Gloria H. Su, 2004*
102. **Autoimmunity:** *Methods and Protocols,* edited by *Andras Perl, 2004*
101. **Cartilage and Osteoarthritis:** *Volume 2, Structure and In Vivo Analysis,* edited by *Frédéric De Ceuninck, Massimo Sabatini, and Philippe Pastoureau, 2004*
100. **Cartilage and Osteoarthritis:** *Volume 1, Cellular and Molecular Tools,* edited by *Massimo Sabatini, Philippe Pastoureau, and Frédéric De Ceuninck, 2004*
99. **Pain Research:** *Methods and Protocols,* edited by *David Z. Luo, 2004*
98. **Tumor Necrosis Factor:** *Methods and Protocols,* edited by *Angelo Corti and Pietro Ghezzi, 2004*
97. **Molecular Diagnosis of Cancer:** *Methods and Protocols, Second Edition,* edited by *Joseph E. Roulston and John M. S. Bartlett, 2004*
96. **Hepatitis B and D Protocols:** *Volume 2, Immunology, Model Systems, and Clinical Studies,* edited by *Robert K. Hamatake and Johnson Y. N. Lau, 2004*
95. **Hepatitis B and D Protocols:** *Volume 1, Detection, Genotypes, and Characterization,* edited by *Robert K. Hamatake and Johnson Y. N. Lau, 2004*
94. **Molecular Diagnosis of Infectious Diseases,** *Second Edition,* edited by *Jochen Decker and Udo Reischl, 2004*
93. **Anticoagulants, Antiplatelets, and Thrombolytics,** edited by *Shaker A. Mousa, 2004*
92. **Molecular Diagnosis of Genetic Diseases,** *Second Edition,* edited by *Rob Elles and Roger Mountford, 2004*
91. **Pediatric Hematology:** *Methods and Protocols,* edited by *Nicholas J. Goulden and Colin G. Steward, 2003*
90. **Suicide Gene Therapy:** *Methods and Reviews,* edited by *Caroline J. Springer, 2004*
89. **The Blood–Brain Barrier:** *Biology and Research Protocols,* edited by *Sukriti Nag, 2003*
88. **Cancer Cell Culture:** *Methods and Protocols,* edited by *Simon P. Langdon, 2003*
87. **Vaccine Protocols,** *Second Edition,* edited by *Andrew Robinson, Michael J. Hudson, and Martin P. Cranage, 2003*
86. **Renal Disease:** *Techniques and Protocols,* edited by *Michael S. Goligorsky, 2003*
85. **Novel Anticancer Drug Protocols,** edited by *John K. Buolamwini and Alex A. Adjei, 2003*

METHODS IN MOLECULAR MEDICINE™

Lymphoma

Methods and Protocols

Edited by

Tim Illidge

CRUK, Paterson Institute for Cancer Research, University of Manchester, Manchester, UK

Peter W. M. Johnson

Cancer Sciences Division, Southampton General Hospital, Southampton, UK

HUMANA PRESS TOTOWA, NEW JERSEY

Softcover reprint of the hardcover 1st edition 2005
999 Riverview Drive, Suite 208
Totowa, New Jersey 07512

www.humanapress.com

This publication is printed on acid-free paper. ∞
ANSI Z39.48-1984 (American Standards Institute) Permanence of Paper for Printed Library Materials.

Production Editor: Nicole E. Furia
Cover design by Patricia F. Cleary

Cover Illustration: Figure 1 from Chapter 14, "Antibody Techniques Used in the Study of Anaplastic Lymphoma Kinase-Positive ALCL," by Karen Pulford, Helen M. Roberton, and Margaret Jones.

For additional copies, pricing for bulk purchases, and/or information about other Humana titles, contact Humana at the above address or at any of the following numbers: Tel.: 973-256-1699; Fax: 973-256-8341; E-mail: orders@humanapr.com; or visit our Website: www.humanapress.com

10 9 8 7 6 5 4 3 2 1

ISBN 978-1-61737-395-4 eISBN 978-1-59259-936-3

Library of Congress Cataloging-in-Publication Data

Lymphoma : methods and protocols / edited by Timothy Illidge, Peter W.M. Johnson.
p. ; cm. — (Methods in molecular medicine, ISSN 1543-1894 ; 115)
Includes bibliographical references and index.

1. Lymphomas—Molecular aspects—Laboratory manuals.
[DNLM: 1. Lymphoma. 2. Clinical Laboratory Techniques. 3. Genetic Techniques. WH 525 L9854 2005] I. Illidge, Timothy. II. Johnson, P. W. M. III. Series.
RC280.L9L9527 2005
616.99'446—dc22

2004026632

Preface

The molecular investigation of hematological malignancies has always forerun that of other cancers. There are a number of potential reasons for this, some of which are more logistical than theoretical, and include the ready access to pathologic material with the presence of malignant cells generally in great excess in comparison with the normal. These factors are combined with a set of diseases for which potentially curative systemic therapies are available, making the precise subclassification for prognostic and therapeutic purposes even more important. In general, studies of the leukemias have first started with immunophenotyping, classical cytogenetics, restriction digest analysis, polymerase chain reaction studies (PCR), fluorescent *in situ* hybridization (FISH), and comparative genomic hybridization. Most recently, gene expression arrays have been tested first in leukemia, closely followed by the application of these techniques to lymphoma.

The different techniques described in *Lymphoma: Methods and Protocols* have evolved in parallel over the last three decades. The first was classical cytogenetics and the identification of consistent structural abnormalities in the chromosomes of malignant cells, with the findings linked to morphologic and immunophenotypic entities. From chromosomal rearrangements, reverse genetics led to the characterization of key genes adjacent to breakpoints, whose function was then related back to the abnormal cellular behavior. The finding that an activating oncogene, c-Myc, was involved in the characteristic chromosome 8 breakpoint in Burkitt's lymphoma was a key moment for this field. Analysis of different breakpoints has yielded other, similarly important insights, such as identification of a failure to undergo apoptosis as a central mechanism in malignancy following the finding of the Bcl-2 gene at the chromosome 18q21 breakpoint in follicular lymphoma. The field of cytogenetics has been enhanced greatly by the development of FISH, in which insights into more sophisticated patterns of chromosomal abnormality can be understood, and there has subsequently been a steady rise in the number of regions for study.

An increase in our understanding of lymphocyte biology, particularly B-cell ontogeny and the germinal center reaction has led to the application of immunoglobulin gene rearrangements as markers of clonality and to patterns of somatic mutation in the variable regions being used as indicators of the stage in development at which transformation occurred. Study of these patterns of mutation in low-grade lymphoma has yielded the fascinating information that follicular types are preferentially mutated at glycosylation sites, suggestive of a ligand-related selection pressure in the germinal center during pathogenesis. In chronic lymphocytic leukemia (CLL) the more "immature" unmutated/nongerminal center types show a considerably more aggressive course than the post-germinal center mutated cases. There are interesting parallels in diffuse large B-cell lymphoma, which is always mutated in the immunoglobulin V genes, but in which a germinal center immunophenotype and pattern of mRNA expression conveys a better prognosis. The application of gene arrays to the question of biological heterogeneity in morphologically similar diseases has been especially rewarding. Different subtypes of large B-cell lymphoma have been clearly defined, and the grey zone between Hodgkin lymphoma and sclerosing mediastinal lymphoma is being steadily illuminated.

Currently gene arrays are not a routine part of the diagnostic investigation for lymphoma, although it seems highly likely that this will be the case for subsequent editions of this book. However, it may be that the gene signatures are sufficiently paralleled by the phenotype to allow immunohistochemistry to be used instead, once a firm correlation has been established. This looks likely to be the case for large B-cell lymphoma with the use of Bcl-6 and CD10 as germinal center markers, and certainly broadens the applicability of the classification when fresh biopsy material is difficult to obtain.

The process of classifying and reclassifying lymphoma has been a source of some frustration for clinicians and pathologists alike for many years, but the advent of the Revised European American Lymphoma (REAL) classification and subsequently its adoption into the new WHO classification have brought unprecedented harmony into this area. The recognition of REAL disease entities has been critical to the assimilation of immunophenotypic and molecular data into the classification, which has been a notable success. The process of subdividing the different entities along biological lines is well underway, with classes of CLL and diffuse large B-cell lymphoma already characterized as described. Other entities such as MALT lymphoma are being split down according to the precise translocation present, and in all these cases the subdivisions seem likely to have relevance to the type of therapy chosen. Thus, gastric MALT lymphoma with a t(11;18)(q21;q21) is much more likely to respond to the eradication of *Helicobacter pylori* than is one with t(1;14)(p22;q32).

The use of such molecular information to guide therapy is slowly gaining ground, although in other areas the benefits remain less clear. The detection of minimal residual disease using PCR techniques has been extensively studied, particularly in follicular lymphoma, with the general conclusion that absence of the pathognomonic t(14;18)(q32;q21) translocation at the time of clinical remission is preferable, but no firm data as to whether the pursuit of such molecular remission actually conveys a survival benefit. Until the advent of rituximab antibody therapy there were few patients in whom molecular remission was achieved with anything less than myeloablative treatment, but now that there is an intervention that can achieve a high rate of conversion from PCR-positive to PCR-negative it may be possible to test the validity of this hypothesis. The use of quantitative PCR to follow progress sequentially has added a further level of refinement to this approach and made it much easier to consider therapy directed by molecular results.

As well as providing prognostic information, molecular analyses have been used to produce novel therapeutics, especially in the area of immunotherapy. Characterization of the lymphocyte cell surface molecules has been used to identify antigens against which vaccines or antibodies may be deployed, and the newer technique of serological identification by expression cloning (SEREX) has provided a wealth of information on this. The idiotype represents the truly unique antigen on a B-cell surface and here once again the application of molecular techniques has been able to provide a highly specific immunogen, in the form of a DNA vaccine with patient-specific sequences derived from the lymphoma.

In conclusion, the aim of this book is to give some practical information on the current molecular approaches being used in the understanding, classification, and therapy of lymphoma. Though it cannot be exhaustive in providing information for every chromosomal translocation and gene rearrangement, we hope that it provides a useful background to the field and a means to get started with the molecular diagnostics of a group of diseases that are both biologically interesting and medically important.

Tim Illidge
Peter Johnson

Contents

Contributors

Gavin Babbage • *Cancer Sciences Division, University of Southampton, Southampton, UK*

Alison H. Banham • *Nuffield Department of Clinical Laboratory Sciences, University of Oxford, Oxford, UK*

Sharon Barrans • *Leeds Teaching Hospitals NHS Trust, Leeds, UK*

David Blythe • *Leeds Teaching Hospitals NHS Trust, Leeds, UK*

Elias Campo • *Department of Pathology, Hospital Clinic, University of Barcelona, Barcelona, Spain*

Claire Dallman • *Cancer Sciences Division, University of Southampton, Southampton, UK*

Angela Darby • *CRUK Oncology Unit, University of Southampton School of Medicine, Southampton University Hospitals NHS Trust, Southampton, UK*

Silvana Debarnardi • *St. Bartholomew's Hospital, London, UK*

Mariella Dono • *División Oncologia Medica C, Instituto Nazionale per la Ricerca Sul Cancro, Genova, Italy*

Martin J. S. Dyer • *Department of Cancer Studies and Molecular Medicine, University of Leicester, Leicester, UK*

Manlio Ferrarini • *Dipartamento Oncologia, Biologia e Genetica, Un. Studi di Genova, Genova, Italy; Instituto Nazionale per la Ricerca Sul Cancro, Genova, Italy*

John G. Gribben • *Department of Medical Oncology, Barts and the London School of Medicine, London, UK*

Barbara A. Guinn • *Guy's, Kings, and St. Thomas' School of Medicine, London, UK*

Susan Harris • *Wessex Immunology Service, Southampton University Hospital NHS Trust, Southampton, UK*

Christine J. Harrison • *Leukaemia Research Fund Cytogenetics Group, Cancer Sciences Division, Southampton University Hospitals NHS Trust, Southampton, UK*

Luis Hernández • *Department of Pathology, Hospital Clinic, University of Barcelona, Barcelona, Spain*

Viktoria Hjalmar • *Karolinska Hospital, Stockholm, Sweden*

Elizabeth Hodges • *Wessex Immunology Service, Southampton University Hospitals NHS Trust, Southampton, UK*

Rachel E. Ibbotson • *Molecular Biology Department, Royal Bournemouth Hospital, Bournemouth, UK*

TIM ILLIDGE • *Patterson Institute for Cancer Research, University of Manchester, Manchester, UK*
ANDREW JACK • *Leeds Teaching Hospitals NHS Trust, Leeds, UK*
PETER W. M. JOHNSON • *Cancer Sciences Division, Southampton University Hospitals NHS Trust, Southampton, UK*
MARGARET JONES • *Nuffield Department of Clinical Laboratory Sciences, University of Oxford, Oxford, UK*
JASPAL S. KAEDA • *Division of Investigative Sciences, Department of Haematology, Imperial College of London, London, UK*
E. LORAINE KARRAN • *Department of Cancer Studies and Molecular Medicine, University of Leicester, Leicester, UK*
KIM LAST • *St. Bartholomew's Hospital, London, UK*
AMANDA P. LIGGINS • *Nuffield Department of Clinical Laboratory Sciences, University of Oxford, Oxford, UK*
T. ANDREW LISTER • *St. Bartholomew's Hospital, London, UK*
KATY MCCANN • *Cancer Sciences Division, Southampton University Hospitals NHS Trust, University of Southampton, Southampton, UK*
DAVID G. OSCIER • *Haematology Department, Royal Bournemouth Hospital, Bournemouth, UK*
CHRISTIAN H. OTTENSMEIER • *Cancer Sciences Division, Southampton University Hospitals NHS Trust, University of Southampton, Southampton, UK*
GRAHAM PACKHAM • *Cancer Sciences Division, University of Southampton, Southampton, UK*
ANTON E. PARKER • *Molecular Biology Department, Royal Bournemouth Hospital, Bournemouth, UK*
KAREN PULFORD • *Nuffield Department of Clinical Laboratory Sciences, University of Oxford, Oxford, UK*
ANDREW RAWSTRON • *Leeds Teaching Hospitals NHS Trust, Leeds, UK*
HELEN M. ROBERTON • *Nuffield Department of Clinical Laboratory Sciences, University of Oxford, Oxford, UK*
FIONA M. ROSS • *Wessex Regional Genetics Laboratory, Salisbury District Hospital, Salisbury, UK and Human Genetics Division, University of Southampton, Southampton, UK*
SURINDER S. SAHOTA • *Cancer Sciences Division, Southampton University Hospitals NHS Trust, University of Southampton, Southampton, UK*
JOHN L. SMITH • *Wessex Immunology Service, Southampton University Hospitals NHS Trust, Southampton, UK*
TAKASHI SONOKI • *Second Department of Internal Medicine, Kumamoto University School of Medicine, Japan*
FREDA K. STEVENSON • *Cancer Sciences Division, Southampton University Hospitals NHS Trust, University of Southampton, Southampton, UK*

Simon D. Wagner • *Division of Investigative Sciences, Department of Haematology, Imperial College London, London, UK*
Anthony P. Williams • *Wessex Immunology Service, Southampton University Hospitals NHS Trust, Southampton, UK*
Niklas Zojer • *Cancer Sciences Division, Southampton University Hospitals NHS Trust, University of Southampton, Southampton, UK*

Color Plate

With thanks to Schering Health Care Ltd (UK) for support
of the color insert in this publication.

Color Plates 1–12 appear as an insert following p. 270.

Color Plate 1: Chapter 1, Figure 2.
Flow cytometric analysis of cell surface markers on purified follicular lymphoma cells. For discussion and full legend, *see* p. 7–9.

Color Plate 2: Chapter 5, Figure 3.
Membrane following primary screening and color development. For discussion and full legend, *see* p. 123–124.

Color Plate 3: Chapter 5, Figure 4.
Membrane following secondary screening and color development. For discussion and full legend, *see* p. 123–124.

Color Plate 4: Chapter 5, Figure 5.
Membrane following tertiary screening and color development. For discussion and full legend, *see* p. 123, 125.

Color Plate 5: Chapter 7, Figure 1.
Flowchart of V gene analysis. For discussion, *see* p. 149.

Color Plate 6: Chapter 9, Figure 2.
PCR analysis of *TCRG* gene rearrangements. For discussion and full legend *see* p. 203–204, 207, 210.

Color Plate 7: Chapter 9, Figure 3.
PCR analysis of *TCRB* gene rearrangements. For discussion and full legend, *see* p. 205–207.

Color Plate 8: Chapter 9, Figure 4.
PCR analysis of *TCRD* gene rearrangements. For discussion and full legend, *see* p. 207–208, 212.

Color Plate 9: Chapter 10, Figure 1.
Schema showing the structure of the rearrangements within the immunoglobulin heavy (*IGH*). For discussion and full legend, *see* p. 219–220.

Color Plate 10: Chapter 14, Figure 1.
Immunolabeling studies on ALK-positive ALCL. For discussion and full legend, *see* p. 280–284.

Color Plate 11: Chapter 11, Figure 1.
FISH for trisomy 12 in peripheral blood from a patient with CLL. For discussion, *see* p. 235–236.

Color Plate 12: Chapter 16, Figure 4.
Quantitative real-time PCR analysis. For discussion and full legend, *see* p. 321–323, 325.

1

Purification of Primary Malignant B-Cells and Immunoblot Analysis of Bcl-2 Family Proteins

Claire Dallman and Graham Packham

Summary

The ability to isolate relatively pure populations of primary normal and malignant lymphocytes has brought studies of lymphoid malignancies to the forefront of cancer research. Apoptosis (programmed cell death) plays a key role in controlling normal B-cell numbers, and resistance to apoptosis contributes to lymphomagenesis and reduces the effectiveness of chemotherapy and radiotherapy. Multiple Bcl-2 family proteins orchestrate key life and death decisions in lymphocytes, and the prototypical family member, Bcl-2, is activated by reciprocal translocation in human lymphoma. Here, we describe an immunomagnetic method to isolate and purify malignant B-cells suitable for in vitro analyses from lymph node biopsies. Methods to analyze the expression of Bcl-2 family proteins by immunoblotting also are described.

Key Words: Bcl-2; apoptosis; lymphoma; purification; immunoblotting.

1. Introduction

Apoptosis is a genetically controlled cell death pathway that plays a key role in controlling normal lymphocyte numbers. B-cell development is characterized by waves of apoptosis that delete unwanted cells with, for example, nonfunctional or self-reactive B-cell receptor rearrangements *(1)*. Given the key role of apoptosis in controlling lymphocyte numbers, it is not surprising that its suppression promotes lymphomagenesis. Moreover, many treatments for lymphoma, such as cytotoxics, act via induction of apoptosis. Analyzing the molecular events that control apoptosis in normal and malignant lymphocytes, therefore, should provide new insights into the mechanisms of lymphoma development and may offer new possibilities for treatment. The molecular control of apoptosis is complex and involves cell surface receptors, such as the B-cell receptor, Fas, and CD40; the p53 tumor suppressor; proteases, such as caspases; and Bcl-2 family proteins. The reader is referred to recent reviews for a detailed consideration of the role of these molecules in controlling cell death *(2–6)*.

From: *Methods in Molecular Medicine, Vol. 115: Lymphoma: Methods and Protocols*
Edited by: T. Illidge and P. W. M. Johnson © Humana Press Inc., Totowa, NJ

The Bcl-2 protein family comprises more than a dozen molecules, some of which, like Bcl-2, suppress apoptosis (e.g., Bcl-X_L, Mcl-1, Bfl-1), whereas others promote cell death (e.g., Bax, Bad, Bik *[7]*). These molecules often localize to the cytoplasmic membrane of various intracellular organelles, most notably mitochondria. Although the precise mechanism of action is not known, Bcl-2 prevents the release of cytochrome c, a key event leading to caspase activation in apoptosis induced by diverse stimuli ***(8,9)***. The expression of some Bcl-2 family proteins is tightly and coordinately regulated during normal B-cell development, and altered expression in mouse models systems (e.g., transgenic and knockout mice) alters lymphocyte repertoire and can promote lymphomagenesis ***(10)***. Bcl-2 is activated by the reciprocal t(14:18) translocation found in the majority of follicular lymphomas and some chronic lymphocytic leukemias ***(10,11)***. This translocation brings the Bcl-2 gene on chromosome 18 under transcriptional control of immunoglobulin regulatory regions on chromosome 14, resulting in constitutive Bcl-2 overexpression. Other lymphoid malignancies express high levels of Bcl-2 without translocation. Recent studies have suggested that the proapoptotic Bax molecule may be inactivated by mutation, at least in lymphoid cell lines ***(12,13)***, and the antiapoptotic Bcl-X_L protein is activated by retroviral insertion in some murine leukemias and often is highly expressed in human lymphoid malignancies ***(14,15)***.

Here, we describe methods to study expression of Bcl-2 family proteins in human lymphoma cells. Although cancer-derived cell lines have been invaluable for many areas of research, there is a growing acceptance that they may not reproducibly reflect the behaviors of freshly isolated tumor cells. The relative ease of access to normal lymphocytes and malignant cells from lymph node biopsies, as well as the range of markers suitable for cell purification, means that studying primary lymphoid cells is relatively straightforward. The first protocol describes the isolation and purification of malignant B-cells from lymph node biopsies. Cells are recovered from biopsy material by physical separation, followed by centrifugation on a Ficoll-Paque gradient, which separates mononuclear cells on the basis of their cell density. The protocol then uses a mixture of commercially available labeled antibodies to "capture" contaminating non-B-cells on magnetic columns, resulting in a very pure population of lymphoma cells (**Fig. 1**). The antibodies used here are against CD2 (T and natural killer [NK] cells), CD4 (predominantly T-helper cells), CD11b (myeloid and NK cells), CD16 (neutrophils, NK cells, macrophages), CD36 (platelets, endothelial cells), and IgE (mast cells). Where the target cell is relatively abundant, this negative selection approach is preferred to positive selection (where antibodies specific for the target cell are used) because the B-cells

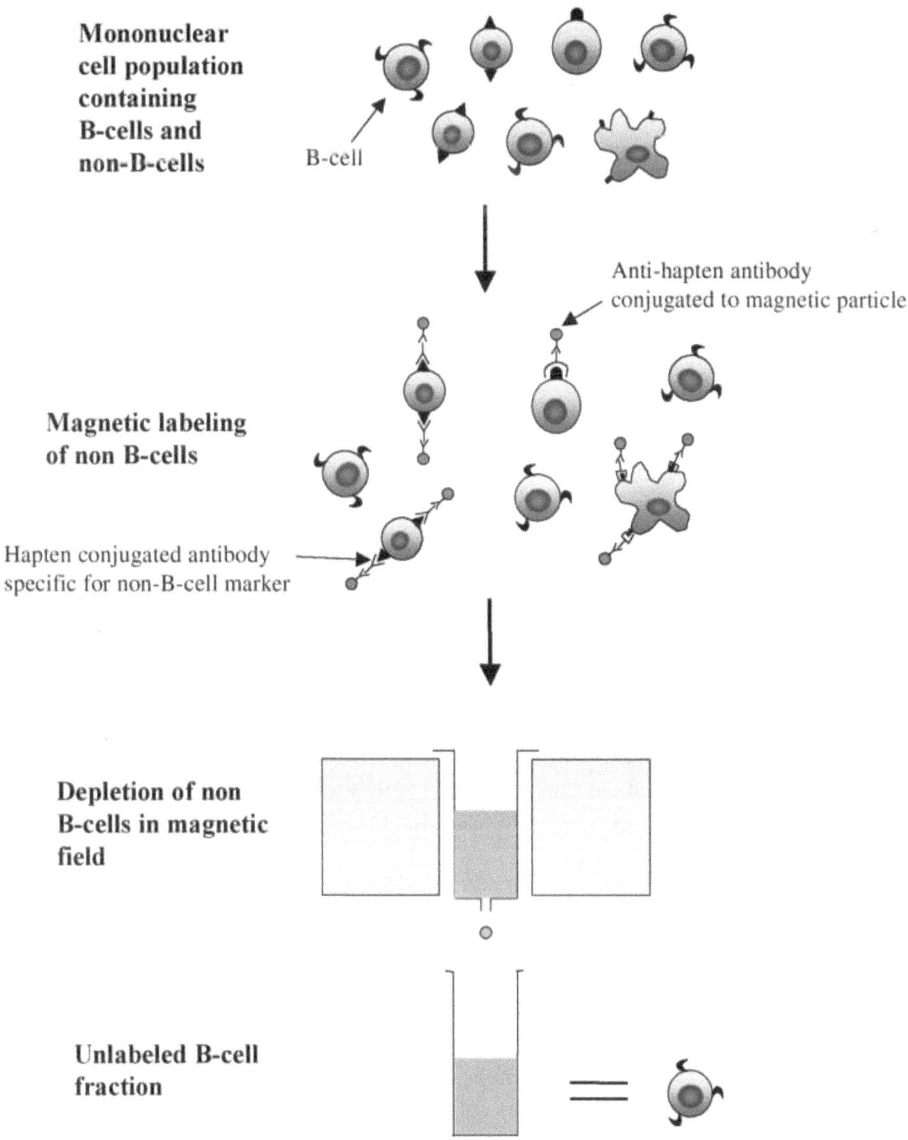

Fig. 1. Negative selection of B-cells using a MACS B-cell isolation kit. Contaminating non-B-cells in a preparation of mononuclear cells are indirectly magnetically labeled using a cocktail of hapten-conjugated antibodies and magnetic beads coupled to an anti-hapten monoclonal antibody. The magnetically labeled non-B-cells are depleted by retention on a column in a magnetic field. Untouched B-cells pass through the column.

are "untouched," that is, not reacted with antibodies that might alter subsequent cell behavior/expression patterns. The purity of the preparation can be assessed by flow cytometry using antibodies specific for B-cell and non-B-cell surface markers. The cells obtained are suitable for direct studies of expression patterns or for in vitro stimulation, for example, via anti-CD40 antibody.

The second protocol describes the analysis of certain Bcl-2 family proteins by immunoblotting (Western blotting). Immunoblotting is an invaluable technique to analyze the steady-state expression of specific proteins in complex cell lysates. Proteins are separated according to their molecular weight by migration through polyacrylamide gels under denaturing conditions ***(16)***. The proteins are transferred to a nitrocellulose membrane and detected using specific antibodies ***(17)***. Some Bcl-2 family protein-specific antibodies are suggested along with recommended conditions for use (**Table 1**); however, the approach can be used to study any protein for which suitable reagents are available. Immunoblotting can be incorporated into further protocols to detect protein modification and interactions. Modifications of the basic procedure are discussed in the Notes.

2. Materials

2.1. Isolation of B-Cells From Lymph Node Biopsies

1. Equipment: Sterile metal scissors and forceps, sterile small metal sieve, magnetic cell separator, and columns (MACS, Miltenyi Biotec, Bisley, UK). The specific separator and columns required would depend on the scale of the experiment; see manufacturer's instructions for details (http://www.miltenyibiotec.com). *See* **Notes 1–3**.
2. Preparation medium: RPMI-1640 medium supplemented with 2 m*M* L-glutamine, 100 µg/mL penicillin G, 100 µg/mL streptomycin, 1 m*M* sodium pyruvate, 1% (v/v) nonessential amino acid solution; and 0.5 µg/mL Fungizone (all from GIBCO, Paisley, UK).
3. B-cell medium: IMDM medium supplemented with 10% (v/v) human serum (Sigma, Poole, UK), 2 m*M* L-glutamine, 20 µg/mL gentamycin, 100 µg/mL penicillin G, and 100 µg/mL streptomycin.
4. MACS buffer: phosphate-buffered saline (PBS; 125 m*M* NaCl, 16 m*M* Na_2HPO_4, 10 m*M* NaH_2PO_4, pH 7.2) supplemented with 10% (v/v) heat inactivated human serum, 0.5% (w/v) bovine serum albumin, and 2 m*M* ethylenediaminetetraacetic acid.
5. Ficoll-Paque Plus (Amersham Pharmacia Biotech, Little Chalfont, UK).
6. B-cell Isolation Kit (MACS, Miltenyi Biotec, Bisley, UK). The kit contains hapten-conjugated CD2, CD4, CD11b, CD16, CD36, and IgE antibodies (antibody cocktail); FcR-blocking reagent; and magnetic microbeads conjugated to a monoclonal antihapten antibody.

Table 1
Recommended Initial Conditions for Using Some Bcl-2 Family Protein Antibodies

Antibody	Source	Concentration (μg/mL) or dilution[a]	Secondary antibody (dilution)	Tertiary antibody (dilution)	Buffer used[b]	Approx Mw (kDa):
Rabbit anti-human Bcl-X_L	R&D Systems (AF800)	0.5	Anti-rabbit HRP (1:5000)	n/a[c]	TBS	30
Rabbit anti-human Mcl-1	Santa Cruz (S-19)	0.5	Anti-rabbit HRP (1:5000)	n/a	TBS	42
Hamster anti-human Bcl-2	Pharmingen (clone 6C8)	0.5	Rabbit anti-hamster (1:1000)	Anti-rabbit HRP (1:5000)	TBS	26
Rabbit anti-human Bax	Santa Cruz (N-20)	0.4	Anti-rabbit HRP (1:5000)	n/a	TBS	21
Goat anti-human Bnip3	Santa Cruz (C-18)	0.4	Anti-goat HRP (1: 2000)	n/a	TBS	60
Rabbit anti-human Actin[d]	Sigma (20–33)	1:500	Anti-rabbit HRP (1:5000)	n/a	TBST	42

[a]The dilution factor used is given where the concentration is not known.
[b]Indicates whether blocking buffer contains TBS or TBST and whether TBS or TBST is used for washing the membrane.
[c]n/a, not applicable.
[d]Analysis of actin expression is a useful way to confirm equivalent loading of intact proteins for each sample.

2.2. Immunoblotting

1. Equipment: Electrophoresis apparatus (e.g., Mini-Protean III Cell, Bio-Rad, Hemel Hempstead, UK), transfer unit (e.g., Mini-Protean II transfer unit, Bio-Rad), chemiluminescent imager (Fluor-S max, Bio-Rad), or autoradiographic film, cassette, and film-developing equipment.
2. Precast sodium dodecylsulfate (SDS)-polyacrylamide gels (e.g., 4–15% gradient ready gels, Bio-Rad).
3. Prestained broad-range protein markers (New England Biolabs, Hitchin, UK).
4. Nitrocellulose membrane (Schleicher and Schuell, Dassel, Germany), 0.2-μm pore size, cut into 9 × 6-cm pieces.
5. Whatman 3MM chromatography paper (Merck, Lutterworth, UK) cut into 10 × 7-cm pieces.
6. Plastic wrap (Saran wrap).
7. SDS sample buffer: 50 m*M* Tris-HCl, pH 6.8, 12% (w/v) SDS, 0.1% (w/v) bromophenol blue, 10% (v/v) glycerol, with 0.1 *M* dithiothreitol added on day of use.
8. Protein running buffer: 25 m*M* Tris base, 200 m*M* glycine, 0.1% (w/v) SDS.
9. Transfer buffer: protein running buffer with 25% (v/v) ethanol.
10. Tris-buffered saline (TBS): 10 m*M* Tris-HCl, pH 8.0, 150 m*M* NaCl.
11. TBST: TBS plus 0.05% (v/v) Tween-20 (BDH, Poole, UK).
12. Blocking buffer: TBS or TBST plus 5% (w/v) non-fat milk powder.
13. Chemiluminescent HRP substrate (Supersignal West Pico, Pierce, Perbio Science, Cheshire, UK).
14. Antibodies: (**Table 1**). All secondary antibodies were supplied by Amersham Pharmacia Biotech, Little Chalfont, UK.

3. Methods

3.1. Isolation of B-Cells From Lymph Node Biopsies (See Notes 4 and 5)

3.1.1. Homogenization

1. Place lymph node in 10 mL of preparation medium.
2. Place sterile sieve in a 10-cm Petri dish and add lymph node and medium to sieve.
3. Hold lymph node with forceps and cut into small pieces with scissors.
4. Use the plunger from a 20-mL syringe to gently force the sample through the sieve in to the Petri dish.
5. Add 5 mL of preparation medium and wash any remaining cells through sieve.
6. Transfer cell suspension from the Petri dish to 50-mL Falcon tube (*see* **Note 6**).

3.1.2. Isolation of Mononuclear Cells

1. Take the cell suspension from **step 6** in **Subheading 3.1.1.** and underlay with 35 mL of Ficoll-Paque by placing the pipette tip at the bottom of the tube and gently releasing the contents so the cell suspension remains above the Ficoll-Paque.

2. Centrifuge at 500*g* for 25 min at room temperature. Use slowest acceleration and deceleration options if available.
3. A white cloudy interface will form, which contains viable mononuclear cells. Above this will be a layer of media and below the interface is a layer of Ficoll-Paque, with a pellet of granulocytes and erythrocytes at the bottom of the tube. Remove as much of the upper layer as possible using a 5-mL pipet, leaving the cloudy interface undisturbed.
4. Collect the entire cloudy mononuclear cell layer using a 1-mL pipet. Gently suck up the cells and a minimum amount of the Ficoll-Paque layer underneath and place in a fresh 50-mL tube.
5. Fill tube with preparation medium.
6. Collect cells by centrifugation at 300*g* for 10 min at room temperature.
7. Discard supernatant and resuspend cells in 10 mL of preparation medium.
8. Count cells using a hemocytometer.

3.1.3. B-Cell Isolation by Magnetic Negative Selection

1. Degas MACS buffer in the refrigerator overnight with the cap loosened by half a turn.
2. Resuspend cells in 60 μL of MACS buffer per 10^7 total cells.
3. Add 20 μL of FcR-blocking reagent per 10^7 total cells.
4. Add 20 μL of Antibody Cocktail per 10^7 total cells.
5. Mix well by pipetting up and down.
6. Incubate in refrigerator for 10 min.
7. Wash cells by adding 10–20 times the volume of labeling buffer, centrifugation at 300*g* for 3 min, and discard supernatant.
8. Repeat **step 7**.
9. Resuspend cells in 80 μL of MACS buffer per 10^7 total cells.
10. Add 20 μL of magnetic microbeads per 10^7 total cells.
11. Mix well by pipetting up and down.
12. Incubate in refrigerator for 15 min.
13. Wash cells as **step 7**.
14. Resuspend cells in 500 μL of MACS buffer per 10^8 total cells (for fewer cells, maintain 500 μL).
15. Place separation column in magnetic field of MACS magnetic cell separator.
16. Prepare column by rinsing with MACS buffer.
17. Apply cells to column.
18. Let the unlabeled cells pass through the column and collect this fraction. This fraction contains the B-cells.
19. Rinse column with MACS buffer and collect column effluent containing B-cells.
20. Dispose of column (non-B-cells are retained on column).
21. B-cell purity can be determined by flow cytometry for B-cell and T-cell markers (e.g., CD20, CD40, CD3) and the clonality of the cells can be determined by analyzing immunoglobulin light chain expression (**Fig. 2**).

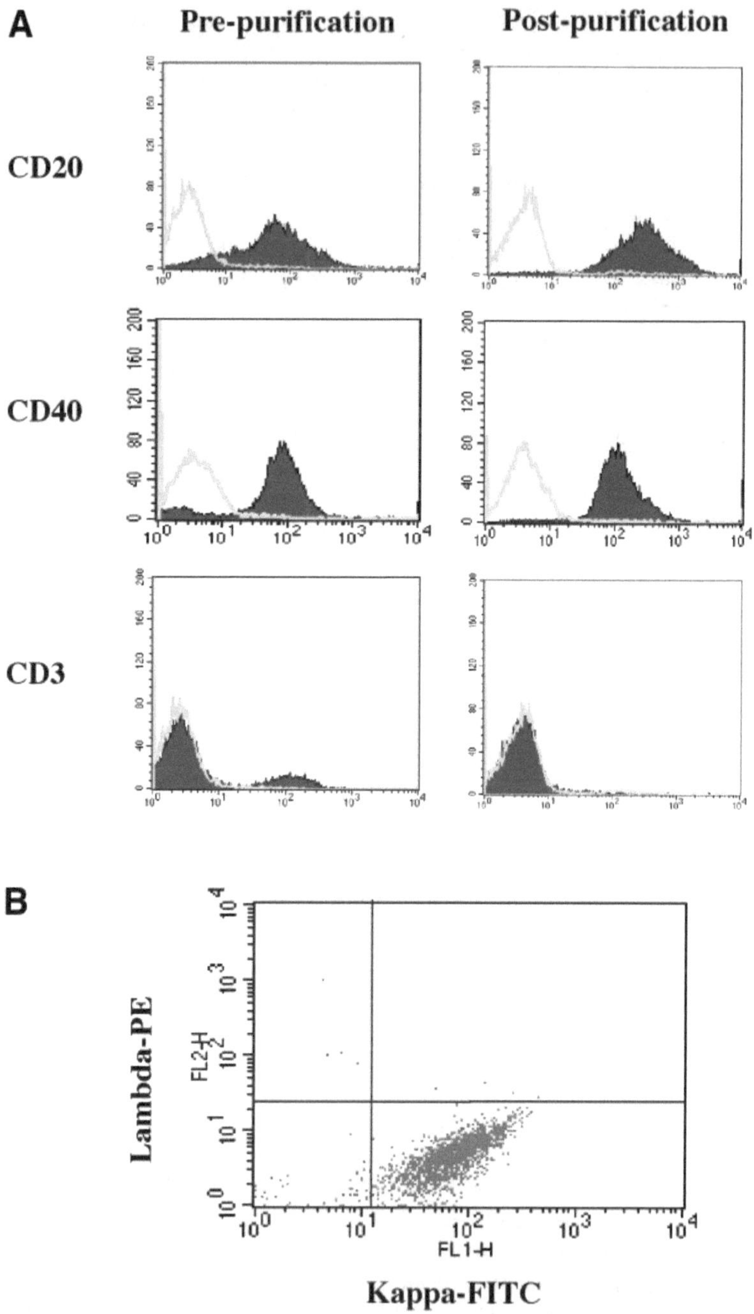
A
Pre-purification
Post-purification
CD20
CD40
CD3
B
Lambda-PE
FL2-H
FL1-H
Kappa-FITC

3.2. Immunoblotting

3.2.1. Preparation of Cell Lysates

1. A minimum of 5×10^5 primary B-cells are recommended per blot (*see* **Note 7**). Collect cells by centrifugation and wash in PBS, transferring cells to an Eppendorf tube. Remove all supernatant and snap freeze pellet in liquid nitrogen. Store pellets at –80°C until ready for analysis (*see* **Note 8**).
2. Solubilize cell pellet in SDS sample buffer at a concentration of 15 µL per 5×10^5 cells. Mix by pipetting up and down. Protein markers should be prepared in parallel but do not require sonication.
3. Sonicate samples to shear genomic DNA.
4. Heat samples and protein markers to 95°C for 5 min. The sample is now ready to be loaded on a SDS polyacrylamide gel (*see* **Note 9**).

3.2.2. Polyacrylamide Gel Electrophoresis

1. Assemble pre-cast gel in electrophoresis equipment and fill tank and wells with protein running buffer.
2. Load 15 µL of sample into each well (*see* **Note 10**).
3. Load 5 µL of prestained protein markers.
4. Run gel at 200 V until dye front reaches the bottom of the gel (*see* **Note 11**).

3.2.3. Transfer of Proteins From Gel to Membrane

1. Wet nitrocellulose membrane in distilled water.
2. Presoak sponges, nitrocellulose membrane and Whatman 3MM paper in transfer buffer.

Fig. 2. (*opposite page*) Flow cytometric analysis of cell surface markers on purified follicular lymphoma cells. **(A)** Assessment of purity. Open histogram: immunostaining with a fluorescently conjugated isotype matched control antibody. Closed histogram: immunostaining with a fluorescently conjugated antibody against CD20, CD40 (B-cell markers), or CD3 (T-cell marker). Cell counts are shown on the *y*-axis, and fluorescence intensity is shown on the *x*-axis. Note that CD3-positive, CD40/CD20-negative T-cells are completely removed by the selection protocol leaving pure B-cells. **(B)** Assessment of clonality. Expression of the two immunoglobulin light chains kappa and lambda is normally approximately equal in a nonclonal population of B-cells, whereas clonal B-cell malignancies show clonal restriction and express a single light chain. Therefore, clonal restriction is a simple measure of the proportion of malignant cells in a B-cell preparation. Light chain expression was analyzed by double staining using FITC (fluorescein isothiocyanate) conjugated anti-kappa (*x*-axis) and PE (phycocoerythrein) conjugated antilambda (*y*-axis) antibodies (Dako, Ely, UK). Note that the negatively selected B-cells studied here are pure B-cells (all cells express light chains) and are clonal (all express kappa) with very few contaminating normal lambda-positive B-cells. *See* **Color Plate 1**, following page 270.

3. Place open cassette in a suitable container with enough transfer buffer so that it just covers the surface of the cassette.
4. Assemble the gel sandwich in the following order: sponge, Whatman 3MM paper, gel, nitrocellulose membrane, Whatman 3MM paper, sponge. Smooth out any air bubbles after addition of each layer and close the cassette.
5. Place cassette in the transfer apparatus ensuring that the nitrocellulose membrane is placed towards the anode.
6. Add the ice block for cooling, fill the tank with transfer buffer and run at 100 V for 1 h.

3.2.4. Probing Membrane With Antibodies

All incubation and wash steps should be conducted with gentle shaking.

1. Block membrane by incubating with the appropriate blocking buffer (i.e., TBS or TBST, *see* **Table 1**) for 1 h at room temperature.
2. Discard blocking buffer and incubate membranes overnight at 4°C with primary antibody in the appropriate blocking buffer (*see* **Note 12**).
3. Wash membrane three times for 5 min in TBS/TBST.
4. Incubate membrane for 1 h at room temperature with the appropriate secondary antibody in the appropriate blocking buffer.
5. Wash membrane three times for 5 min in TBS/TBST.
6. If a tertiary antibody is required, incubate the membrane for 1 h at room temperature with the appropriate antibody, in the appropriate blocking buffer. Then wash membrane three times for 5 min in TBS/TBST.
7. Incubate filter with chemiluminescent reagents, following the manufacturer's instructions.
8. Wrap membrane in plastic wrap and detect bands using a chemiluminescent imager or exposure to film. Representative results are shown in **Fig. 3** (*see* **Note 13**).

4. Notes

1. All work with patients' material must be performed in accordance with current ethical requirements.
2. All work with patients' material must be considered hazardous (at least Cat 2 containment). All requirements must be met for containment and disposal of material.
3. Lymph node biopsy samples can be stored overnight in preparation medium at 4°C before processing.
4. The B-cell isolation procedure can also be applied to spleen biopsies.
5. After homogenization of lymph nodes (**Subheading 3.1.1.**) cells can be frozen for later use. Centrifuge cells at 300*g* for 5 min, aspirate supernatant and resuspend cells in fresh freezing medium (40% preparation medium, 50% human serum, 10% dimethylsulfoxide) at 1×10^7 to 1×10^8 cells/mL. Place 1 mL of cell suspension in 1.5-mL cryovials and place tubes in an isopropanol freezing box (Nalgene, Merck, Lutterworth, UK). Place the freezing box at –80°C overnight and then transfer vials to liquid nitrogen storage. To revive cells from liquid ni-

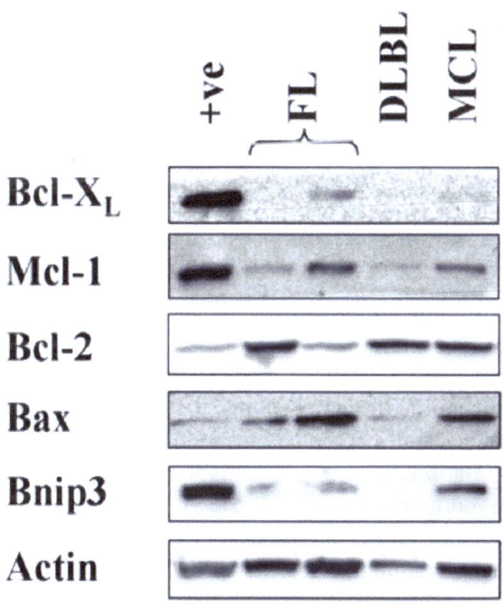

Fig.3. Immunoblot analysis of Bcl-2 family proteins in purified lymphoma cells. B-cells were purified from four primary samples: two follicular lymphomas (FL), a diffuse large B-cell lymphoma (DLBL), and a mantle cell lymphoma (MCL). Proteins were separated by SDS polyacrylamide gel electrophoresis and detected using the antibodies listed in the table. Actin is shown as a loading control. +ve, positive control, a Burkitt's lymphoma cell line.

trogen storage, place cryovials in a 37°C water bath until thawed. Immediately pipet contents of one vial very slowly into 10 mL of IMDM medium that contains 10 µg/mL DNase (Sigma, Poole, UK), at room temperature. Invert tube twice and centrifuge at 250*g* for 3 min. Remove supernatant and resuspend cell pellet in 5 mL of B-cell medium. Transfer cell suspension to a cell culture flask and place in a humidified incubator set at 37°C and 5% CO_2 for 3 h to allow the cells to recover. Proceed to **Subheading 3.1.2.**

6. Isolated B-cells can be cultured in B-cell medium for up to 72 h in a humidified incubator at 37°C with 5% CO_2, at a concentration of 1×10^6 cells/mL. There may be extensive spontaneous cell death over this period, although the extent is dependent on the lymphoma type.
7. Where larger numbers of B-cells are available for immunoblotting, cell lysates can be prepared using RIPA buffer (0.15 *M* NaCl; 0.05 *M* Tris-HCl, pH 8.0; 1% [v/v] Nonidet-P40; 0.5% [w/v] deoxycholate), which allows the determination of precise protein concentrations using the Bio-Rad Protein Assay .
8. Cell lysates prepared in Subheading 3.2.1. can be stored at –80°C until use. Boil samples for 3 min at 95°C prior to loading on an SDS gel.

9. See standard laboratory manuals of recipes for "homemade" polyacrylamide gels.
10. Where available, include appropriate positive and negative control cell lysates on the SDS-polyacrylamide gel. An Epstein–Barr virus-transformed lymphoblastoid cell line would be expected to express all of the proteins listed in **Table 1**.
11. Appropriate safety measures should be consider for all protocols. The hazards of unpolymerized acrylamide solutions and high electric fields deserve special mention.
12. All antibody concentrations given in **Table 1** are guidelines. All antibodies should be titrated to determine optimal concentrations. It is very important to confirm the specificity of commercial antibodies and not simply assume that they will detect the protein of interest.
13. Immunoblotting can be used for further studies. For example, a number of phospho-specific antibodies are available that recognize proteins phosphorylated on specific residues and these can be used to monitor protein modification ***(18)***. Some phosphorylations alter migration is SDS polyacrylamide gels and this is a simple way to monitor phosphorylation ***(19)***. Protein:protein interactions are important for regulating Bcl-2 family protein and can be monitored by using antibodies to immunoprecipitate a protein followed by immunoblotting to determine the presence of an interacting partner in the complex ***(20)***.

References

1. Cohen, J. J. (1991) Programmed cell death in the immune system. *Adv. Immunol,* **50,** 55–85.
2. Ashkenazi, A. and Dixit, V. M. (1998) Death receptors: signaling and modulation. *Science* **28,** 1305–1308.
3. Thornberry, N. A., and Lazebnik, Y. (1998) Caspases: enemies within. *Science* **28,** 1312–1316.
4. Evan, G. and Littlewood, T. (1998) A matter of life and cell death. *Science* **28,** 1317–1322.
5. Adams, J. A. and Cory, S. (1998) The Bcl-2 protein family: arbiters of cell survival. *Science* **28,** 1322–1326.
6. Zorning, M., Heuber, A., and Baum, W. (2001) Apoptosis regulators and their role in tumorigenesis. *Biochim. Biophys. Acta.* **1551,** F1–F37.
7. Gross, A., McDonnell, J. M., and Korsmeyer, S. J. (1999) Bcl-2 family members and the mitochondria in apoptosis. *Genes Dev.* **13,** 1899–1911.
8. Kroemer, G. and Reed, J. C. (2000) Mitochondrial control of cell death. *Nat. Med.* **6,** 513–519.
9. Tsujimoto, Y. and Shimizu, S (2000) Bcl-2 family: life-or-death switch. *FEBS Lett.* **466,** 6–10.
10. Korsmeyer, S. J. (1999) BCL-2 gene family and the regulation of programmed cell death. *Cancer Res.* **59,** 1693–1700.
11. Adachi, M., Tefferi, A., Greipp, P.R., Kipps, T. J., and Tsujimoto, Y. (1990) Preferential linkage of bcl-2 to immunoglobulin light chain gene in chronic lymphocytic leukemia. *J. Exp. Med.* **171,** 559–564.

12. Brimmell, M., Mendiola, R., Mangion, J., and Packham, G. (1998) BAX frameshift mutations in cell lines derived from human haemopoietic malignancies are associated with resistance to apoptosis and microsatellite instability. *Oncogene* **16,** 1803–1812.
13. Meijerink, J. P., Mensink, E. J., Wang, K., et al. (1998) Hematopoietic malignancies demonstrate loss-of-function mutations of BAX. *Blood* **91,** 2991–2997.
14. Packham, G., White, E. L., Eischen, C. M., et al. (1998) Selective regulation of Bcl-XL by a Jak kinase-dependent pathway is bypassed in murine hematopoietic malignancies. *Genes Dev.* **12,** 2475–2487.
15. MacCarthy-Morrogh, L., Mouzakiti, A., Townsend, P., Brimmell, M., and Packham, G. (1999). Bcl-2-related proteins and cancer. *Biochem. Soc. Trans.* **27,** 785–789.
16. Laemmli, U. K. (1970) Cleavage of structural proteins during the assembly of the head of bacteriophage T4. *Nature* **227,** 680–685.
17. Towbin, H., Staehelin, T., and Gordon, J. (1979) Electrophoretic transfer of proteins from polyacrylamide gels to nitrocellulose sheets: procedure and some applications. *Proc. Natl. Acad. Sci. USA* **76,** 4350–4354.
18. Wolfman, J. C. and Wolfman, A. (2000). Endogenous c-N-Ras provides a steady-state anti-apoptotic signal. *J. Biol. Chem.* **275,** 19315–19323.
19. Haldar, S., Jena, N., and Croce, C. M. (1995) Inactivation of Bcl-2 by phosphorylation. *Proc. Natl. Acad. Sci. USA* **92,** 4507–4511.
20. Oltvai, Z. N., Milliman, C. L., and Korsmeyer, S. J. (1993) Bcl-2 heterodimerizes in vivo with a conserved homolog, Bax, that accelerates programmed cell death. *Cell* **74,** 609–619.

2

Molecular Diagnosis of Lymphoma

Outcome Prediction by Gene Expression Profiling in Diffuse Large B-Cell Lymphoma

Kim Last, Silvana Debarnardi, and T. Andrew Lister

Summary

This chapter describes the illness diffuse large B-cell lymphoma (DLBCL) and why research has and continues to focus on creating accurate predictors of response to treatment to allow individual risk assessment for a patient and individualization of treatment choice to maximize the chances of cure. Microarray technology has the promise to bring these objectives within reach. The first papers attempting to identify molecular signatures of response and outcome using microarray technology were generated using DLBCL samples and are described. The different types of microarray platform and data analysis tools are reviewed followed by a detailed step-by-step guide to data generation using the Affymetrix chip system from RNA extraction to laser scanning of the hybridized and stained chips.

Key Words: Diffuse; lymphoma; microarray; Affymetrix; expression profiling; outcome; prediction.

1. Introduction

1.1. A Clinical Summary of Diffuse Large B-Cell Lymphoma

Diffuse large B-cell lymphoma (DLBCL) is the most common form of non-Hodgkin's lymphoma *(1)* and follows an aggressive course, resulting in the death of patients within months without treatment *(2)*. Researchers, when using anthracycline-based combination chemotherapy, have found that 80 to 85% of patients respond, with more than 50 to 76% achieving a complete response, that is, no disease identifiable 4 or more weeks after the end of treatment *(3,4)*. Unfortunately, in nearly half of responders, their lymphoma returns, with only a minority being cured by more intensive retreatment *(5)*. Thus, at 5 yr from the diagnosis of DLBCL, less than 50% of patients remain alive, disease-free *(1)*. The best, validated predictor of response and outcome to treatment to date is a crude index based upon five clinical variables termed the International

From: *Methods in Molecular Medicine, Vol. 115: Lymphoma: Methods and Protocols*
Edited by: T. Illidge and P. W. M. Johnson © Humana Press Inc., Totowa, NJ

Prognostic Index (IPI *[6]*). The IPI stratifies patients into low-, intermediate-, high-intermediate, and high-risk groups, with the respective 5-yr overall survival of each group being 73, 51, 46, and 32%. Because most patients fall into the intermediate group, the IPI fails to define their risk any better than the risk for all patients considered together. Therefore, the ability to predict which patients will respond to treatment and be cured of their lymphoma and which will ultimately die of their DLBCL still cannot be performed accurately for the majority.

The variability in clinical response and course of DLBCL and the recognition of morphological subtypes and nuances has led to the hypothesis that DLBCL is in fact composed of several distinct subtypes with differing outcomes to treatment. Because such subtypes cannot be successfully reproduced on the basis of morphological appearance alone, the search for molecular methods of subdividing DLBCL into meaningful clinical subtypes has long been the goal of lymphoma clinicians and scientists.

1.2. An Introduction to Microarray Technology

The means of discovery of molecular signatures of response, long-term outcome, and subtype definition took a great leap forward with the advent of microarray technology *(7,8)*. By allowing the simultaneous measurement of the mRNA expression of 100s to 1000s of genes from across the genome, array technology offered the potential to screen thousands of genes without the need for preconceived hypotheses.

Microarrays can investigate mitochondrial RNA (mRNA) or genomic deoxyribonucleic acid (DNA). Genomic DNA arrays can reveal large-scale gains and losses or mutations and polymorphisms, whereas mRNA targeted arrays allow gene-expression to be studied. An array is constructed on a solid substrate, often termed the "platform," made of either glass (microarray) or nitrocellulose or nylon (macroarrays). Two types of array dominate the expression profiling field: "chips" where oligonucleotide probes are grown out from the substrate surface, and "dot-blot" slides or membranes, where tiny dots of probe solution are blotted on to the substrate. A third type "oligonucleotide ink-jet/piezo" arrays, has been developed more recently and will be described briefly. For a list of commercial suppliers of arrays, visit http://www.lab-on-a-chip.com and http://ihome.cuhk.edu.hk/~b400559/array.html.

On the substrate, 100s (macroarrays) to 1000s (microarrays) of complimentary DNA (cDNA) amplicons or oligonucleotides are immobilized in an ordered, grid pattern. Confusingly, the arrayed cDNA amplicons or oligonucleotides are called "targets" in most systems but "probes" in Affymetrix chips. Because this chapter refers to the use of the Affymetrix system, the cDNA amplicons or oligonucleotides will be referred to as "probes" henceforth. To the "probes," labeled complementary (c)RNA, cDNA, or genomic DNA are hybridized in a manner similar to that of Southern and Northern blotting. (In most systems, the labeled cRNA, cDNA, or genomic DNA is referred to as the "probe," whereas in the Affymetrix system, and the remainder of this chapter, it is referred to as the "target.") Each of the immobilized "probes" acts as an assay for its specific partner strand in the complex nucleic acid mixture of the target. The target labels can be fluorophores, biotin, or radioactive phosphorus. Arrays designed for radioactive labeled target (macroarrays) require as little as 50 ng RNA (5000 cells), compared with the minimum of 5 μg (500,000 cells) required for fluorescent systems. ^{33}P-based arrays, however, produce reliable readouts only for highly expressed genes, which are the minority. Fluorescence-dependent arrays allow the detection of low- and medium-abundance genes, which are the majority, as well as those genes highly expressed at the mRNA level. It is the fluorescence-dependent arrays that have been used to great effect in the study of DLBCL and that will now be described in more detail.

1.3. "Dot-Blot" Arrays

The probes for "dot-blot" slides are created from cDNA clone libraries using the polymerase chain reaction to amplify part of the cDNA clone insert of each bacteriophage in the library. The "arrayer," a robot, arrays 0.25–1 nL of probe cDNA solution in the same place on the 20 or more chemically treated slides under production. As many as 40,000 different probes can be arrayed per standard size slide. After the probe solutions have dried, the probes are covalently fixed to the slide using ultraviolet light. Excess probe is then washed off using 0.1% sodium dodecyl sulfate) Depending on the number of probes held, a batch of slides takes anywhere from 1 to 8 h to make. Maintaining the clone libraries required for dot-blot slides makes slide manufacture too expensive for all but the largest noncommercial organizations, unless the number of probes arrayed is compromised, and has sensibly lead to the establishment of core facilities capable of providing arrays to a network of labs. Nonetheless, the resultant slides are cheaper to produce than oligonucleotide arrays. A concern with cDNA arrays is the clone error rate, that is, when a clone transpires not to contain the plasmid sequence it is meant to. In one quality-control study, of the 1189 clones sequenced, only 62% were uncontaminated and contained cDNA inserts that had significant sequence identity to published data for the ordered clones *(9)*.

Because the volume of each probe spot deposited can vary, apparent expression changes could be produced by spot differences alone. To compensate for this artifact, two target samples are used: a test sample and a control or reference RNA, usually created from pooled cell lines in sufficient quantity to be used with all the test samples in a particular experiment. The test sample RNA is converted into labeled cDNA target using one fluorophore whereas the reference RNA is converted into labeled cDNA target using a different fluorophore. Equal amounts of test and control target are added to each array, allowing the test and reference cDNA fragments to compete to hybridize with the probes. If a test cDNA is in excess the resultant signal will come from its fluorophore, whereas if the control cDNA dominates, the fluorescence detected will come from the control cDNA. Thus, the problem of dot variability is overcome by using a competitive hybridization method. For a comprehensive guide to the manufacture of dot-blot arrays see the protocol pages of http://www.microarrays.org/index.html. cDNA arrays can be purchased from Agilent (http://www.chem.agilent.com/) as well as other suppliers.

1.3.1. Oligonucleotide Ink Jet/Piezo Arrays

A development from dot-blot arrays, oligonucleotide ink jet/piezo arrays use no-contact, less-wasteful piezo electric pulse or ink-jet technology to propel a tiny volume of synthesized oligonucleotide solution on to the platforms. Oligomers of 60 base-pair lengths were found to offer optimal sensitivity and specificity ***(10)***. Sensitivity down to one transcript per cell can be achieved. Standard and custom-made 25- or 60-mer oligonucleotide arrays are available from Agilent (http://www.chem.agilent.com/) and Amersham Biosciences (http://www4.amershambiosciences.com/). Whether the additional cost (compared with standard cDNA arrays) is truly outweighed by more informative data production remains to be decided.

1.4. Chip Arrays

Chip arrays consist of oligonucleotide probes that are synthesized *in situ* on silica wafers under the control of photolithographic chemistry ***(11)***. The lengths of both the probes and targets are critical to the sensitivity and specificity of the hybridization reactions. Probe oligomers between 20 and 60 bases in length provide the best balance between discriminant and sensitive hybridization. As well as the correct oligonucleotides, "missense" oligonucleotides are created in parallel for each probe, which allow the specificity of the hybridization reaction to be determined by comparison of the extent of hybridization to the missense and sense probes, as well as background noise reduction by subtraction of missense from sense signal. In the Affymetrix system (see www.affymetrix.com/), the sense probes are 25 mers (high specificity but reduced sensitivity compared with longer oligomers) and are referred to as "perfect matches" (PM), whereas the missense probes are termed "mismatches" (MM), differing from their sense probe by just their middle, 13th base. The lower the value of the missense:sense signal ratio, the better. For each gene, a set of 11–20 PM and MM probe pairs is laid down, thereby increasing the sensitivity for detecting a gene transcript to, at best, 1 in 300,000 transcripts. Through the reduction in feature size, as many as 54,000 gene probes can now be included on one chip. As with dot-blot slides, the target for oligonucleotide chips is created from test sample RNA. The RNA is reverse transcribed into cDNA followed by transcription back to RNA, as cRNA. Because this two-step procedure results in amplification of the mRNA, less RNA is required for chip arrays compared with dot-blot arrays (5–10 μg vs 30 μg). To produce the labeled target, biotin-conjugated bases are used in the synthesis of the cRNA. The labeled cRNA requires fragmentation into lengths of 20 to 200 base pairs, followed by denaturing before application to the array. Unlike dot-blot arrays, competitive hybridization with a reference RNA is not required for interchip array expression profile comparison because the oligonucleotide synthesis of each feature is so precisely controlled that interchip variation is minimal. The cost of commercially available generic chips has reduced substantially since their introduction, making the technology affordable to an increasing number of research facilities. Furthermore, customized chips can be ordered that contain only the gene features of interest from previous experiments or known to be critical to a particular illness, tissue, or set of experimental conditions.

1.5. Expression Profiling in DLBCL

The two major platforms for expression profiling have been used in DLBCL and have produced remarkable and reproducible expression signatures that reveal molecularly defined subtypes of DLBCL and predict for response to treatment and long-term outcome ***(12–14)***.

In an article by Shipp et al. ***(14)***, diagnostic, pretreatment, frozen biopsy material was studied from 58 patients with DLBCL and 19 patients with follicular lymphoma, a closely related germinal centre malignancy. The expression profile, or "signature," of each biopsy was created using the Affymetrix 7800 gene chip, which consisted of probe features representing 7817 known and putative genes. The resulting gene expression data was analyzed using supervised learning techniques ***(15)***. The first distinction attempted, based on expression variance, was between the DLBCL and follicular lymphoma samples. This proved possible, and the resulting 30-gene model's reproducibility was confirmed by the "leave-one-out" cross-validation technique. Next, subdivision of the DLBCL samples into different subtypes based upon outcome to treatment was examined, again using a weighted-voting algorithm ***(16)***. A recurring subset of genes was indeed discovered that were highly associated with the distinction between those patients that had a good outcome (i.e., alive and cured yr after treatment) and those with a bad outcome (i.e., dead from lymphoma or DLBCL unresponsive to treatment) A model using just 13 genes could predict outcome for the 58 patients, with 70% of the patients stratified in the good-risk group being alive at 5 yr vs just 12% of the patients placed in the bad-risk group remaining alive at 5 yr ($p = 0.00004$).

An interesting discovery was that the 13-gene model could subdivide the patients contained within the different IPI subgroups into "cured" and "dead/ refractory" subgroups with significantly different outcomes, revealing that the gene expression-based outcome predictor contained additional information to the clinical prognostic model, the IPI. For example, when the 37 patients defined as low/low-intermediate risk according to the IPI were sorted by the 13-gene model, those displaying a "cured" gene-expression signature had a 5-yr overall survival of 75% compared with a 5-yr overall survival of 32% for the patients displaying the "fatal/refractory" signature ($p = 0.02$) The combination of clinical and molecular variables suggests a possible strategy for further individualization of patient treatment decisions. Nevertheless, additional information still remains to be captured because the use of both models in series failed to produce groups with 100% and 0% 5-yr overall survivals. Finally, the 13-gene model suggested novel therapeutic targets and strategies. Whether therapeutic leads suggested by expression profiling will prove useful and result in molecularly determined individualization of treatment remains to be seen.

In the other two articles, the clustering analysis was performed using a different approach termed hierarchical clustering ***(17)***. Alizadeh et al. ***(12)*** demonstrated that molecular subclassification of DLBCL on the basis of gene expression was possible. The two subtypes had expression profiles similar to those of different putative cells of origin. This finding was confirmed and extended in the much larger series of Rosenwald et al. ***(13)***, in which DLBCL was divided into three subtypes termed germinal center-like, activated B-cell-like and type 3 DLBCL. In both articles, the patients with lymphomas subclassified as germinal center-like fared better than the patients with lymphoma subclassified as activated B-cell-like, suggesting clinical relevance to DLBCL subclassification according to the putative cell of origin.

1.6. The Stages of a Gene Expression Profile Experiment

The procedures fall into three stages: (1) sample preparation; (2) array hybridization and image acquisition; and (3) data handling and interpretation. Each of these stages is outlined herein.

1.6.1. Sample Preparation: From Living Tissue to Labeled Target

Control of RNA quality and quantity extracted from cell-lines is straightforward, as the sample is 100% interesting and fresh. However, from human body tissues guaranteeing excellent quality and quantity of RNA is more difficult. First, obtaining sufficient human tissue of interest is often problematic. Although radioactive systems, using phosphorus-32, can use very small amounts of RNA

(50 ng) retrievable from a 16-gage needle core biopsy, they are reliable only for high-abundance genes, which are the minority. For fluorescent systems, considerably more tissue is required, necessitating an open biopsy. Second, minimizing the time in which RNA degradation can occur from collection to freezing or processing of the material is critical. Considerable resources and co-operation between many individuals, not least the patients who allow the samples to be taken, are required to overcome these obstacles. Once obtained, verification of sufficient tumor infiltration of each sample must be undertaken. If the tumor infiltrate is too low, conventionally taken as less than 50%, the expression profile obtained will relate more to the nonmalignant cell population, such as fibroblasts and nonmalignant lymphocytes than the tumor itself. In such cases, purification of the tumor cells may be required by cell sorting or microdissection ***(18)***. Cell sorting may change the tumor's expression profile because of the cells' response to processing. If microdissection is undertaken, additional polymerase chain reaction (PCR) amplification of the RNA will be needed if a fluorescent, as opposed to a radioactive, array system is to be used ***(19)***. This in turn carries the risk of differential signal amplification, distorting the expression pattern being sought, a problem that is being actively addressed ***(20,21)***.

Once the RNA has been extracted, it requires cleaning of protein and other impurities to maximize the efficiency of the transcription reactions and target hybridization to probe. The cleaned RNA is reverse transcribed into cDNA, followed by transcription back into labeled cRNA using biotinylated ribonucleotides. The two-step procedure of first- and second-strand cDNA/RNA synthesis uses a poly T primer to anneal to the poly-A tail present at the 5' end of all mRNA. Before synthesizing the second cDNA strand, the original RNA is destroyed to prevent its continued replication. As already mentioned, to make an efficient target out of the labeled cRNA, it must be fragmented into small pieces and then denatured.

To summarize, sample preparation consists of the following steps:

1. RNA extraction (2 h)
2. RNA purification (1 h)
3. First-strand cDNA synthesis (1 h)
4. Second-strand cDNA synthesis (2 h)
5. Clean-up of double-stranded complementary DNA (ds-cDNA) (1 h)
6. In vitro transcription: cRNA synthesis (5 h)
7. Fragmentation of biotinylated cRNA (1 h)

1.6.2. Array Hybridization and Image Acquisition

Hybridization of the fragmented target to the array requires overnight incubation at 45°C. After removal of the target solution from the chip, unbound target is removed by performing several washes. Staining of the biotin-labeled, hybridized target fragments is achieved using streptavidin, which strongly binds to biotin. The streptavidin is made visible by virtue of its conjugation to the dye phycoerythrin, which fluoresces under laser light. To amplify the streptavidin–phycoerythrin (SAPE) signal, a biotinylated antibody against streptavidin is incubated with the array after the first exposure to SAPE. A second incubation with SAPE solution is then performed, followed by washing to remove unbound SAPE. The expression profile on the array is read by measuring the fluorescence produced by scanning the array with a laser at 570 n*M*. Once captured, the fluorescent intensity of each target-probe hybrid is converted into a numerical value to produce quantitative gene expression levels for each feature of the array.

To summarize, array hybridization and image acquisition involves the following steps:

1. Hybridization of the fragmented target to the probe array in the cartridge/chip (overnight).

The "Fluidics" steps: (2 h)

2. Washing to remove nonspecifically bound target.
3. First SAPE staining.
4. Signal enhancement by addition of a biotinylated antibody against streptavidin.
5. Second SAPE staining.

Post-Fluidics: (10 min)

6. Laser scanning.

1.6.3. Data Analysis

Data analysis has, for the first time in biomedical science, become the bottleneck in experiment completion, as the acquisition of data outstrips the capacity to find meaning within it. Data analysis involves the following steps:

1. Confirmation of successful, specific hybridization across the chip.
2. Data transformation and normalization.
3. Exclusion of nonvarying genes.
4. Performance of cluster analyses/data mining.
5. Cluster reproducibility testing.

The raw data from each chip require interrogation by Microarray Suite (Affymetrix) to confirm successful hybridization. The sensitivity of an array can be gauged by ascertaining the lowest concentration of control oligonucleotide in the hybridization cocktail and through assessing PM to MM ratios across each probe set.

Precluster analysis, the data require elimination of background signal, filtration, and normalization. Microarray suite subtracts background automatically by taking the MM from PM signal intensity for each probe and probe set. High background implies that impurities, cell debris, and salts, as well as target are binding to the probe array surface in a nonspecific manner and fluorescing at 570 nm (the scanning wavelength) This nonspecific binding causes a low signal-to-noise ratio (SNR), meaning that genes for transcripts present at very low levels in the sample may incorrectly be called absent and excluded from further analysis. High background creates an overall loss of sensitivity in the experiment. The purer the starting RNA, and later the ds-DNA and cRNA, the less background produced.

In order for the data from each chip in a series to be compared with the data of the others, adjustments need to be made. Low-quality readings are removed, or "filtered." These are predominantly low intensity readings (in which the signal is close to background, causing relative error to increase) and the highest intensity readings (in which saturation of the probe feature occurs) necessitating application of a "floor" and "ceiling" to exclude such observations. For the remaining features, their intensities require adjustment to account for variations in target labeling efficiency and hybridization, producing false expression changes on comparison with other chip intensities. This involves two processes called "scaling" and "normalization." "Scaling" involves the setting of a scaling factor to be applied to all the intensities on a chip. By applying the same scaling factor to each chip in a data set, a source of false expression variation is prevented. "Normalization" involves the removal of systematic variation, such as variable hybridization labeling efficiency and starting quantity of RNA, that affects the measured gene expression levels to differing extents for each array. Generation of "normalization" factor adjusts signal intensities on each chip so that the intensities of each are readily comparable with the rest in the data set. Using the Affymetrix software, "Normalization" involves generation of a factor that allows the average intensity of an experimental array to be adjusted to the average intensity of the baseline array. The normalization factor for a particular array will therefore change when the comparison baseline array is changed. For detailed reviews and methods on "normalization," see http://www.dnachip.org/mged/normalization.html ***(22,23)***.

A further form of necessary data filtering is the removal of genes with no or minimal variance across the data set. Such filtering greatly aids identification of the most interesting differentially expressed genes by reducing false groupings and clustering on use of the different data mining tools ***(24)***. The simplest method to eliminate stable genes is application of an expression fold-difference threshold, usually of twofold. Only those genes with greater than twofold expression changes are taken forward for data analysis. More sophisticated methods of identifying differentially expressed genes involve calculation of intensity-independent and -dependent Z scores for the data set, so allowing the variably expressed genes to be defined as those lying outside of the 95% confidence intervals derived *(25)* and use of analysis of variance techniques *(26)*.

After these steps, two principal methods of data analysis are used, unsupervised and supervised. In an unsupervised analysis, no preconditions are applied to the data set under scrutiny. The program used is merely asked to split the data set into varying numbers of groups or clusters using the profiles for all or a selected group of gene probes. This can be a powerful way of discovering unexpected similarities and differences between samples but can also result in groups of little obvious clinical or scientific relevance. In a supervised analysis, gene profiles are sought that associate with a prescribed distinction between the different samples, be it the time points of samples in a drug exposure experiment or the outcome to treatment of the patients the samples came from.

Numerous programs and tools are used to perform unsupervised and supervised analyses. Frequently used analysis methods include hierarchical clustering *(17)*, self-organizing maps *(15)*, k-nearest neighbor *(27)*, principal components analysis *(28)*, support vector machines *(29)*, and weighted voting *(16)*.

Hierarchical clustering is the most commonly used unsupervised analysis tool. It involves the creation of a phylogenetic tree, where the branching lengths represent the degree of similarity between the data sets. Hierarchical clustering can produce groupings with clinical correlation but can also miss many of the ways in which data varies by being too rigid a structuring tool. The resultant cluster pictures are referred to as "dendrograms."

The self-organizing maps (SOMs) algorithm is a neural-network based method that allows extraction of "executive summaries" from the data by defining the n most important groupings. Different numbers of nodes or partitions are suggested to the program by the operator to group the most variable genes. The relationship of individual data points to each node is then computed, and all the data points are shuffled one by one. Eventually, the grouping of the gene data points is maximized, just as if a vase were reconstructed from the millions of shards of glass produced when broken. One of the advantages of SOMs is imposition of partial, rather than complete, structure on the data set. In addition, SOMs can be refined or reorganized as discoveries are made. One of the problems with SOMs is the need to remove all genes with stable expression across the majority of samples in the data set. If these low-variability genes are included in the analysis, false clusters are produced.

K-nearest neighbor organizes the data into similar groupings in k dimensional "gene expression" space. The means of defining the vector, or expression distance, between data points distinguishes k-nearest neighbor clustering from that of SOMs. Both techniques are adept at "training" an algorithm using provided data, be it histology type or extent of T-cell infiltration, to recognize biologically meaningful patterns in the data set.

Multidimensional scaling can be used to reduce complex data sets to a few specified dimensions so that relationships between groups can be more effectively visualized, in effect cutting down most of the trees in the forest to see the most interesting. Multidimensional scaling is not a clustering technique ***(30)***. Principal component analysis works similarly, revealing the dominant themes within the data set by elimination of less significant variation trends. It is best used in conjunction with a supervised learning technique such as k nearest neighbor or SOMs as it lacks definition when used alone ***(31,32)***.

Cluster reproducibility testing is essential after the generation of supervised and unsupervised analyses. Because the expression variance of large numbers of genes has been mined, false positive results can easily be produced. Such testing can be performed using the discriminating gene subset defined by the same analysis tool on a separate group of allied samples, or where further samples are not available, by using the "leave-one-out" method. This method involves re-examining each sample in turn using the analysis tool gene subset to see whether the sample will be reassigned to the same cluster or a different one. Once all samples have been reviewed, the true positive and type 1 and 2 error rates can be calculated. By varying the number of genes used in the assignment process, the optimal number can be defined. Two others means of assessing the robustness of groupings and clustering are by applying different analysis tools to see if the results of the first analysis are reproduced, and by performing permutation testing, whereby the strengths of randomly generated clusters are compared to those derived by the chosen data mining tool ***(33)***. If the permuted clusters transpired to have less strength than the observed clusters, the latter are considered to be of statistical significance.

In an ideal world, each sample should be prepared and analyzed more than once to eliminate or contain the variability in the data due to technical factors. Because of the constraints of RNA availability and cost, this is rarely done. Criteria for determining the quality of data sets are still evolving, as are the best methods and practices for data analysis and mining.

It is important to ensure that you are quite clear as to what question(s) you are attempting to answer through expression profiling and whether you are in fact going to be arraying the right material in sufficient quantities to come close to meaningful insights into cancer biology and clinical heterogeneity. The following reference gives guidance on minimal sample size ***(34)***. Finally, data storage, which initially is manageable using Excel and Filemaker Pro, rapidly becomes a major logistic issue as your experiment files expand. Guidance on best practice for data storage (required by several journals for article publication) has been created by the MIAME consortium (Minimum information about a microarray experiment) See http://www.mged.org/Workgroups/MIAME/miame.html for details.

2. Materials

When working with chemicals, always wear a suitable laboratory coat, disposable gloves, and protective goggles. Keep away from food and drink. Avoid contact with skin and with eyes. In case of contact with eyes, rinse immediately with plenty of water and seek medical advice. If swallowed, seek medical advice immediately and show the container or label. Use a fume hood when handling chemicals.

2.1. Preventing RNA Degradation and Contamination

RNA degradation is one of the principal problems and frustrations of gene expression profiling. To prevent RNase contamination, always wear latex or vinyl gloves and use diethyl pyrocarbonate (DEPC)-treated distilled water (see below), sterile RNase-free disposable pipet tips, and Microfuge tubes throughout the procedure. Avoid sources of dust or other contaminants, which can interfere with the multiple procedures you will be undertaking.

1. 2-, 20-, 200-, and 1000-μL pipets.
2. RNAse-free tips for 2-, 20-, 200-, and 1000-μL pipets.
3. RNAse-free 0.5-, 1.5-, and 2-mL Microfuge tubes.

2.2. DEPC-Treated Distilled Water

1. Distilled water.
2. DEPC (Sigma-Aldrich; cat. no. 15922). Store at 4–8°C; stable for 2 yr. Safety information: DEPC is a suspected carcinogen and should be handled with great care. Toxic if inhaled, in contact with skin, and if swallowed. Keep away from food and drink. Irritating to eyes, respiratory system. Combustible.)

To prepare DEPC H_2O, add 0.1 mL of DEPC to 100 mL of distilled water or 1 mL of DEPC to 1000 mL of distilled water. Shake vigorously to bring DEPC into solution, then incubate for 12 h at 37°C. Autoclave for 15 min to remove any trace of DEPC. Store, shielded from light at room temperature (RT). Stable for months.

2.3. RNA Extraction, Concentration, and Purification

It is essential to produce highly purified RNA free of proteins, polysaccharide, cell debris, and particularly RNAses. The former contaminants can interfere with the efficiency of synthesis of biotinylated cRNA and also can bind nonspecifically to probes, resulting in increased background and the masking of low frequency target signals.

2.3.1. RNA Extraction

1. TRIzol Reagent (Invitrogen; cat. no. 15596) Store at 4°C, stable for 6 mo. Safety information: toxic in contact with skin and if swallowed. TRIzol causes burns (*see* **Note 1**).

2. Chloroform (BD; cat. no. 10077). Store at RT, stable for minimum of 5 yr. Safety information: harmful by inhalation and if swallowed. Irritating to skin. Possible risk of irreversible effects exists. Danger of serious damage to health by prolonged exposure.
3. DEPC H_2O (*see* **Subheading 2.2.**).
4. 100% Ethanol (BD; cat. no. 10107). Store at RT, stable for minimum of 5 yr. Safety information: highly flammable. Keep away from sources of ignition. Keep container tightly closed.
5. 75% Ethanol (make up using 100% ethanol and DEPC H_2O).
6. 1.5-mL Microfuge tubes.
7. Heating block or waterbath suitable for 1.5-mL Microfuge tubes.
8. Microfuge.

2.3.2. Thawing of Suspended Cryopreserved Cells

Although most lymphoma samples are solid pieces of tissue, usually lymph node, some are derived from body fluids, from which the cells have been concentrated and cryopreserved in suspension.

1. RPMI 1640 media (Invitrogen; cat. no. 21875-034). Store at 4°C.
2. Fetal calf serum (Invitrogen; cat. no. 26140-095). Store at 4°C.
3. Sterile trypan blue solution (0.4%; Sigma; cat. no. T8154). Store at 4°C.
4. Cell counter.
5. Cover slips.
6. Microscope.

2.3.3. Concentration and Cleaning of Total RNA by Ethanol Precipitation

1. Isopropanol (BD; cat. no. 10224). Store at room temperature; stable for minimum 5 yr. Safety information: highly flammable. Keep away from sources of ignition. Keep container tightly closed. May cause harm to the unborn child. Irritating to eyes.
2. 3 *M* sodium acetate, pH 5.2 (Sigma-Aldrich; cat. no. 57899). Store at RT; stable for 1 yr. Safety information: avoid contact and inhalation.
3. 100% ethanol (BD; cat. no. 10107). Store at RT; stable for minimum 5 yr. Safety information: highly flammable. Keep away from sources of ignition. Keep container tightly closed.)
4. DEPC H_2O (*see* **Subheading 2.2.)**
5. 80% ethanol (make up using 100% Ethanol and DEPC H_2O)
5. 1.5-mL Microfuge tubes.
6. Microfuge.

2.3.4. Concentration and Clean-Up of Total RNA Using the RNeasy Mini Kit

The purpose of the total RNA clean-up is to eliminate protein and polysaccharide contamination that can inhibit the transcription and hybridization reactions and increase background noise on the hybridized array by causing nonspecific hybridization to the glass surface.

1. 100% ethanol (BD; cat. no. 10107) Store at RT; stable for minimum 5 yr. Safety information: highly flammable. Keep away from sources of ignition. Keep container tightly closed.
2. DEPC H_2O (*see* **Subheading 2.2.**)
3. Microfuge suitable for 2-mL Microfuge tubes.
4. RNeasy mini kit (X50; Qiagen; cat. no. 74104) Store at RT; stable for 1 yr)

The kit contains:

1. RLT buffer. (Safety information: RLT buffer contains guanidine isothiocyanate, harmful by inhalation, in contact with skin and if swallowed. Contact with acids liberates very toxic gas.)
2. RPE buffer. (Supplied as a concentrate. Before using for the first time add 4 volumes of ethanol [96–100%] as indicated on the bottle. Safety information: Flammable.)
3. RNeasy mini spin columns (silica gel-based membranes, binding up to 100 µg of RNA longer than 200 bases)
4. 1.5-mL collection tubes.
5. 2.0-mL collection tubes.

2.4. Quantity and Quality Assessment of Total RNA

2.4.1. Assessing the Quantity of Total RNA by Spectrophotometry

1. Absorbance spectrometer (e.g., GeneQuant II; Pharmacia Biotech)
2. DEPC H_2O (*see* **Subheading 2.2.**)

2.4.2. Assessing the Quality of Total RNA by Gel Electrophoresis

1. Agarose (Invitrogen; cat. no. 15510-027) Store in a cool and dry place at RT; stable for minimum 5 yr.
2. Heating block suitable for 0.5-mL tubes.
3. Gel loading tank.
4. Power pack.
5. Ultraviolet light box.
6. Photographic equipment.
7. Denaturing loading buffer (*see* **Subheadings 2.4.2.1.** and **2.4.2.2.**).
8. DNA ladder/marker 200 base pairs (bp) to 3 kbp: ϕX174 DNA/*Hae*III (Promega; cat. no. G1761; store at –20°C; stable for 1 yr) and 1-kb DNA ladder (Promega; cat. no. G5711; store at –20°C, stable for 1 yr).
9. Ethidium Bromide tablets (Sigma-Aldrich; cat. no. E-2515) Store at RT; stable for minimum 5 yr. Safety Information: harmful if swallowed; very toxic by inhalation. Irritating to eyes, to respiratory system, and to skin. Keep container tightly closed and in a well-ventilated place.

10. 10X TBE stock solution (*see* **Subheadings 2.4.2.3.** and **2.4.2.4.**). Alternatevely (Invitrogen; cat. no. 15581-028). Store at RT. Safety information: toxic. Harmful by inhalation and in contact with skin. Irritating to eyes and to skin.

2.4.2.1. Denaturing Loading Buffer

1. 10X MOPS (3[*N*-Morpholino]propanesulfonic acid; Sigma-Aldrich; cat. no. M-8899) Store at RT; stable for 3 yr. Safety Information: Irritating to eyes, to respiratory system, and to skin.
2. *N,N*-Dimethylformamide (Sigma-Aldrich; cat. no. D-4551) Store at RT; stable for minimum 5 yr. Safety Information: combustible. Teratogen, target organs: liver and kidneys. May cause harm to the unborn child. Harmful by inhalation and in contact with skin. Irritating to eyes and to skin.
3. Mixed-Bed Resin (Sigma-Aldrich; cat. no. M-8032) Store at RT, stable for minimum 3 yr.
4. Formaldehyde 37% (BDH; cat. no. 43753) Store at RT, stable for minimum 5 yr. Safety Information: toxic by inhalation, in contact with skin, and if swallowed. Causes burns. Danger of very serious irreversible effects. May cause sensitization by skin contact.
5. Glycerol (BDH; cat. no. 10118) Store at RT, stable for minimum 5 yr.
6. Bromophenol Blue (Sigma-Aldrich; cat. no. B-8026) Store at RT, stable for minimum 5 yr. Safety Information: avoid contact and inhalation.
7. DEPC H_2O (*see* **Subheading 2.2.**).

2.4.2.2. Method for Preparing Denaturing Loading Buffer

1. Prepare 10X loading buffer (50 % glycerol, 0.1 mg/mL bromophenol blue sodium salt) as follows:
2. Add 0.2 mg of bromophenol blue sodium salt to 500 µL of DEPC H_2O and mix.
3. Add 500 µL of glycerol and mix thoroughly.
4. Store at RT.
5. Prepare deionized formamide as follows:
6. Add 1 g of mixed bed resin to 50 mL of formamide.
7. Stir for 1 h.
8. Filter through filter paper.
9. Store at –20°C.
10. Prepare in bulk 10 µL of loading buffer for each 1–1.5 µg/µL sample of total RNA, cRNA, or fragmented cRNA as follows:

DEPC H_2O	1.75 µL
10X MOPS	0.50 µL
Deionized formamide	5.00 µL
Formaldehyde 37%	1.75 µL
10X loading buffer (50% glycerol, 0.1 mg/mL Bromophenol Blue)	1.00 µL
Final volume	10.0 µL

11. Freeze in 100- to 200-μL aliquots and keep at –20°C.
12. Make a 10mg/mL ethidium bromide solution when ready to add buffer to samples.
13. Add 0.5 μL of ethidium bromide (10 mg/mL)/100 μL defrosted denaturing loading buffer just before adding the buffer to the samples.

2.4.2.3. 10X TBE Stock Solution

1. DEPC H_2O (*see* **Subheadings 2.2.** and **3.**).
2. TRIS base (Invitrogen; cat. no. 15504-020). Store at RT; stable for minimum of 2 yr. Safety Information: toxic by inhalation, in contact with skin, and if swallowed. Irritating to eyes, respiratory system.
3. Boric acid (BD; cat. no. 100583R). Store at 15–30°C; stable for minimum of 2 yr. Safety Information: irritating by inhalation, in contact with skin, and if swallowed.
4. Ethylenediamine tetra-acetic acid (EDTA) di-Sodium Salt, pH 8.0 (Sigma-Aldrich; cat. no., E-7889). Store at RT, stable for 1 yr.

2.4.2.4. Method for Preparing 10X TBE Stock Solution

1. Make a solution of: (1) 108 g TRIS, (2) 55 g boric acid, (3) 40 mL 0.5 *M* EDTA, and (4) DEPC H_2O to 1000 mL.
2. Filter through a 0.2-μm vacuum filter unit. Store at 4°C and shield from light.

2.4.3. Assessing the Quality of Total RNA Using the 2100 Agilent Bioanalyzer

1. Agilent 2100 Bioanalyser System (Agilent Technologies; cat. no. G2940CA). Includes 2100 bioanalyzer equipped with bayonet electrode cartridge, HP Compaq EvoD510 SFF (Pentium IV, Windows 2000), 17" monitor, HP DeskJet color printer, bioanalyzer system software, vortex mixer with chip adapter, and startup accessories.
2. RA 6000 Nano LabChip Kit (cat. no. 5065-4476).

The kit contains:

1. RNA chips.
2. Electrode cleaners.
3. RNA dye concentrate. (Molecular Probes; Shield from light to prevent degradation by light exposure. Store at 4°C. Stable for 3 mo. Safety Information: toxicity unknown, as it contains dimethyl sulfoxide, which facilitates organic molecule entry through the skin, wear double gloves.)
4. RNA 6000 Nano Marker. (Store at 4°C and shield from light.)
5. RNA Gel Matrix. (Store at 4°C and shield from light.)
6. 1-mL syringe.
7. Chip Priming Station (Agilent Technologies; cat. no. 5065-4401).
8. Vortex Mixer IKA.
9. RNA 6000 ladder (Ambion; cat. no. 7152) Aliquot and store at –80°C.

10. RNAseZAP (Ambion; cat. no. 9780) Store at RT, stable for minimum 5 yr. Safety Information: avoid contact and inhalation.
11. DEPC H_2O (*see* **Subheading 2.2.**).
12. 0.5- and 1.5-mL Microfuge tubes.
13. Microfuge.
14. Timer.
15. Heating block suitable for 0.5-mL Microfuge tubes.

2.4.3.1. Method for Preparing Gel-Dye Mix

This resultant 132 µL of gel-dye mix is stable for 1 wk if kept at 4°C and shielded from light. This volume is sufficient for 4 RNA chips.

1. Pipet 400 µL of gel matrix (red dot on lid) into a spin filter receptacle.
2. Place the spin filter into a 1.5-mL Microfuge tube.
3. Centrifuge at RT, 1500*g* for 10 min.
4. Pipet 130 µL of the filtered gel matrix into a fresh 1.5-mL Microfuge tube.
5. Add 2 µL of RNA Dye Concentrate (blue dot on lid) and vortex for 1 min to mix.
6. Store at 4°C, shield from light, and use within 1 wk.
7. Store the remaining filtered gel matrix at 4°C and use within 1 mo.

2.5. ds-cDNA Synthesis

2.5.1. First-Strand cDNA Synthesis

1. Oligo (dT)23 (Sigma, cat. no. 04387). Store at –20°C; stable for 1 yr).
2. 10 m*M* dNTP. Mix (10 m*M* each dATP, dGTP, dCTP, and dTTP at neutral pH; Invitrogen; cat. no. 18427-013). Store at –20°C; stable for 6 mo.
3. 500-µL Microfuge tubes.
4. Microfuge.
5. Two heating blocks suitable for 500-µL Microfuge tubes, one with a heated lid or a water bath.
6. SuperScript TM II RNase H- Reverse Transcriptase Kit (Invitrogen; cat. no. 18064-014). Store at –20°C; stable for 6 mo.

The kit contains:

1. 5X First Strand Buffer: 250 m*M* Tris-HCl, pH 8.3, 375 m*M* KCl, 15 m*M* $MgCl_2$.
2. 0.1 *M* dithiothreitol (DTT). Safety information: irritating to eyes, skin, and respiratory system.
3. SuperScript TM II Reverse Transcriptase (200 U/µL).

2.5.2. Second-Strand cDNA Synthesis

1. 5X Second-Strand Buffer (100 m*M* Tris-HCl, pH 6.9; 450 m*M* KCl; 23 m*M* $MgCl_2$; 50 m*M* $(NH_4)2SO_4$, 0.75 m*M* β-NAD+; (Invitrogen; cat. no. 10812-014). Store at –20°C; stable for 6 mo.
2. 10 m*M* dNTP Mix (10 m*M* each dATP, dGTP, dCTP, and dTTP at neutral pH; Invitrogen; cat. no. 18427-013). Store at –20°C; stable for 6 mo.

3. *E. coli* DNA Ligase (10 U/μL; Invitrogen; cat. no. 18052-019). Store at –20°C; stable for 6 mo.
4. *E. coli* DNA Pol I (10 U/μL; Invitrogen; cat. no. 18010-025). Store at –20°C, stable for 6 mo.
5. *E. coli* RNase H (2 U/μL; Invitrogen; cat. no. 18021-071). Store at –20°C, stable for 6 mo.
6. T4 DNA Polymerase (5 U/μL; Invitrogen; cat. no. 18005-025). Store at –20°C; stable for 6 mo.
7. Ethylenediamine tetra-acetic acid (EDTA) di-Sodium Salt, pH 8.0 (Sigma-Aldrich; cat. no. E-7889). Store at RT, stable for 1 yr.
8. 500-μL Microfuge tubes.
9. Microfuge.
10. Refrigerated water bath.

Or

11. Refrigerated PCR block with heated lid and wells for 500-mL Microfuge tubes.

2.6. Clean-Up and Concentration of ds-cDNA

2.6.1. Clean-Up of ds-cDNA

1. Phase Lock Gel tubes (2 mL, light; Eppendorf; cat. no. 0032 005101). Store at RT, stable for 1 yr.
2. Phenol:chloroform:isoamyl alcohol, 25:24:1, pH 6.6, buffered pH 7.9 (Ambion; cat. no. 9732). Store at 4°C or –20°C; stable for 6 mo. Accompanied by a separate pre-made Alkaline Buffer solution to be added just prior to use (10 m*M* Tris-HCl, 1 m*M* EDTA, pH 8.0). Safety Information: toxic in contact with skin and if swallowed; causes burns.)
3. 1.5-mL Microfuge tubes.
4. Microfuge suitable for 2-mL tubes.

2.6.2. Precipitation of ds-cDNA

1. 7.5 *M* ammonium acetate (Sigma-Aldrich; cat. no. A-2706). Store at RT, stable for 1 yr. Safety Information: irritant to eyes, skin and respiratory system.
2. Glycogen (5 mg/mL; Ambion; cat. no. 9510). Store at –20°C, stable for 1 yr.
3. 100 % Ethanol (BD; cat. no. 10107). Store at RT, stable for minimum 5 yr. Safety information: highly flammable. Keep away from sources of ignition. Keep container tightly closed.

2.7. In Vitro Transcription–Synthesis of Biotinylated cRNA

1. DEPC H_2O (*see* **Subheading 2.2.**).
2. BioArray High Yield RNA Transcript Labeling Kit (Enzo Biochem; cat. no. 900182). Store at –20°C; stable for 3 mo.

The kit contains:

10X HY reaction buffer.
10X Biotin-labeled ribonucleotides (ATP, GTP, CTP, UTP with Bio-UTP and Bio-CTP).
10X DTT.
10X RNase inhibitor mix.
20X T7 RNA Polymerase (*see* **Note 2**).

2.7.1. Clean-Up of cRNA

This step is performed to eliminate unincorporated biotin-labeled ribonucleotides.

1. 100 % ethanol (BD; cat. no. 10107). Store at RT, stable for minimum 5 yr. Safety information: highly flammable. Keep away from sources of ignition. Keep container tightly closed.
2. DEPC H_2O (*see* **Subheading 2.2.**).
3. RNeasy Mini Kit (X50; Qiagen; cat. no. 74104). Store at RT, stable for 1 yr.

The kit contains:

RLT buffer. (Safety Information: RLT Buffer contains guanidine isothiocyanate, harmful by inhalation, in contact with skin and if swallowed. Contact with acids liberates very toxic gas.)
RPE buffer. (The buffer is supplied as a concentrate. Before using for the first time, add 4 volumes of ethanol (96–100%) as indicated on the bottle. Safety information: flammable.)

4. RNeasy mini spin columns. (The columns contain a silica-gel-based membrane, which binds up to 100 mg of RNA longer than 200 base pairs.)
5. 1.5-mL collection tubes.
6. 2.0-mL collection tubes.
7. Microfuge suitable for 2-mL tubes.

2.8. Assessing the Quantity and Quality of the Purified cRNA

2.8.1. Assessing the Quality of Purified cRNA by Spectrophotometry

See **Subheading 2.4.1.**

2.8.2. Assessing the Quality of the Purified cRNA by Gel Electrophoresis

See **Subheading 2.4.2.**

2.8.3. Assessing the Quality of the Purified cRNA Using the Agilent Bioanalyzer

See **Subheading 2.4.3.**

2.9. Increasing cRNA Concentration by Ethanol Precipitation

1. 7.5 *M* ammonium acetate (Sigma-Aldrich; cat. no. A-2706). Store at RT, stable for 1 yr. Safety information: irritant to eyes, skin and respiratory system.
2. 100% ethanol (BD; cat. no. 10107). Store at RT, stable for minimum 5 yr. Safety information: highly flammable. Keep away from sources of ignition. Keep container tightly closed.
3. DEPC H_2O.
4. 80% ethanol (made from 100% ethanol and DEPC H_2O).

2.10. cRNA Fragmentation

1. TRIZMA Base (Sigma-Aldrich; cat. no. T-1503). Store at RT, stable for 3 yr. Safety Information: Irritating to eyes, to respiratory system and to skin.
2. Magnesium acetate (Sigma-Aldrich; cat. no. M-2545). Store at RT, stable for 3 yr.
3. Potassium Acetate (Sigma-Aldrich; cat. no. P-5708). Store at RT, stable for 3 yr. Safety Information: Irritating to eyes, to respiratory system and to skin.
4. Glacial acetic acid (Sigma-Aldrich; cat. no. A-6283). Store at RT, stable for minimum 5 yr. Safety Information: Flammable. Harmful in contact with skin; causes severe burns. Keep away from sources of ignition.
5. DEPC H_2O (*see* **Subheading 2.2.**).
6. pH meter.

2.10.1. Method for Preparing 5X Fragmentation Buffer

Composition: 200 m*M* Tris-acetate, pH 8.1, 500 m*M* KOAc, 150 m*M* MgOAc.

Adjust an adequate volume of Trizma base to pH 8.1 using glacial acetic acid. Combine the following components to a total volume of 20 mL:

1 *M* Tris acetate, pH 8.1	4.0 mL
Magnesium acetate	0.64 g
Potassium acetate	0.98 g
DEPC H_2O to	20 mL

Mix thoroughly and filter through a 0.2-mm vacuum filter unit. Aliquot as 1 mL volumes and store at RT or 4°C (stable for 1 yr)

2.10.2. Assessing the Quality of the Fragmented cRNA

It is not possible to meaningfully assess the quantity of fragmented cRNA. Instead, use the concentration of purified cRNA to calculate the amount of fragmented cRNA.

2.10.3. Assessing the Quality of the Fragmented cRNA by Gel Electrophoresis

See **Subheading 2.4.2.**

2.10.4. Assessing the Quality of the Fragmented cRNA by 2100 Agilent Bioanalyzer

See **Subheading 2.4.3.**

2.11. Probe Hybridization Cocktail

The eukaryotic hybridization controls are added to allow the sensitivity achieved on each chip to be assessed, whereas the control oligonucleotide B2 is added to allow the demarcation and orientation of the array grid to be determined in the scanned image. If the control oligonucleotide B2 is accidentally left out, the chip(s) in question will be unreadable.

1. Fragmented cRNA (15 µg).
2. GeneChip hybridization control kit (Affymetrix cat. no. 9900454). The kit contains: 20X eukaryotic hybridization controls (bioB 30 p*M*, bioC 100 p*M*, bioD 500 p*M*, cre 2000 p*M*. Store at –20°C; stable for 6 mo. 3 n*M* control oligonucleotide B2.
3. 2X hybridization buffer (*see* **Subheadings 2.13.3.** and **2.13.4.**).
4. Acetylated bovine serum albumin (50 mg/mL; Invitrogen; cat. no. 15561-020). Store at –20°C; stable for 6 mo.
5. Herring sperm DNA (10 mg/mL; Promega; cat. no. D1811). Store at –20°C aliquotted; stable for 6 mo.
6. DEPC H_2O.
7. 500-µL Microfuge tubes.

2.12. Denaturing the Fragmented Target in the Hybridization Cocktail

Two heating blocks suitable for 500-µL Microfuge tubes.

2.13. Hybridizing the Target to the Probe Array

1. Probe array chip(s) (*see* **Note 3**).
2. GeneChip Hybridization Oven 640 (Affymetrix).
3. 12X MES stock solution (*see* **Subheadings 2.13.1.** and **2.13.2.**).
4. 2X Hybridization buffer (*see* **Subheadings 2.13.3.** and **2.13.4.**).
5. Analytical-grade water (e.g., from a bench-top unit such as Simplicity® Personal Ultrapure Water System, Millipore; cat. no. SIMS 600 00; *see* **Note 4**).

2.13.1. 12X MES Stock

1. MES free acid monohydrate (4-morpholineethanesulfonic acid monohydrate 2-(*N*-morpholino)ethanesulfonic acid; Sigma-Aldrich; cat. no. M-5287). Store at RT, shield from light, stable for 1 yr. Safety Information: irritating to eyes, to respiratory system, and to skin.
2. MES sodium salt (2-morpholinoethanesulfonic acid sodium salt; Sigma-Aldrich; cat. no. M3058). Store at RT, shield from light, stable for 1 yr.
3. Analytical-grade water (e.g., from a bench-top unit such as Simplicity® Personal Ultrapure Water System, Millipore; cat. no. SIMS 600 00).

4. 0.2-µm filters.
5. Vacuum filter unit.

2.13.2. Method for Preparing 1 L of 12X MES Stock

The final 1X concentration will be 1.22 M MES, 0.89 M NaCl

1. Make a solution of: (1) 70.4 g MES free acid monohydrate; (2) 193.3 g MES sodium salt; and (3) analytical-grade water to 1000 mL.
2. Filter through a 0.2-µm vacuum filter unit. Store at 4°C and shield from light (*see* **Note 5**).

2.13.3. 2X Hybridization Buffer

2X concentration: 200 m*M* MES, 2 *M* NaCl, 40 m*M* EDTA, and 0.02% Tween-20.

1. 12X MES stock (*see* **Subheadings 2.13.1.** and **2.13.2.**).
2. Analytical-grade water (e.g., from a bench-top unit such as Simplicity® Personal Ultrapure Water System, Millipore; cat. no. SIMS 600 00).
3. 5 *M* sodium chloride (Sigma-Aldrich; cat. no. S-S150). Store at RT, stable for 1 yr.
4. EDTA di-Sodium Salt, pH 8.0 (Sigma-Aldrich; cat. no. E-7889). Store at RT, stable for 1 yr.
5. Tween-20 (Sigma-Aldrich; cat. no. P-9416). Store at RT, stable for minimum 1 yr.
6. 0.2-µm filters.
7. Vacuum filter unit.

2.13.4. Method for Preparing 50 mL of 2X Hybridization Buffer

2X hybridization buffer is used to make the hybridization cocktail and as a 1X solution to prime the array chips ready for the denatured hybridization cocktail. 50 mL is sufficient to make the necessary hybridization cocktail and 1X priming solution for a mini (e.g., Test 3) and standard chip (e.g., HG-U133) for 100 samples. The final 1X concentration will be 100 m*M* MES, 1 *M* NaCl, 20 m*M* EDTA, and 0.01% Tween-20.

1. Make a solution of the following:

12X MES Stock	83.3 mL
5 *M* sodium chloride	17.7 mL
0.5 *M* EDTA	4.0 mL
10% Tween-20	0.1 mL
Analytical-grade water	19.9 mL
Final volume	50.0 mL

2. Filter through a 0.2-µm vacuum filter unit. Store at 4°C, and shield from light (*see* **Note 6**).

2.14. Fluidics Station Procedures

1. GeneChip Fluidics station 400 or 450 (Affymetrix). (*See* **Note 7**).

2. Microarray Suite 5.1 (Affymetrix).
3. 1.5-mL Microfuge tubes.

2.14.1. Fluidics Washing Solutions

1. 12X MES Stock (*see* **Subheadings 2.13.1.** and **2.13.2.**).
2. 20X SSPE (Invitrogen; cat. no. 15591-043). Store at RT, stable for 1 yr.
3. 5 *M* sodium chloride (Sigma-Aldrich; cat. no. S-S150). Store at RT, stable for 1 yr.
4. Tween 20 (Sigma-Aldrich; cat. no. P-9416). Store at RT, stable for minimum 1 yr.
5. Analytical-grade water (e.g., from a bench-top unit such as Simplicity® Personal Ultrapure Water System, Millipore; cat. no. SIMS 600 00).
6. 0.2-µm filters.
7. Vacuum filter unit.

2.14.2. Method for Preparing 1 L of Nonstringent Wash Buffer (Solution A)

The final concentration will be 6X SSPE, 0.01% Tween-20.

1. Make a solution of the following:

20X SSPE	300 mL
10% Tween-20	1.0 mL
Analytical-grade water	698 mL
Final volume	1000 mL

2. Filter through a 0.2-µm vacuum filter unit. Store at 4°C, and shield from light.
3. Use within 1 wk.

2.14.3. Method for Preparing 1 L of Stringent Wash Buffer (Solution B)

The final concentration will be 100 mM MES, 0.1 M NaCl, 0.01% Tween-20

1. Make a solution of the following:

12X MES stock	8.3 mL
5 *M* sodium chloride	5.2 mL
10% Tween-20	1.0 mL
Analytical-grade water	910.5 mL
Final volume	1000 mL

2. Filter through a 0.2-µm vacuum filter unit. Store at 4°C, and shield from light.
3. Use within 1 wk.

2.14.4. Fluidics Staining Solutions

1. R-Phycoerythrin streptavidin (Molecular probes; cat. no. S-866). Store at 2–8°C and shield from light; stable for 3 mo.
2. Biotinylated, goat, anti-streptavidin antibody (Vector laboratories; cat. no. BA-0500). Store at 2–8°C, stable for 6 mo. For long-term storage, keep aliquots at –20°C.
3. Goat IgG (Sigma-Aldrich; cat. no. I-5256). Store at 2–8°C, stable for 6 mo. For long-term storage, keep aliquots at –20°C.
4. Acetylated bovine serum albumin (50 mg/mL; Invitrogen; cat. no. 15561-020). Store at –20°C; stable for 6 mo.

5. 12X MES Stock (*see* **Subheadings 2.13.1.** and **2.13.2.**).
6. 5 *M* sodium chloride (Sigma-Aldrich; cat. no. S-S150). Store at RT, stable for 1 yr.
7. Tween-20 (Sigma-Aldrich; cat. no. P-9416). Store at RT, stable for at least 1 yr.
8. Analytical-grade water (e.g., from a bench-top unit such as Simplicity® Personal Ultrapure Water System, Millipore; Cat No SIMS 600 00).
9. 0.2-µm filters.
10. Vacuum filter unit.

2.14.5. Method for Preparing 250 mL of 2X Stain Buffer

The final 1X concentration will be 100 m*M* MES, 1 *M* NaCl, and 0.05% Tween-20.

1. Make a solution of the following:

12X MES stock	41.7 mL
5 *M* sodium chloride	92.5 mL
10% Tween-20	2.5 mL
Analytical-grade water	112.8 mL
Final volume	250 mL

2. Filter through a 0.2-µm vacuum filter unit. Store at 4°C, and shield from light.
3. Use within 1 mo.

2.15. Laser Scanning the Array

1. Microarray Suite 5.1 (Affymetrix).
2. GeneArray scanner (Agilent Technologies).

OR

3. GeneChip Scanner 3000 enabled for high-resolution scanning if using HG-U133 Plus 2.0 or HG-U133A 2.0 (Affymetrix; cat. no. 00-0074).

We recommend training and supervision when you start using the following equipment or else delays, errors, and faults will occur:

GeneChip Fluidic Station 400 or 450 (Affymetrix)
GeneArray scanner (Agilent Technologies)
GeneChip Scanner 3000 (Affymetrix)

2.16. Data Analysis and Storage

Microarray Suite 5.1 (Affymetrix)

2.16.1. Data-Storage Systems

Careful storage of the masses of information you will soon acquire is imperative. Commercial and academic options are available. One popular free web-based storage site is AMAD (Another MicroArray Database; visit http://www.microarrays.org/AMADFaq.html for details and registration). With AMAD, a researcher with no prior UNIX or database skills can rapidly and cheaply set up a database system capable of storing thousands of gene expression experiments.

2.16.2. Data Analysis Packages

Considerable time and resources will be required to confidently produce and validate gene clusters. If you are unable to collaborate with an experienced bioinformatics person, at least attend a training course to ease some of the inevitable frustrations that will come if you attempt analysis alone. An increasing number of evolving free and commercially available packages are available from which to choose. None is easy to use for a novice with little statistical experience, but all are a lot more user friendly than pure statistical packages or methodologies alone. One advantage of a commercial software package is some back up if you don't have easy access to a bioinformatics expert. Most of the free-to-academic-user packages can be accessed via the commendably comprehensive web pages at http://www.microarrays.org/index.html and http://ihome.cuhk.edu.hk/~b400559/array.html.

The major two noncommercial data packages are listed below:

- "Cluster" and "Treeview": Created by the team at Stanford University, California, these complimentary programs allow processing and visualization of large data sets using hierarchical clustering, self-organizing maps, k-means clustering, and principal component analysis (http://rana.lbl.gov/EisenSoftware.htm)
- GeneCluster2 GeneCluster 2.0: provides the tools to perform supervised classification, gene selection, and permutation test methods. It includes algorithms for building and testing supervised models using weighted voting (WV) and k-nearest neighbours (KNN) algorithms, batch self-organizing maps clustering, and a visualization module. (http://www-genome.wi.mit.edu/cancer/software/genecluster2/gc2.html)
- The pre-eminent commercial package is GeneSpring 7: Contains normalization tools as well as visualization and analysis programs for performing hierarchical clustering, experiment trees, self-organizing maps, k-means clustering, support vector machines, and principal components analysis (PCA) to aid characterization of the most significant patterns in a given experiment (http://www.silicongenetics.com/cgi/SiG.cgi/Products/GeneSpring/index.smf)

3. Methods

Use the following time scale to help plan what you can realistically do on a given day and by when you will need to have prepared the stock solutions detailed in the Materials subsections above.

3.1. A Time-Scale: From Tumor to Chip to Data Analysis

RNA extraction, clean-up, and assessment, 3 h	(Day 1)
First-strand cDNA synthesis, 2 h	(Day 2)
Second-strand cDNA synthesis, 2 h	(Day 2)

Clean-up of ds-cDNA, 1 h	(Day 2)
In vitro transcription	
~ Biotinylated cRNA synthesis, 5 h	(Day 3)
Clean-up and assessment of biotinylated cRNA, 1 h	(Day 3)
Fragmentation and assessment of biotinylated cRNA, 2 h	(Day 4)
Hybridization onto chips, overnight 16 h	(Day 4/5)
Fluidics: 1st SAPE, antibody, and 2nd SAPE staining, 2 h	(Day 5)
Laser scanning, 10 min	(Day 6)
Data processing	(Day 6+)

3.2. RNA Extraction

Good-quality RNA is essential to the overall success of the analysis. We strongly recommend that you work on as few as two samples at a time and no more than eight to avoid excessive delays and errors. In the absence of an established protocol, use one of the commercially available kits or reagents designed for RNA isolation (e.g., Qiagen RNA/DNA Kits; TRIzol Reagent).

3.2.1. RNA Extraction

1. Warm a heat block or water bath to 55°C and chill 75% and 100% ethanol tubes to –20°C and a centrifuge to 4°C.
2. Place TRIzol on ice and fresh 1.5-mL Microfuge tubes and vials of tissue stored in liquid nitrogen on dry ice.
3. Working on dry ice, use a sterile blade to cut slivers of tissue from each lymph node piece, adding no more than 2 mm^3 to each chilled Microfuge tube.
4. To each tube in turn, add 1 mL of TRIzol and homogenize using sterile plastic pestle supplied with each tube (*see* **Note 8**).
5. Incubate for 5 min at RT.
6. Add 0.2 mL of chloroform per 1 mL of TRIzol, shake vigorously for 15 s.
7. Incubate for 2 to 3 min at RT (*see* **Note 9**).
8. Centrifuge samples for 15 min at 4°C and ≤12,000*g*.
9. After centrifuging, the mixture separates into a lower red, phenol-chloroform phase, an interphase, and a colorless upper aqueous phase. Recover this upper phase into a new set of labeled tubes, which contains the RNA, avoiding the interphase.
10. Precipitate the RNA by mixing with 0.5 mL of isopropanol per 1 mL of TRIzol used for the initial homogenization.
11. Incubate samples at RT for 10 min.
12. Centrifuge at ≤12,000*g* for 10 min at 4°C. The RNA precipitate will have formed into a gel-like pellet on the side and bottom of the tube.
13. Carefully remove the supernatant and wash the RNA pellet once by adding ≥ 1 mL of ethanol 75% per 1 mL of TRIzol used.
14. Mix by vortexing and centrifuge at ≤7500*g* for 5 min at 4°C.
15. Remove the supernatant and allow samples to air dry.

16. Resuspend in 40–50 µL of DEPC H_2O.
17. Incubate samples at 55°C for 5 min to aid RNA dissolution.
18. Read a 1:2 to 1:5 dilution on a spectrophotometer as described in **Subheading 3.3.1.**
19. Proceed to either "Concentration & Clean-up of Total RNA by Ethanol Precipitation" (**Subhheading 3.2.3.**) or "Concentration and Clean-up of Total RNA Using the RNeasy mini Kit" (**Subheading 3.2.4.**) to concentrate and purify further the RNA obtained (*see* **Notes 10** and **11**).

3.2.2. RNA Extraction From Suspended Cryopreserved Cells

3.2.2.1. Thawing of Suspended Cryopreserved Cells

1. Prepare 10 mL RPMI 1640 medium with 10% fetal calf serum per vial of cells to be thawed.
2. Remove vials from liquid nitrogen and immediately thaw in 37°C water bath.
3. Empty contents of each vial into separate sterile 10 mL tubes.
4. Add medium one drop every 10–15 s for 2 min, then two drops every 10–15 s for 2 min, then gradually increase numbers of drops to 5 mL level.
5. Top up to 10 mL then spin at 800*g* for 5 min.
6. Resuspend pellet in 2 mL medium and perform a cell count (10 µL 0.1% Trypan Blue + 10 µL cells; (*see* **Note 12**).

3.2.2.2. RNA Extraction From Suspended Cryopreserved Cells

1. Split cells in 2 mL tubes to a maximum of 15 million cells per tube.
2. Spin at 800*g* (17 cm rota arm) for 5 min to remove the medium.
3. Add 0.1 mL of TRIzol per million cells.
4. Proceed with RNA extraction as detailed in **Subheading 3.2.1.** from **step 6** above.
5. After isopropanol precipitation and wash, allow samples to air dry.
6. Resuspend in 40–50 µL of DEPC H_2O.
7. Leave samples at 55°C for 5 min.
8. Read a 1:2 to 1:5 dilution at the spectrophotometer as described in the next section (*see* **Note 13**)

3.2.3. Concentration and Clean-Up of Total RNA by Ethanol Precipitation

Much better yields of labeled cRNA are obtained from the in vitro transcription and labeling reaction when inhibitors of transcription are removed from the total RNA. Perform either this procedure or the next, **Subheading 3.2.4.** (*see* **Note 14**).

1. Chill 80% and 100% ethanol tubes to –20°C. To each sample, add 1/10 volume 3 *M* sodium acetate, pH 5.2, and 2.5 volumes of cold 100% ethanol.
2. Mix and incubate at –20°C for at least 1 h to overnight.
3. Centrifuge at 12,000*g* and 4°C for 20 min.
4. Wash pellet twice with cold 80% ethanol.
5. Air dry pellet. Check for dryness before proceeding.

6. Resuspend the RNA in DEPC H_2O RNA to give a final minimal concentration of >1 μg/μL, (to be able to use 10 μg of RNA for first- and second-strand reaction) Incubate samples at 55°C for 5 min to aid RNA dissolution (*see* **Note 15**).

3.2.4. Clean-Up of Total RNA Using the RNeasy Mini Kit

This is an alternative to the procedure detailed in **Subheading 3.2.3.**

1. Warm to RT reagents listed in **Subheading 2.2.4.**
2. All steps of the protocol should be performed at RT.
3. Do not add β-mercaptoethanol to RLT buffer because it can increase background signal.
4. Label the lid of a set of RNeasy spin columns and a set of 1.5-mL collection tubes with each RNA sample's identifier (*see* **Note 16**).
5. For each 10 μL, RNA add the following:

DEPC H_2O	15 μL
RLT buffer	87.5 μL
Final volume	112.5 μL

6. Mix thoroughly by pipetting.
7. Then, add 62.5 μL of 100% ethanol for each 10 μL of RNA to give a total volume per 10 μL of RNA of 175 μL.
8. Mix thoroughly by pipetting.
9. Transfer the entire contents of each RNA tube to the corresponding spin column placed inside the first set of 2-mL collection tubes.
10. Centrifuge for just 15 s at 8000*g*.
11. Transfer the spin column to the second set of 2-mL collection tubes.
12. Add 500 μL of RPE buffer to each spin column.
13. Transfer this second set of collection tubes containing the spin columns back to the centrifuge and again centrifuge for 15 s at 8000*g*.
14. Transfer the spin column to the third set of 2-mL collection tubes.
15. Add 500 μL of RPE buffer to each spin column.
16. Centrifuge for 2 min at maximum speed.
17. Transfer the spin column to the fourth and final set of 2-mL collection tubes.
18. Centrifuge for 1 min at maximum speed to ensure that the spin column membrane is quite dry.
19. Transfer the spin columns to the correspondingly labeled set of 1.5-mL RNase-free collection tubes.
20. Resuspend the RNA in DEPC H_2O RNA to give a final minimal concentration of >1 μg/μL (to be able to use 10 μg of RNA for first and second strand reaction)
21. Allow 2 min for the RNA to dissolve.
22. Collect the cleaned RNA solution by centrifuging for 1 min at 8000*g*.
23. Perform a second elution (*see* **Subheading 3.2.5.**) if you are worried that the RNA yield will not yet be 10 μg, or move on to **Subheading 3.3.** (*see* **Note 17**).

3.2.5. Second Elution to Maximize Total RNA Recovery

1. Add a further 30–50 µL of DEPC H_2O to the spin column still inserted in the 1.5-mL collection tube.
2. Centrifuge at 8000*g* for 1 min.
3. Quantitate and qualitate the RNA according to the next stage (*see* **Note 18**).

3.3. Quantity and Quality Assessment of Total RNA

3.3.1. Assessing the Quantity of Total RNA by Spectrophotometry

1. Turn on the spectrophotometer 15 min before use.
2. Calibrate the meter using a DEPC H_2O control according to the machine's specific instructions.
3. Quantify RNA yield by spectrophotometric analysis at 260 and 280 nm for sample concentration and purity(*see* **Note 19**).

3.3.2. Assessing the Quality of Total RNA by Gel Electrophoresis

1. Make a 1% agarose gel using 1X TBE solution (*see* **Subheadings 2.4.2.3.** and **2.4.2.4.**).
2. Warm a heating block to 65–70°C.
3. Cover gel in tank with 1X TBE solution.
4. Defrost a DNA reference ladder covering 200 to 3 kbp.
5. Mix 0.5 µg to 1 µg of each total RNA with 10 µL of denaturing loading buffer, prepared as described in **Subheading 2.4.2.2.**
6. Denature samples by heating to 65–70°C for 2 min.
7. Place samples on ice for a minute. Spin briefly.
8. Load samples into the 1% agarose gel along with the DNA ladder.
9. Run for 30–40 min at 70 volts.
10. View and photograph gel under ultraviolet light using usual protective gear (*see* **Note 20**).

3.3.3. Assessing the Quality of Total RNA Using the 2100 Agilent Bioanalyzer

Refer to the detailed and well-illustrated accompanying manual for further details to those below. For total RNA, the concentration range that can be quantified is between 25 and 500 ng/µL.

1. Therefore, for most of your samples you will need to make a diluted aliquot. Warm the reagents, including an aliquot of RNA 6000 ladder, to RT and a heating block to 70°C.
2. Turn on the Bioanalyzer and its workstation 15 min before use. Start the Agilent 2100 Bioanalyzer software by double clicking on the Bioanalyzer desktop icon.
3. Prepare 3 µL of each total RNA to be measured with a concentration <500 ng/µL using DEPC H_2O.
4. Denature the RNA samples and a 3-µL aliquot of RNA 6000 ladder by heating to 70° for 2 min.
5. Place denatured ladder and samples on ice (*see* **Note 21**).

3.3.3.1. Decontaminating the Electrodes

1. Fill the first electrode cleaner chip via one of its wells with 350 µL of RNAseZAP.
2. Open the lid of the Agilent 2100 Bioanalyzer and insert the first electrode cleaner.
3. Close the lid; leave for 1 min and then remove the first electrode cleaner chip.
4. Add 350 µL of DEPC H_2O to the second electrode cleaner chip.
5. Insert the second electrode cleaner chip in the Bioanalyzer and leave for just 10 s before removing.
6. Allow the Bioanalyser electrodes to dry for 10 s before closing the lid.

3.3.3.2. Loading the RNA Chip

1. Set the Chip Priming Station base plate to position C, insert the syringe (1 mL) into the syringe holder and set the adjustable syringe clip to the highest position.
2. Place a new RNA chip on the chip priming station with the writing towards you and the "cut off" corner top right.
3. Dispense 9 µL of gel-dye mix into the bottom of the third well marked with a "G" from the top of the chip (*see* **Note 22**).
4. Raise the syringe plunger to the 1 mL mark and close the chip priming station.
5. Depress the plunger until it is held by the syringe clip.
6. Keep well "G" pressurized for exactly 30 s then release the plunger and return it to the 1 mL mark.
7. Open the chip priming station and ensure that no bubbles are present in the chip channels by hold the chip to the light.
8. If bubbles are present in the channels repeat **steps 4** to **7** above (*see* **Note 23**).
9. Dispense 9 µL of gel-dye mix into the bottom of the other two wells marked with a "G."
10. Pipet 5 µL of RNA 6000 Nano Marker (green dot on lid) into each sample well you will use and the ladder well.
11. Pipet 6 µL of RNA 6000 Nano Marker (green dot on lid) into each sample well not to be used.
12. Add 1 µL of denatured RNA 6000 ladder to the bottom of the well with the ladder symbol (bottom right)
13. Add a 1 µL of each denatured sample into each sample wells, loading from top left to bottom right (1 through 12; *see* **Note 24**).
14. Vortex the chip for 1 minute at the recommended speed (IKA vortexer set-point)
15. Place the chip in the Bioanalyzer and close the lid. Begin the run within 5 minutes to avoid deleterious evaporation (*see* **Note 25**).
16. Return to the workstation, where the chip icon will now be displayed top left, indicating that a chip has been inserted and the lid successfully closed.
17. From the "Assay" menu, select "RNA" and then the type of RNA assay you wish to perform (usually Eukaryote Total RNA nano)
18. Click on the "Start" icon to bring up the "Start" dialog box.
19. Add your desired file prefix. The data will be saved to a file of this name.
20. Adjust the number of samples to be run and ensure that the "Edit samples after start" box is ticked.

21. Click on the "Start" button.
22. As desired, add the identifiers for each sample in the "Samples Information" window of the "General Chip Information" dialogue box (*see* **Notes 26** and **27**).

3.4. Production of ds-cDNA

3.4.1. First-Strand cDNA Synthesis

1. Chill a Microfuge to 4°C and warm a heating block to 65–70°C and a water bath or a heating block with heated lid to 42°C.
2. Defrost the reagents listed in the **Subheading 2.5.1.**, vortex, spin and keep on ice.
3. For each sample, working on ice, add to a labeled 500 µL Microfuge tube (*see* **Notes 28** and **29**).

Total RNA (minimum of 5 µg[a] and maximum of 20 µg[b])	x* µL
T7-(dT)24 primer (100 pmol/µL)	1 µL
DEPC H_2O	y* µL
[a]Final volume	12 µL

OR

[b]Final volume	11 µL

*The volumes will depend on both the concentration and total volume of RNA that is added to the reaction.

4. Pipet to mix and briefly spin in the Microfuge.
5. Incubate at 65–70°C for 10 min.
6. Whilst the RNA tubes are incubating, make a master mix according to the following volumes, multiplying by the number of tubes + 0.5 to cover losses.

10 m*M* dNTPs mix	1 µL
0.1 *M* DTT	2 µL
5X First-strand buffer	4 µL
Final volume	7 µL

7. Vortex and briefly spin the master mix.
8. After incubation, place sample tubes on ice for no more than a couple of minutes, then spin briefly.
9. Add 7 µL of master mix to each sample. Spin briefly if necessary.
10. Incubate at 42°C for 2 min.
11. Keeping tube at 42°C, add 1 µL of Superscript II reverse transcriptase (200 U/µL) if 5 µg of total RNA per tube or 2 µL if 10–20 µg total RNA per tube. Final volume 20 µL.
12. Incubate at 42°C for 1 h.
13. Remove tubes and keep on ice ready for second-strand cDNA Synthesis (**Subheading 3.4.2.**).
14. Alternatively, store the tubes at –80°C.

3.4.2. Second-Strand cDNA Synthesis

1. Chill a water bath to 16°C in a cold room or program a refrigerated PCR block with heated lid and wells for 500 µL Microfuge tubes; chill a Microfuge to 4°C.
2. Defrost, on ice, the reagents listed in **Subheading 2.5.2.** and the first-strand cDNA synthesis products to be used if frozen, vortex and short spin in the chilled centrifuge and keep on ice.
3. Make a master mix on ice as follows. Multiply each reagent volume by the number of 1st strand cDNA synthesis tubes + 0.5 for losses.

DEPC H_2O	91 µL
5X second-strand buffer	30 µL
10 m*M* dNTPs	3 µL
E. coli DNA Ligase (10 U/µL)	1 µL
E. coli DNA *Pol* I (10 U/µL)	4 µL
E. coli RNase H (2 U/µL)	1 µL
Final volume	130 µL

4. Vortex to mix and short spin.
5. Add 130 µL of master mix to each first-strand cDNA synthesis tube to give a new total volume of 150 µL.
6. Vortex to mix and short spin.
7. Incubate the tubes at 16°C for 2 h.
8. Add 2 µL of T4 DNA polymerase (10 units) to each tube.
9. Incubate at 16°C again for just 5 min.
10. On ice, add 10 µL of 0.5 M EDTA, pH 8.0, to inactivate enzymes. New final volume 162 µL.
11. Either freeze the tubes down to –80°C for continuation another day within 2 wk or proceed to the next stage, ds-cDNA clean-up in **Subheading 3.5.1.** (*see* **Note 30**).

3.5. Clean-Up and Concentration of ds-cDNA

3.5.1. Clean-Up of ds-cDNA

This procedure is performed to remove enzymes and salts from the ds-cDNA, which can interfere with cRNA transcription.

1. Calculate volume of buffer saturated phenol solution needed to provide 162 µL for each tube of ds-cDNA plus losses (*see* **Note 31**).
2. Add 65 µL of the alkaline buffer solution to each 1mL of phenol–chloroform–isoamylalcohol mix.
3. Vortex for a minute and briefly centrifuge. Keep at RT once made.
4. Defrost the cDNA tubes on ice if frozen; otherwise, keep on ice until ready.
5. Label a set of phase-lock tubes and a set of 1.5-mL Microfuge tubes.
6. Spin the phase-lock tubes at RT and maximum speed for 30 s to ensure the separating gel is collected at the bottom of each tube.
7. Add an equal volume of buffer saturated phenol mix to each ds-cDNA tube, i.e., 162 µL if above-mentioned methodology has been followed. Draw up the lower organic phase of the buffer saturated phenol solution, being careful to avoid the upper aqueous phase.

8. Vortex the tubes for a minute but do not spin.
9. Carefully pipette all the buffered phenol and ds-cDNA mix into the corresponding, spun, phase-lock tube for each sample. At all costs, avoid scratching the membrane/gel. Centrifuge the phase-lock tubes at maximum speed and RT for 2 min (*see* **Note 32**).

For each sample, carefully transfer the aqueous, upper phase into the corresponding1.5-mL Microfuge tube. The new volume will be approx 150 μL.

3.5.2. Precipitation of ds-cDNA

The precipitation is undertaken to concentrate the cleaned ds-cDNA ready for efficient in vitro transcription.

1. Chill tubes of 80 and 100% ethanol to –20°C.
2. Precipitate each cleaned ds-cDNA sample, with the following reagents:

2.5X volumes 100% cold ethanol	375 μL
0.5X volume of 7.5 *M* ammonium acetate	75 μL
5 mg/mL glycogen	4 μL

3. Mix by tapping tubes or vortex briefly.
4. Centrifuge immediately at RT and maximum speed for 20 min.
5. A pellet of precipitated ds-cDNA will have formed at the bottom of the tubes. Keeping samples on ice, carefully remove the supernatant.
6. Wash the ds-cDNA pellet from salts by adding 500 μL of cold 80% ethanol and then centrifuge at maximum speed for 5 min. Remove the supernatant (*see* **Note 33**).
7. Repeat cold 80% ethanol wash of **step 6** once.
8. Carefully pipet away the ethanol, ensuring the ds-cDNA pellet is left intact. Briefly spin the tubes to pool the residual ethanol and use a pipette to remove.
9. Air dry the ds-cDNA pellets. This will take between 5 to 10 min (*see* **Note 34**).
10. Add 12 mL of DEPC H_2O to each pellet, resuspending by gentle pipetting.
11. Either proceed to the next stage, in vitro transcription (**Subheading 3.6.**), or freeze the cleaned, ds-cDNA by placing tubes on dry ice and then storing in a –80°C freezer (*see* **Notes 35** and **36**).

3.6. In Vitro Transcription ~ Synthesis of Biotinylated cRNA

1. Warm a water bath or a heating block with heated lid to 37°C.
2. Defrost the reagents listed in **Subheading 2.7.** to RT and the cleaned, concentrated ds-cDNA samples, if frozen.
3. Vortex and briefly spin tubes at RT to ensure uniform mixing.
4. Make a master mix of the cRNA synthesis ingredients in a 0.5 or 1.5 mL Microfuge tube at RT, as follows. Multiply each reagent volume by the number of samples + 0.5 for losses:

DEPC H_2O	10 μL
10X HY reaction buffer	4 μL
10X Biotin-labeled ribonucleotides	4 μL
10X DTT	4 μL

10X RNase inhibitor mix	4 µL
20X T7 RNA polymerase	2 µL
Final volume	28 µL

5. Vortex and briefly spin the master mix tube at RT.
6. Add 28 µL of master mix to each ds-cDNA sample (12 µL).

   New final volume 40 µL
7. Vortex and briefly spin.
8. Incubate the samples at 37°C for 5 h. Vortex and spin the tubes hourly to maximize the cRNA yield.
9. Either freeze the newly synthesized cRNA by placing the tubes on dry ice and storing in a –80°C freezer, or keep on ice and proceed to the next stage, cleaning-up of biotinylated cRNA (**Subheading 3.7.1.**; *see* **Notes 37–39**).

3.6.1. Clean-Up of Biotinylated cRNA

It is essential to remove unincorporated dNTPs so that the quantity of cRNA can be accurately determined using 260 nm absorbance.

1. As necessary, defrost the cRNA and warm to RT reagents listed in **Subheading 2.8.**
2. All steps of the protocol should be performed at RT.
3. Do not add beta-mercaptoethanol to RLT buffer, as it can increase background signal.
4. Label the lid of a set of RNeasy spin columns and a set of 1.5-mL collection tubes with each cRNA sample's identifier (*see* **Notes 40** and **41**).
5. To each cRNA tube (40 µL content) add the following:

DEPC H_2O	60 µL
RLT buffer	350 µL
Final volume	450 µL

6. Mix thoroughly by pipetting.
7. Then add 250 µL of 100% ethanol to each tube, to give a total volume of 700 µL.
8. Mix thoroughly by pipetting.
9. Transfer the entire contents of each cRNA tube to the corresponding spin column placed inside the first set of 2-mL collection tubes.
10. Centrifuge for just 15 s at 8000*g*.
11. Transfer the spin column to the second set of 2-mL collection tubes.
12. Add 500 µL of RPE buffer to each spin column.
13. Transfer this second set of collection tubes containing the spin columns back to the centrifuge and again centrifuge for 15 s at 8000*g*.
14. Transfer the spin column to the third set of 2-mL collection tubes. Add 500 µL of RPE buffer to each spin column.
15. Centrifuge for 2 min at maximum speed.
16. Transfer the spin column to the fourth and final set of 2-mL collection tubes.
17. Centrifuge for 1 min at maximum speed to ensure that the spin column membrane is quite dry.

18. Transfer the spin columns to the correspondingly labeled set of 1.5 mL RNase-free collection tubes.
19. Add 40–50 μL of DEPC H_2O to each spin column avoiding membrane contact.
20. Allow 2 min for the cRNA to dissolve.
21. Collect the cleaned cRNA solution by centrifuging for 1 minute at 8000*g*.
22. Perform a second elution if you are worried the cRNA yield will not yet be adequate or move on to quantitate and qualify the cRNA according to the stages below (*see* **Note 42**).

3.6.2. Second Elution to Maximize cRNA Recovery

Add a further 30–50 μL of DEPC H_2O to the spin column still inserted in the 1.5-mL collection tube.

Centrifuge at 8000*g* for 1 min. Quantitate and qualitate the cRNA.

3.7. Assessing the Quantity and Quality of the Purified cRNA

3.7.1. Assessing the Quantity of the Purified cRNA by Spectrophotometry

1. Turn on the absorbance spectrophotometer 15 min before use.
2. Calibrate the meter using a DEPC H_2O control according to the machine's specific instructions.
3. Quantify RNA yield by spectrophotometric analysis at 260 and 280 nm for sample concentration and purity.
4. Dilute 1 μL of the cleaned cRNA in 4–9 μL of DEPC H_2O (1:5 to 1:10 dilutions)
5. Measure the RNA concentration of each diluted cRNA.
6. Calculate the cRNA content in the undiluted sample multiplying by the dilution factor.
7. Apply the convention that 1 absorbance unit at 260 nm = 40 μg RNA (*see* **Note 43**).

3.7.2. Assessing the Quality of the Purified cRNA by Gel Electrophoresis

Gel electrophoresis of the IVT product is done to estimate the yield and size distribution of labeled transcripts. Follow **steps 1** to **10** of **Subheading 3.3.2.** using cRNA instead of total RNA. In addition please perform an 11th step: View and photograph the gel under ultraviolet light using usual protective gear (*see* **Note 44**).

3.7.3. Assessing the Quality of the Purified cRNA Using the 2100 Agilent Bioanalyzer

Refer to the detailed and well-illustrated accompanying manual for further details to those below. For cRNA, the concentration range that can be quantified is between 25 and 250 ng/μL. Therefore, for most of your samples you will need to make a diluted aliquot.

1. Warm the reagents, including an aliquot of RNA 6000 ladder, to RT and a heating block to 70°C.

2. Turn on the Bioanalyzer and its workstation 15 min before use.
3. Start the Agilent 2100 Bioanalyzer software by double clicking on the Bioanalyzer desktop icon.
4. Prepare 3 μL of each cRNA to be run with a concentration <500 ng/μL using DEPC H_2O.
5. Denature the RNA samples a 3-μL aliquot of RNA 6000 ladder by heating to 70°C for 2 min.
6. Place denatured ladder and samples on ice (*see* **Note 45**).

3.7.3.1. Decontaminating the Electrodes

1. Fill the first electrode cleaner chip via one of its wells with 350 μL of RNAseZAP.
2. Open the lid of the Agilent 2100 Bioanalyzer and insert the first electrode cleaner.
3. Close the lid; leave for 1 min and then remove the first electrode cleaner chip.
4. Add 350 μL of DEPC H_2O to the second electrode cleaner chip.
5. Insert the second electrode cleaner chip in the Bioanalyzer and leave for just 10 s before removing.
6. Allow the Bioanalyzer electrodes to dry for 10 s before closing the lid.

3.7.3.2. Loading the RNA Chip

1. Set the Chip Priming Station base plate to position C, insert the syringe (1 mL) into the syringe holder, and set the adjustable syringe clip to the highest position.
2. Place a new RNA chip on the chip priming station with the writing towards you and the 'cut off' corner top right.
3. Dispense 9 μL of gel-dye mix (**Subheading 2.3.3.1.**) into the bottom of the 3rd well marked with a "G" from the top of the chip (*see* **Note 46**)
4. Raise the syringe plunger to the 1 mL mark and close the chip priming station.
5. Depress the plunger until it is held by the syringe clip.
6. Keep well "G" pressurized for exactly 30 s, then release the plunger and return it to the 1-mL mark.
7. Open the chip priming station and ensure that no bubbles are present in the chip channels by hold the chip to the light.
8. If bubbles are present in the channels, repeat **steps 4** to **7** above (*see* **Note 47**).
9. Dispense 9 μL of gel-dye mix into the bottom of the other two wells marked with a "G."
10. Pipet 5 μL of RNA 6000 Nano Marker (green dot on lid) into each sample well you will use and the ladder well.
11. Pipet 6 μL of RNA 6000 Nano Marker (green dot on lid) into each sample well not to be used.
12. Add 1 μL of denatured RNA 6000 ladder to the bottom of the well with the ladder symbol (bottom right).
13. Add a 1 μL of each denatured sample into each sample wells, loading from top left to bottom right (1 through 12; *see* **Note 48**).
14. Vortex the chip for 1 min at the recommended speed (IKA vortexer set-point)
15. Place the chip in the Bioanalyzer and close the lid. Begin the run within 5 minutes to avoid deleterious evaporation (*see* **Note 49**).

16. Return to the workstation, where the chip icon will now be displayed top left, indicating that a chip has been inserted and the lid successfully closed.
17. From the "Assay" menu, select "RNA" and then the type of RNA assay you wish to perform (usually Eukaryote Total RNA nano)
18. Click on the "Start" icon to bring up the "Start" dialog box.
19. Add your desired file prefix. The data will be saved to a file of this name.
20. Adjust the number of samples to be run and ensure that the "Edit samples after start" box is ticked.
21. Click on the "Start" button.
22. As desired, add the identifiers for each sample in the "Samples Information" window of the "General Chip Information" dialog box.

3.8. Increasing cRNA Concentration by Ethanol Precipitation

1. Chill the 80% and 100% ethanol tubes to –20°C and a Microfuge to 4°C.
2. To each sample to be concentrated, add the following:

   0.5X volume of 7.5 *M* ammonium acetate
   2.5X volume of 100% cold ethanol

3. Precipitate the cRNA at –20°C for a minimum of 1 h to overnight.
4. Centrifuge for 30 min at 4°C and maximum speed.
5. While centrifuging tubes, calculate the volume of DEPC H_2O to add to each sample to give a final concentration of 1–2 µg/µL using the pre-precipitation cRNA weight.
6. Carefully remove the supernatant from each cRNA pellet.
7. Wash the cRNA pellet with 500 µL of cold 80% ethanol followed by centrifuging at maximum speed for 5 min (*see* **Note 33**).
8. Repeat **step 7** once.
9. Carefully remove the supernatant, ensuring the cRNA pellet is left intact. Briefly spin the tubes to pool the residual ethanol and use a pipet to remove.
10. Air dry the pellets for no longer than 5–10 min.
11. Resuspend in the precalculated volumes of DEPC H_2O to achieve a final concentration of 1–2 µg/µL.
12. Either store tubes by freezing on dry ice followed by transfer to a –80°C freezer or proceed to the next stage, cRNA fragmentation (**Subheading 3.9.**).

3.9. cRNA Fragmentation

Fragment an appropriate amount of cRNA for making hybridization cocktail and performing a gel/Bioanalyzer analysis. The fragmentation buffer has been optimized to break down full-length cRNA to 35–200 base fragments by metal-induced hydrolysis.

1. Calculate volume of each sample to give a weight of 20 µg cRNA.
2. Warm a heating block to 94°C or use a PCR machine with a heated lid and a base plate for 0.5-mL tubes.
3. As necessary, defrost your cleaned, concentrated cRNA samples.

4. To each in a set of labelled of 0.5-mL microfuge tubes, add the following:

20 µg of the corresponding cRNA	1–32 µL
5X fragmentation buffer (*see* **Subheading 2.10.1.**)	8 µL
DEPC H_2O to final volume	40 µL

5. Vortex and briefly spin.
6. Incubate at 94°C for 35 min.
7. After the incubation, place tubes on ice.
8. Take a 2 µL (1 µg) aliquot of each fragmented cRNA to run on an agarose gel or RNA nano chip and store the rest at –80°C (*see* **Note 52**).

3.10. Assessing the Quality of Fragmented cRNA

3.10.1. Assessing the Quality of Fragmented cRNA by Gel Electrophoresis

It is not possible to meaningfully assess the quantity of fragmented cRNA. Instead, use the concentration of purified cRNA to calculate the amount of fragmented cRNA. At least 1 µg of fragmented cRNA is needed if using ethidium bromide. Follow **steps 1** to **10** of **Subheading 3.3.2.** using fragmented cRNA instead of total RNA. In addition please perform an 11th step: view and photograph the gel under ultraviolet light using usual protective gear (*see* **Note 53**).

3.10.2. Assessing the Quality of the Fragmented cRNA Using the 2100 Agilent Bioanalyzer

See **Subheading 3.7.3.** and **Note 54.**

3.11. Preparation of the Hybridization Cocktail

300 µL of hybridization mix will be needed per sample for high density array: 80 µL for a mini chip (e.g., Test 3) and 200 µL for a standard array chip (e.g., U95Av2).

1. Calculate the volume (x µL) of each fragmented cRNA to provide 15 µg. If the above method has been followed and a 0.5 µg/µL solution created, the volume required will be 30 µL.
2. Calculate the volume of analytical-grade water needed to give a final volume of 300 µL using: analytical-grade water = 300 – 176–x µL.
3. Warm a heating block to 65°C.
4. Defrost and warm to RT the reagents listed in **Subheading 2.11.** and defrost, on ice, the fragmented cRNA samples to be processed.
5. Once fully thawed, heat the 20X Eukaryotic Hybridization Controls vial and the Control Oligonucleotide B2 vial to 65°C for 5 min. Vortex and briefly spin to ensure complete mixing. This step is performed to ensure that the control cRNA is fully redissolved before use.

6. Make up a master mix at RT, as follows (multiply each reagent volume by the number of samples + 0.5 for losses):

2X hybridization buffer (*see* **Subheading 2.13.**)	150 µL
20X Eukaryotic hybridization controls	15 µL
Control Oligonucleotide B2	5 µL
Acetylated bovine serum albumin (50 mg/mL)	3 µL
Herring sperm DNA (10 mg/mL)	3 µL
Final volume (*see* **Note 55**)	176 µL

7. Aliquot 15 µg of each fragmented cRNA (x µL calculated in **step 1** above) into a correspondingly labelled 500-µL Microfuge tube.
8. Add 176 µL of the master mix to each sample.
9. Add analytical-grade water to each sample to give a final volume of 300 µL, as calculated in **step 2** above.
10. Mix by vortexing followed by a brief, fast spin and keep on ice.
11. Store the hybridization cocktails at –20°C if you are not proceeding immediately to the next stage, denaturing the fragmented target in the hybridization cocktail (**Subheading 3.12.**).

3.12. Denaturing the Fragmented Target in the Hybridization Cocktail

Remember that only four chips can be run simultaneously in each fluidics station you have access to. Because the post target-probe hybridization chip can only be kept for 3 h after completion of the hybridization procedure, don't denature more sample hybridization cocktails than can be taken through the fluidics stages in two consecutive batches (each run will take about 2 h); *see* **Note 56**).

1. Turn on two heating blocks set at 99°C and 45°C.
2. Defrost any frozen hybridization cocktails.
3. Incubate the hybridization cocktails for 5 min at 99°C.
4. Transfer the cocktails immediately to the heating block set at 45°C for 5 min.
5. Spin at maximum for 5 min to precipitate any insoluble material.

3.13. Hybridizing the Target to the Probe Array

If good quality total and purified cRNA have been shown using the Agilent Bioanalyzer, there is no need to run a test chip. Instead proceed straight to using your preferred standard chip.

1. Warm the probe array chip(s) to RT and label appropriately.
2. Make enough 1X hybridization buffer from 2X stock (*see* **Subheadings 2.13.3.** and **2.13.4.**) using analytical-grade water (80 µL for each mini chips, e.g., Test 3 array, and 200 µL for each standard chips e.g., U95Av2 array).
3. Fill each chip with the appropriate volume of 1X hybridization buffer (*see* **Note 57**).
4. Place probe array chips in the hybridization oven at 45°C and 60 rpm rotation for 10 min.

5. Remove the buffer solution from the probe array cartridges and fill with the appropriate volume of the corresponding denatured hybridization cocktail, being careful to avoid any debris at the bottom of the tubes (*see* **Note 58**).
6. Place probe array cartridges back in the hybridization oven, with the settings kept at 45°C and 60 rpm. Hybridize for 16 h (*see* **Note 59**).
7. Make up the non- and stringent wash buffer solutions and the 2X staining solution, as detailed in **Subheadings 2.14.1.** to **2.14.5.**, before the hybridization is completed.
8. After hybridization, recover the hybridization cocktail and keep it at –80°C, as at can be reused (*see* **Note 60**).
9. Completely fill the chips with non-stringent wash buffer solution A.

3.14. Using the Fluidics Station

We highly recommended that a member of staff is trained in the use of the fluidics station and is given day to day responsibility for the running and maintenance of the fluidics station and GeneArray scanner. This will minimize errors and equipment failures.

The GeneChip 400 fluidics station will perform the following actions:

1. Wash the array repeatedly with a non- and then stringent solution at selected temperatures to reduce the extent of non-specific hybridization of targets to probes.
2. Draw the solutions with R-phycoerythrin streptavidin and biotinylated anti-streptavidin antibody from the "sample" vial into the cartridge and mix it by alternately draining and filling the cartridge at a selected temperature.
3. Fill the cartridge with wash solution ready for scanning.

However, you will still need to manually change the "sample" vial to the first SAPE solution, to staining solution, and to second SAPE solution according to the prompts on the workstation.

Follow the detailed instructions in the accompanying manual to set up your experiments and to prepare the machine for use.

You will need to:

1. Make up the nonstringent and stringent wash buffer solutions and the 2X staining solution as detailed in Subheadings **2.14.1.** to **2.14.5.**
2. Prepare the SAPE staining solution. In a separate 1.5-mL Microfuge tube for each array to be washed and stained, make SAPE staining solution the as follows:

2X stain buffer	600 µL
Analytical-grade water	540 µL
Acetylated bovine serum albumin (50 mg/mL)	48 µL
SAPE (1 mg/mL)	12 µL
Final volume	1200 µL

3. Split the SAPE solution into two equal aliquots of 600 μL and label the tubes 1 and 3. Store shielded from light at 4°C.
4. Prepare the antibody solution in a separate 1.5-mL Microfuge tube for each array, as follows:

2X stain buffer	300 μL
Analytical-grade water	266.4 μL
Acetylated bovine serum albumin (50 mg/mL)	24 μL
Normal goat IgG (10 mg/mL)	6 μL
Biotinylated goat antibody (0.5 mg/mL)	3.6 μL
Final volume	600 μL

5. Label the tubes 2 (*see* **Note 61**).
6. When the "fluidics" procedures have finished, hold each array to a light to see if any large bubbles that could interfere with the laser scanning are present.
7. If no large bubbles are present shield the arrays from light and store at 4°C.
8. If large bubbles are present, either manually vent the array and top up with nonstringent wash buffer (solution A) or return the cartridge to its module in the fluidics station for it to be automatically drained and refilled with solution A (*see* **Note 62**).
9. If you have a second batch of arrays ready for processing, you will need to clean the fluidics station (as detailed in the manual), before proceeding as for the first batch of arrays.
10. Once all your arrays have been processed, follow the procedure in the manual for closing down the fluidics station.

3.15. Laser Scanning the Array

After staining and washing the Agilent GeneArray or GeneChip Scanner 3000 scans the probe array cartridges using laser light to obtain the fluorescence intensity data for each feature. For detailed instructions on the operation of the relevant laser scanner see the manual for the instrument provided by Affymetrix or Agilent.

We highly recommended that a member of staff is trained in the use of the laser scanner and is given day to day responsibility for the running and maintenance of the fluidics station and GeneArray scanner. This will minimize errors and equipment failures.

Three points of note:

1. Allow the laser scanner to warm up for at least 15 min before scanning your first chip and warm any refrigerated arrays back to RT, as always shielded from light.
2. Wipe any dirt from the glass surface with a disposable lens cloth.
3. Use the same scanner for all arrays in a given experimental set to avoid systematic variation in expression profiles caused by subtle differences in scanner performance.

3.16. Data Analysis

Follow the instructions and manual accompanying Microarray Suite 5.1 (Affymetrix) to acquire, store, and perform pre-analysis data checks and refinements. Use your chosen data analysis package to filter your data prior to beginning data mining. Remember to validate your findings by performing sufficient replication of experiments and analyses. Good Luck!

4. Notes

1. Alternatively you can use a kit such as the QIAGEN RNA/DNA Kits (see http://www.qiagen.com) or RNA Extraction Kit (extracts RNA from up to 4 g tissue Amersham-Biosciences; cat. no. 27-9270-01).
2. Alternative kit: MEGAscript T7 (Ambion; cat. no.1334) Store at –20°C, stable for 6 mo.
3. Different Chip types available. *See* **Table 1.**
4. For the remaining solutions, the more convenient bench-top produced analytical grade water can be used instead of DEPC-H_2O.
5. Discard 12X MES stock if it starts to turn yellow.
6. Discard 2X hybridization buffer if it starts to turn yellow.
7. An alternative is the newer GeneChip Fluidics station 450, which automatically changes the "sample" vials from first SAPE solution to antibody solution to second SAPE solution, so by allowing the user to leave the station unattended throughout a run.
8. Alternatively, scale up the volume of tissue and TRIzol processed and use an homogenizer to rapidly and thoroughly homogenize your sample in a 50-mL tube.
9. If you have used a homogenizer and therefore have more than 1 mL, transfer to several 1.5-mL tubes to ease RNA retrieval.
10. Avoid drawing up any of the interphase to reduce protein contamination of the RNA.
11. RNA pellets can be overdried. If this happens, dissolving the pellet fully can be very difficult.
12. If less than 75% cells are viable, discard sample!
13. If the RNA concentration is less than 1 μg/μL use either "Concentration and Clean-up of Total RNA by Ethanol Precipitation" (**Subheading 3.2.3.**) or "Clean-up of Total RNA" (**Subheading 3.2.4.**) to concentrate your RNA.
14. To minimize loss of RNA during this procedure, don't add extra salt or ethanol and ensure that the sodium acetate is at the correct pH. Make up fresh sodium acetate when salt from your current stock starts to precipitate around the bottle mouth. When removing the supernatant from the pellet begin with a 1000-μL pipet tip but change to a 200- or 20-μL tip to reduce the rate of fluid removal and so the risk of dislodging the pellet in the currents generated in the supernatant as it is drawn off. If the RNA pellet produced is small, don't risk dislodging and losing it by vortexing after addition of each ethanol wash. Instead, proceed straight to microfuging, replace tube in the same orientation as during the first spin so that the side of tube the pellet is adherent to is again facing outermost.

Table 1
Specifications of Affymetrix Chips for Human mRNA

	TEST 3	HG-UI33 A+B	HG-U133A 2.0	HG-U133 PLUS
Number of probe sets		45,000	22,000	54,000
Number of transcripts		39,000	18,000	47,000
Number of genes[a]	24[a]	33,000	14,500	38,000
Feature size	20 µm	18 µm	11 µm	11 µm
Probe length	25 mer	25 mer	25 mer	25 mer
Probe pairs/sequence	16–20	11	11	11

[a]There are more genes but belonging to other species.
For more details see http://www.affymetrix.com.

15. After homogenization and before addition of chloroform, samples can be stored for at least 1 mo at –80°C. The RNA precipitated with isopropanol (**step 12** above) can be stored in 75% ethanol for at least 1 wk at 4°C, or at least 1 yr at –20°C. After second precipitation, the RNA can be stored for yr at –80°C. in 100% ethanol.
16. Do not write on the side of the RNeasy spin columns, as the writing will be removed by the ethanol washes. The three sets of 2-mL collection tubes do not need labeling as all are discarded after single use.
17. It is imperative that the pipette tips do not scratch the membrane in the spin columns during fluid introduction, as membrane damage will compromise the filtration properties of the membrane. If you think you have scratched a membrane, draw up the introduced fluid from the damaged spin column and reintroduce to new column (once labeled)

    All steps of the protocol should be performed at RT. During the procedure, work without interruption. A second elution can be performed to maximize the RNA recovery. This will result in an increased yield but a reduced concentration. An alternative is to perform the second elution into a separate tube for each sample and measure the RNA yield in the first and second elutions to see whether the second elution is needed and whether it is sufficient to give you the required minimum of 10 µg of total RNA. Save an aliquot of the unpurified IVT product for analysis by gel electrophoresis.
18. Creating a final minimal concentration of RNA of 1 µg/µL allows use of 10 µg of total RNA for first- and second-strand cDNA reactions.
19. Aim for an A260/A280 ratio close to 2.0 for pure RNA (ratios between 1.9 and 2.1 are acceptable). The concentration is determined by absorbance at 260 nm, where 1 absorbance unit = 40 µg RNA.
20. The ribosomal RNA bands should be clear without any obvious smearing patterns.
21. A maximum of 12 samples can be run per chip.
22. Dispense to the bottom of the wells and not the sides to avoid introducing bubbles, which will adversely affect the chip's performance.

23. Small bubbles will be present in the wells. These bubbles will be burst by vortexing the chip.
24. The chip will not run properly if any sample well is left empty, that is, filled with a total of 6 µL.
25. Don't try and force the lid closed because this will damage the electrodes. If the lid will not close effortlessly, you need to reinsert the chip or the RNA cartridge.
26. The run will take approx 20 min.
27. Two sharp and prominent peaks (corresponding to ribosomal 18 and 28S) with a low level of signal across the rest of the image will be present on the gel and time trace for each well containing good quality total RNA. Discard samples where the 18 & 28 S peaks are diminished, absent or the background signal contains many small peaks indicating RNA degradation.
28. High-quality, high-performance liquid chromatography-purified T7-(dT)24 primer is essential not only for ds-cDNA synthesis but also for the in vitro transcription (IVT) reaction. Insufficiently purified primer may appear to produce double-stranded cDNA efficiently (since the 5' end of the primer is not critical for the priming step), but still result in poor IVT yields if the primer is contaminated with shorter sequences (missing the 5' end, which contains the promoter region for the IVT reaction).
29. Work on ice at all times and minimize contact with tubes at RT. Make batches of no more than 8 tubes at once to shorten times tubes are standing idle. This maximizes synthesis of longer length cDNA, by preventing secondary structure reformation once strands are denatured.
30. By using a heated lid with the refrigeration block in **step 7** above, condensation is reduced, ensuring that the contents stay at the bottom of the tube and incubate at the correct temperature. To rapidly freeze the tubes to –80°C, place them in an ice bucket containing dry ice for 5 min, and then transfer them to a prechilled holder or a bag containing several chips of dry ice before transferring to a –80°C freezer.
31. The final mixed, buffer-saturated phenol solution is not stable, so prepare it just before use.
32. The resultant upper phase is the aqueous phase containing the ds-cDNA and the lower phase is the phenol phase containing the unwanted organic impurities.
33. Minimize loss of ds-cDNA by not adding extra salt or ethanol and ensuring that the sodium acetate is at the correct pH. Make up fresh sodium acetate when salt from your current stock starts to precipitate around the bottle mouth. When removing the supernatant from the pellet begin with a 1000-µL pipet tip but change to a 200- or 20-µL tip to reduce the rate of fluid removal and so the risk of dislodging the pellet in the currents generated in the supernatant as it is drawn off. Don't vortex the ds-cDNA pellet after addition of each ethanol wash. Instead proceed straight to microfuging, replace tube in the same orientation as during the first spin so that the side of tube the pellet is adherent to is again facing outermost.
34. An over-dried pellet is hard to resuspend.

35. Addition of glycogen (5 mg/mL) to nucleic acid precipitations aids the visualization of the pellet and may increase recovery. The glycogen does not appear to affect the outcome of subsequent steps in this protocol.
36. Quantifying the amount of ds-cDNA by absorbance at 260 nm is not recommended. The primer can contribute significantly to the absorbance. Subtracting the theoretical contribution of the primer based on the amount added to the reaction is not practical.
37. DTT can precipitate if the solution is cold; therefore, allow adequate time for all reagents to reach RT before commencing the mix and incubation.
38. Condensation on the inside of the tube lids during incubation at 37°C reduces the efficiency of the cRNA transcription reaction. Reduce condensation formation by using a heated lid, if using a heating block, or a closed incubator and remove any condensation hourly by re-vortexing and spinning the tubes.
39. Don't try using less than one volume's worth of cleaned, concentrated cDNA (12 μL) as the efficiency of the cRNA synthesis is variable.
40. Don't write on the side of the RNeasy spin columns because the writing will be erased by the ethanol washes.
41. The three sets of 2-mL collection tubes do not need labeling because all are discarded after single use.
42. It is imperative that the pipet tips do not scratch the membrane in the spin columns during fluid introduction because membrane damage will compromise the filtration properties of the membrane. If you think you have scratched a membrane, draw up the introduced fluid from the damaged spin column and reintroduce to a new column (once labeled) All steps of the protocol should be performed at RT. During the procedure, work without interruption. A second elution can be performed to maximize the cRNA recovery. This will result in an increased yield but a reduced concentration. An alternative is to perform the second elution into a separate tube for each sample and measure the cRNA yield in the first and second elutions to see whether this second is needed and whether it is sufficient to give you the required minimum of 40 μg of cRNA. Save an aliquot of the unpurified IVT product for analysis by gel electrophoresis.
43. If the cRNA yield for any sample is less than 40 μg,where 10 μg of original total RNA was used, a serious failure of cDNA or cRNA synthesis and amplification has occurred and the cRNA sample should not be taken further. Aim for an A260/A280 ratio close to 2.0 for pure RNA (ratios between 1.9 and 2.1 are acceptable)
44. The cRNA smear produced on the 1% agarose gel should have a highlight between 500 and 1000 bp and span 100–2000 bp. If a smear is abnormal do not take the corresponding cRNA sample further. The RNA used in the fragmentation procedure should be sufficiently concentrated to maintain a small volume during the procedure. This will minimize the amount of magnesium in the final hybridization cocktail. The cRNA must be at a minimum concentration of 0.6 μg/μL. If less, the concentration will need to be increased by ethanol precipitation.
45. A maximum of 12 samples can be run per chip.
46. Dispense to the bottom of the wells and not the sides to avoid introducing bubbles, which will adversely affect the chip's performance.

47. Small bubbles will be present in the wells. These bubbles will be burst by vortexing the chip.
48. The chip will not run properly if any sample well is left empty, that is, filled with a total of 6 μL.
49. Don't try and force the lid closed because this will damage the electrodes. If the lid will not close effortlessly, you need to reinsert the chip or the RNA cartridge.
50. The run will take about 20 min.
51. Each sample run lasts 84 s. On the fluorescence vs time graph a bell-shaped curve will be seen between 20 and 40 s with the peak between 30–34 s.
52. The final concentration of RNA in the fragmentation mix must range between 0.5-2 μg/μL. This method will result in a final fragmented cRNA concentration of 0.5 μg/μL.
53. A smear between 20 and 200 bp will be seen on the gel if fragmentation has been successful. Discard abnormal/suboptimal samples.
54. Each sample run lasts 84 s. On the fluorescence vs time graph a large peak will be seen between 20 and 24 s.
55. The eukaryotic hybridization controls are added to allow the sensitivity achieved on each chip to be assessed, whereas the control oligonucleotide B2 is added to allow the demarcation and orientation of the array grid to be determined in the scanned image. If the control oligonucleotide B2 is accidentally left out, the chip(s) in question will be unreadable.
56. Begin the next procedure just before or during this stage to minimize the time the denatured hybridization cocktails are idle before injection into the arrays.
57. To fill an array cartridge pierce one of the two septa on the back of the chip with a micropipette tip to act as a vent for the air in the cartridge that will be displaced upon hybridization buffer introduction. Inject the buffer solution via a second micropipette tip inserted into the other septa. The maximum volumes that the mini and standard chips can hold are 100 and 250 μL, respectively. Filling to less than capacity for the hybridization reaction allows optimal fluid movement across the array features during chip rotation.

    Avoid contact with the outer surface of the glass on which the probes are sited. If the glass becomes scratched or dirty the scan fidelity can be affected. Wipe off any dirt from the glass using a disposable microscope lens cloth.
58. To empty an array cartridge pierce one of the two septa on the back of the chip with a micropipette tip to act as a vent for air to enter the cartridge as the hybridization buffer is withdrawn via a second micropipette tip inserted into the other septa.
59. Extending the hybridization time beyond 16 h will result in excessive sample evaporation with the risks of altering the stringency of the hybridization reaction, dry spots developing on the array causing altered hybridization and inadequate sample to repeat the hybridization process on another chip.
60. Ensure that the chips are symmetrically arranged in the oven as in a centrifuge to avoid unnecessary mechanical strain. The hybridization cocktail can be reused in

a different probe array cartridge. If this is done, repeat all steps of **Subheading 3.13.** The volume to completely fill a mini array is 100 µL, whereas for a standard chip it is 250 µL.

The arrays can be left for a maximum of 3 h at 4°C before commencing the fluidic station procedures.

61. The mini chip protocol with antibody amplification is called Mini_euk2 and the standard chip protocol with antibody amplification is called EukGE-WS2v4. The Mini_euk2 protocol suitable for the Test 3 chip consists of the following steps:
    a. 10 cycles of 2 mixes/cycle using Solution A at 25°C.
    b. 8 cycles of 15 mixes/cycle using Solution B at 50°C.
    c. 10 min array staining with preantibody SAPE solution (vial 1) at 25°C.
    d. 10 cycles of 4 mixes/cycle using Solution A at 30°C.
    e. 10 min array staining biotinylated antibody solution (vial 2) at 25°C.
    f. 10 min array staining with post-antibody SAPE solution (vial 3) at 25°C.
    g. 15 cycles of 4 mixes/cycle using Solution A at 35°C.
    h. Return to 25°C until array is removed from its module.
62. Repeatedly refilling a chip will reduce the signal intensity.

References

1. A clinical evaluation of the International Lymphoma Study Group classification of non-Hodgkin's lymphoma. The Non-Hodgkin's Lymphoma Classification Project. *Blood* **89,** 3909–3918.
2. Armitage, J. O. (1993) Treatment of non-Hodgkin's lymphoma. *N. Engl. J. Med.* **328,** 1023–1030.
3. Fisher, R. I., Gaynor, E. R., Dahlberg, S., Oken, M. M., Grogan, T. M., Mize, E. M., et al. (1993) Comparison of a standard regimen (CHOP) with three intensive chemotherapy regimens for advanced non-Hodgkin's lymphoma. *N. Engl. J. Med.* **328,** 1002–1006.
4. Coiffier, B. (2003) Immunochemotherapy: the new standard in aggressive non-Hodgkin's lymphoma in the elderly. *Semin. Oncol.* **30(1 Suppl 2),** 21–27.
5. Philip, T., Guglielmi, C., Hagenbeek, A., Somers, R., Van der Lelie, H., Bron, D., et al. (1995) Autologous bone marrow transplantation as compared with salvage chemotherapy in relapses of chemotherapy-sensitive non-Hodgkin's lymphoma. *N. Engl. J. Med.* **333,** 1540–1545.
6. The International Non-Hodgkin's Lymphoma Prognostic Factors Project. (1993) A predictive model for aggressive non-Hodgkin's lymphoma. *N. Engl. J. Med.* **329,** 987–994.
7. Pease, A. C., Solas, D., Sullivan, E. J., Cronin, M. T., Holmes, C. P., and Fodor, S. P. (1994) Light-generated oligonucleotide arrays for rapid DNA sequence analysis. *Proc. Natl. Acad. Sci. USA* **91,** 5022–5026.
8. Schena, M., Shalon, D., Davis, R. W., and Brown, P. O. (1995) Quantitative monitoring of gene expression patterns with a complementary DNA microarray. *Science* **270,** 467–470.

9. Halgren, R. G., Fielden, M. R., Fong, C. J., and Zacharewski, T. R. (2001) Assessment of clone identity and sequence fidelity for 1189 IMAGE cDNA clones. *Nucleic Acids Res.* **29,** 582–588.
10. Hughes, T. R., Mao, M., Jones, A. R., Burchard, J., Marton, M. J., Shannon, K. W., et al. (2001) Expression profiling using microarrays fabricated by an ink-jet oligonucleotide synthesizer. *Nat. Biotechnol.* **19,** 342–347.
11. Lockhart, D. J., Dong, H., Byrne, M. C., Follettie, M. T., Gallo, M. V., Chee, M. S., et al. (1996) Expression monitoring by hybridization to high-density oligonucleotide arrays. *Nat. Biotechnol.* **14,** 1675–1680.
12. Alizadeh, A. A., Eisen, M. B., Davis, R. E., Ma, C., Lossos, I. S., Rosenwald, A., et al. (2000) Distinct types of diffuse large B-cell lymphoma identified by gene expression profiling. *Nature* **403,** 503–511.
13. Rosenwald, A., Wright, G., Chan, W. C., Connors, J. M., Campo, E., Fisher, R. I., et al. (2002) The use of molecular profiling to predict survival after chemotherapy for diffuse large-B-cell lymphoma. *N. Engl. J. Med.* **346,** 1937–1947.
14. Shipp, M. A., Ross, K. N., Tamayo, P., Weng, A. P., Kutok, J. L., Aguiar, R. C., et al. (2002) Diffuse large B-cell lymphoma outcome prediction by gene-expression profiling and supervised machine learning. *Nat. Med.* **8,** 68–74.
15. Tamayo, P., Slonim, D., Mesirov, J., Zhu, Q., Kitareewan, S., Dmitrovsky, E., et al. (1999) Interpreting patterns of gene expression with self-organizing maps: methods and application to hematopoietic differentiation. *Proc. Natl. Acad. Sci. USA* **96,** 2907–2912.
16. Golub, T. R., Slonim, D. K., Tamayo, P., Huard, C., Gaasenbeek, M., Mesirov, J. P., et al. (1999) Molecular classification of cancer: class discovery and class prediction by gene expression monitoring. *Science* **286,** 531–537.
17. Eisen, M. B., Spellman, P. T., Brown, P. O., and Botstein, D. (1998) Cluster analysis and display of genome-wide expression patterns. *Proc. Natl. Acad. Sci. USA* **95,** 14863–14868.
18. Bonner, R. F., Emmert-Buck, M., Cole, K., Pohida, T., Chuaqui, R., Goldstein, S., and Liotta, L. A. (1997) Laser capture microdissection: molecular analysis of tissue. *Science* **278,** 1481,1483.
19. Luo, L., Salunga, R. C., Guo, H., Bittner, A., Joy, K. C., Galindo, J. E., et al. (1999) Gene expression profiles of laser-captured adjacent neuronal subtypes. *Nat. Med.* **5,** 117–22.
20. Kitahara, O., Furukawa, Y., Tanaka, T., Kihara, C., Ono, K., Yanagawa, R., et al. (2001) Alterations of gene expression during colorectal carcinogenesis revealed by cDNA microarrays after laser-capture microdissection of tumor tissues and normal epithelia. *Cancer Res.* **61,** 3544–3549.
21. Xiang, C. C., Chen, M., Ma, L., Phan, Q. N., Inman, J. M., Kozhich, O. A., and Brownstein, M. J. (2003) A new strategy to amplify degraded RNA from small tissue samples for microarray studies. *Nucleic Acids Res.* **31,** e53.
22. Quackenbush, J. (2002) Microarray data normalization and transformation. *Nat. Genet.* **32(Suppl),** 496–501.

23. Yang, Y. H., Dudoit, S., Luu, P., Lin, D. M., Peng, V., Ngai, J., and Speed, T. P. (2002) Normalization for cDNA microarray data: a robust composite method addressing single and multiple slide systematic variation. *Nucleic Acids Res.* **30,** e15.
24. DeRisi, J. L., Iyer, V. R., and Brown, P. O. (1997) Exploring the metabolic and genetic control of gene expression on a genomic scale. *Science* **278,** 680–686.
25. Yang, I. V., Chen, E., Hasseman, J. P., Liang, W., Frank, B. C., Wang, S., et al. (2002) Within the fold: assessing differential expression measures and reproducibility in microarray assays. *Genome Biol.* **3,** 00262.
26. Kerr, M. K., Martin, M., and Churchill, G. A. (2000) Analysis of variance for gene expression microarray data. *J. Comput. Biol.* **7,** 819–837.
27. Tavazoie, S., Hughes, J. D., Campbell, M. J., Cho, R. J., and Church, G. M. (1999) Systematic determination of genetic network architecture. *Nat. Genet.* **22,** 281–285.
28. Raychaudhuri, S., Stuart, J. M., and Altman, R. B. (2000) Principal components analysis to summarize microarray experiments: application to sporulation time series. *Pac. Symp. Biocomput.* 455–66.
29. Brown, M. P., Grundy, W. N., Lin, D., Cristianini, N., Sugnet, C. W., Furey, T. S., et al. (2000) Knowledge-based analysis of microarray gene expression data by using support vector machines. *Proc. Natl. Acad. Sci. USA.* **97,** 262–267.
30. Meyer, J. M., Heath, A. C., and Eaves, L. J. (1992) Using multidimensional scaling on data from pairs of relatives to explore the dimensionality of categorical multifactorial traits. *Genet. Epidemiol.* **9,** 87–107.
31. Alter, O., Brown, P. O., and Botstein, D. (2000) Singular value decomposition for genome-wide expression data processing and modeling. *Proc. Natl. Acad. Sci. USA* **97,** 10101–10106.
32. Alter, O., Brown, P. O., and Botstein, D. (2003) Generalized singular value decomposition for comparative analysis of genome-scale expression data sets of two different organisms. *Proc. Natl. Acad. Sci. USA* **100,** 3351–3356.
33. Tusher, V. G., Tibshirani, R., and Chu, G. (2001) Significance analysis of microarrays applied to the ionizing radiation response. *Proc. Natl. Acad. Sci. USA* **98,** 5116–5121.
34. Hwang, D., Schmitt, W. A., and Stephanopoulos, G. (2002) Determination of minimum sample size and discriminatory expression patterns in microarray data. *Bioinformatics* **18,** 1184–1193.

3

Demonstration of a Germinal Center Immunophenotype in Lymphomas by Immunocytochemistry and Flow Cytometry

Andrew Jack, Sharon Barrans, David Blythe, and Andrew Rawstron

Summary

The germinal center plays an important role in the pathogenesis of B-cell lymphomas, and evidence exists to suggest that most cases are germinal center or postgerminal center derived. Burkitt lymphoma and follicular lymphoma are derived from the germinal center stage of differentiation. It has been shown that diffuse large B-cell lymphomas with a germinal center-type pattern of RNA expression or a germinal center cell phenotype using immunocytochemistry have a more favorable outcome compared with those with a postgerminal center/activated profile. Microarray technology may not be available in many diagnostic laboratories, and antibody-based methods are much simpler and cheaper and are therefore more applicable to the routine setting. Immunocytochemistry has the advantage that the cells of interest are identified morphologically, and it is applicable retrospectively to fixed tissue. The main disadvantage is that only single-color staining is currently used in the routine setting. Flow cytometry allows one to obtain a more precise definition of individual cell types. The cells of interest are identified by a combination of physical characteristics and by the use of multiple antibodies labeled with different fluorochromes. Flow cytometry has the major advantage of being able to analyze very large numbers of cells, and results can be obtained within a few hours of the specimen being taken. The methods described allow B-cell lymphomas to be crudely divided into two groups, those with a germinal center phenotype and those that are mainly postgerminal center tumors. As knowledge of the normal biology of the germinal center develops, it will become possible to use immunophenotypic methods to more precisely classify all types of mature B-cell malignancies.

Key Words: Germinal center; flow cytometry, immunohistochemistry; TSA; follicular lymphoma; diffuse large B-cell lymphoma; Burkitt lymphoma.

1. Introduction

1.1. What Is the Germinal Center?

The function of the germinal center and the central role this structure plays in the normal B-cell response to antigen has become clear during the past decade.

From: *Methods in Molecular Medicine, Vol. 115: Lymphoma: Methods and Protocols*
Edited by: T. Illidge and P. W. M. Johnson © Humana Press Inc., Totowa, NJ

Understanding the germinal center reaction at a cellular level has provided the basis for the observation that during a secondary immune response, the affinity of the antibody increases, and there is a switch from immunoglobulin M (IgM) to IgG or IgA production. The germinal center is a transient structure that forms within primary B-cell follicles when B-cells responding to antigen receive appropriate signals from antigen-stimulated helper T-cells. A small number of such cells differentiate into centroblasts and enter a phase of rapid cell division. During the cell cycle, mutation of the rearranged immunoglobulin genes takes place, leading to intraclonal diversity within the expanding centroblast population of the germinal center. The mechanism of immunoglobulin gene mutation is not completely understood but appears to require the cells to be in cycle and for there to be active transcription of the relevant genes. The process involves double-stranded DNA breaking and subsequent DNA repair. The protein AID (activation-induced cytidine deaminase) recently has been shown to be essential for mutation to occur *(1,2)*. As clonally expanded and mutated cells exit from the germinal center, they differentiate into centrocytes. These cells are screened for the expression of high-affinity surface immunoglobulin through contact with antigen presented on follicular dendritic cells. The majority of cells die at this stage by apoptosis. The remaining cells that are able to bind antigen with high affinity respond to cytokine and T-cell interactions and undergo further differentiation into memory B-cells or long lived bone marrow plasma cells. Cells that leave the germinal center to become memory B-cells may re-enter the germinal center after a subsequent encounter with antigen, in which they may undergo additional rounds of somatic hypermutation. Cells that are destined to become plasma cells initiate class switching of their immunoglobulin gene constant (Cm) coding region which is exchanged for Cg or Ca, leading to the expression of IgG or IgA rather than IgM. These cells differentiate into plasma cells as they leave the lymph node and migrate to the bone marrow.

1.2. Why Is the Germinal Center Important in the Classification of Lymphomas?

It is now becoming clear that the germinal center plays an important role in the pathogenesis of lymphomas and that tumors derived from cells at the germinal center stage of differentiation are pathologically and clinically distinctive. The presence of immunoglobulin gene mutation can be used as a marker to determine whether B-cells have passed through a germinal center, and the presence of intraclonal diversity indicates that the mutational process remains active. With the exception of acute lymphoblastic leukemia, mantle cell lymphoma and some cases of B-chronic lymphocytic leukemia (CLL), immunoglobulin gene mutation is found in almost all B-cell malignancies *(3,4)*, suggesting that the majority of B-cell malignancies are germinal center or post-germinal center derived and consist of germinal center B-cells, memory B-cells, or plasma cells. It has been recognized for many years that mature B-cell neoplasms arc a much morc common occurrence than their T-cell counterparts, and a reasonable hypothesis to explain this difference is that the mutation and genetic recombination that occurs in the normal germinal center is responsible for an excess of oncogenic genetic abnormalities in germinal center and postgerminal center B-cells. Three distinct type of abnormalities have been demonstrated. Balanced translocations involving the immunoglobulin genes may result from deoxyribonucleic acid (DNA) breaks caused by the normal function of the mutator mechanism. The t(14;18) is an important example of this type of abnormality ***(5)***. Balanced translocations involving the immunoglobulin switch region, which presumably arise through aberrant class switching, are associated with c-*MYC* rearrangements in Burkitt lymphoma. These are almost invariably present in the postgerminal center plasma cells in monoclonal gammopathy of uncertain significance ***(6–9)***. Recently, it has been found that genes other than immunoglobulin genes are also mutated in germinal center B-cells. The best described is *BCL*-6 ***(10)***; however, mutations of a wider range of genes, some of which may be pathogenically important are described in B-cell lymphomas ***(10,11)***. In some cases of Hodgkin lymphoma, a mutation may inactivate expression of the immunoglobulin genes ***(12,13)***.

1.3. Germinal Center-Derived Lymphomas

1.3.1. Follicular Lymphoma

Follicular lymphoma is the archetypal germinal center-derived lymphoma. In almost every case the tumor shows evidence of follicle formation, and the tumor cells morphologically resemble centrocytes and centroblasts. The tumor cells have a germinal center phenotype and, in more than 90% of cases, the t(14;18) is present. The demonstration of the translocation or aberrant bcl-2 expression and a germinal center phenotype is an essential component in the diagnosis of follicular lymphoma. This is required to make an accurate distinction between follicular lymphoma and reactive lymphoid hyperplasia. In addition, several types of tumor, including mantle cell lymphoma, marginal zone lymphoma, and lymphocyte predominant nodular Hodgkin lymphoma, can have an apparently follicular or nodular growth pattern, and it is important to be able to accurately differentiate these from follicular lymphoma. In some follicular lymphomas, the tumor may have a substantial interfollicular component, and these tumors may show partial loss of the germinal center phenotype ***(14,15)***.This may also be the case with follicular lymphoma involving the bone marrow and can lead to difficulties in establishing a diagnosis in which marrow infiltration is the patient's only presenting feature. This diagnosis can be resolved by the routine use of polymerase chain reaction (PCR) or fluorescence *in situ* hybridization (FISH) to demonstrate the t(14;18) in all bone marrow infiltrates of lymphoma that do not have the immunophenotype of CLL or mantle cell lymphoma. Recently, a subgroup of follicular lymphomas with large cell morphology have been recognized that have a follicular growth pattern, but a significant proportion lack a germinal center phenotype and t(14;18). It is possible that these also have a different clinical outcome ***(16)***.

1.3.2. Diffuse Large B-Cell Lymphoma

Diffuse large B-cell lymphoma (DLBCL) is considered as a single disease entity in the REAL and WHO classification but has long been recognized to be heterogeneous in its clinical behavior. Approximately 40% of patients are cured by CHOP (cyclophosphamide, doxorubicin, vincristine, and prednisone)-type combination chemotherapy, with most of the remainder dying of their disease. A minority of high-risk, poor-prognosis patients can be identified using clinical features alone, and this has led to a search for biological factors that can be used to assess the intrinsic malignancy or treatment resistance of the tumor cells at the cellular level. A key observation in this regard was the demonstration, using the Lymphochip DNA microarray, that DLBCL with a germinal center type pattern of RNA expression had a more favorable clinical outcome ***(17)***. This result has also been confirmed using immunocytochemistry to demonstrate a germinal center cell phenotype ***(18)***. This is important because micoarray technology may not be available in many diagnostic laboratories. Antibody-based methods are much simpler and cheaper and are therefore more applicable to the routine setting. Flow cytometry in particular allows more precise definition of individual cell types. Although germinal center type DLBCL has been shown to be a better prognostic group compared with other types of DLBCL, this is an oversimplification and is potentially misleading. Within the group of germinal center-type DLBCL there is a wide range of genetic abnormalities, including t(14;18), leading to abnormal bcl-2 expression, p53 mutations and deletion, and deregulation of *BCL*-6 by translocation or mutation. These abnormalities all affect the apoptotic mechanisms within the cell and hence the ability of chemotherapy to eliminate the tumor. Germinal center-type lymphomas with bcl-2 expression have a poor prognosis, and there is some evidence that this group can be better defined by demonstration of the t(14;18) ***(20)***. Inactivation of p53 by mutation or deletion or abnormalities of *BCL*-6 may act synergistically with bcl-2 to block apoptosis, further impairing the prognosis of the patient ***(21–23)***. When these factors are taken into account, it can be seen that DLBCL with a germinal center phenotype can be divided into two groups. Those without genetic abnormalities that inhibit apoptosis appear to have an excellent clinical outcome. In contrast, when the apoptotic pathway is abnormal, particularly where multiple abnormalities are present, the outcome often is very poor. Taking these variables into account, it is perhaps a little surprising that the initial studies using gene array techniques were able to show a significant difference in outcome in a relatively small and unselected series.

1.3.3. Burkitt's Lymphoma

Burkitt's lymphoma is the third type of germinal center cell-derived lymphoma. Burkitt's lymphoma was initially defined by its morphological features; however, morphology is altered by the effects of fixation and interobserver agreement can be poor. It is now apparent that all cases of Burkitt's lymphoma have a germinal center phenotype, and this alone can improve the level of diagnostic accuracy ***(24,25)***. However, the distinction between Burkitt's lymphoma, particularly those with atypical morphology, and germinal center-type DLBCL, remains a problem. The gold standard diagnostic feature is the rearrangement and activation of c-*MYC*, but suitable material is not always available to demonstrate these abnormalities. For this reason, it has been suggested that nearly 100% expression of the cell cycle marker Ki67 can be used as a surrogate for the activation of c-*MYC*. The specificity can be further enhanced by the demonstration of p53 inactivation, which appears to be an essential component of c-*MYC*-induced tumors in both mice and humans ***(26–28)***. A further useful feature is the absence of bcl-2 expression in most cases of Burkitt's lymphoma. At present, there are few data on the correlation among morphology, phenotype, and cytogenetics in Burkitt's lymphoma. Resolving these problems of definition is important because there are a proportion of cases of DLBCL with very aggressive clinical behavior and poor outcome when treated with CHOP. These patients may be successfully treated using high-intensity chemotherapy regimens ***(29,30)***.

2. Materials

2.1. Choice of Antibody Panels

Most of the antibodies currently used to define the germinal center phenotype have been selected on a purely empirical basis as a result of screening panels of monoclonal antibodies against normal and tumor cells. This strategy is now changing, and it is likely that, in the future, molecules identified through studies of normal germinal center B-cell development will be used to define phenotypes. The use of gene expression microarrays will provide an overview of the profile of germinal center B-cells and lead to the ability to select novel discriminatory molecules for use in antibody panels.

2.1.1. CD10

CD10 is an endopeptidase that is involved in growth factor modulation. In normal peripheral lymphoid tissue, CD10 is confined to expression on cells of the germinal center and is therefore important in antibody panels designed to identify tumor cells with a germinal center phenotype. Unfortunately, CD10 is not specific for normal and neoplastic germinal center B-cells but also can be expressed in a variety of epithelial cell tumors and carcinomas. This should not normally be a major diagnostic problem because a diagnosis of B-cell lymphoma is extremely unlikely to be made in the absence of other lineage-specific markers. CD10 expression recently has been described in the neoplastic T-cells in angioimmunoblastic type T-cell lymphoma ***(31)***. Because some neoplastic T-cells also express CD20; in some cases there may be a possibility of confusion between angioimmunoblastic T-cells lymphoma and a T-cell rich B-cell lymphoma with a germinal center phenotype. In practice, this is likely to be a problem that is encountered rarely. The heterogeneity of expression of CD10 also can result in problems with interpretation. Within a lymph node that is determined to have follicular lymphoma, CD10 is almost invariably expressed on the follicular component but not on the interfollicular or bone marrow components of the tumor. This can make it difficult to definitely characterize a bone marrow infiltrate and also suggests that some diffuse large B-cell lymphomas of germinal center type could be negative with CD10. A further problem is that normal bone marrow B-cell precursor cells express CD10 and these must not be mistaken for tumor infiltration of the bone marrow. These cells are identified by flow cytometric analysis by coexpression of very high levels of CD38, weak or absent CD20, and the absence of surface immunoglobulin.

2.1.2. Bcl-6

Bcl-6 is a nuclear transcription factor that has been shown to play a vital role in the development of the germinal center. Knockout mice that lack expression of this molecule do not have germinal centers and do not mount a secondary immune response ***(32)***. In immunocytochemical preparations of normal lymphoid tissue, bcl-6 appears to be expressed in most, if not all, germinal center cells ***(33)***. Bcl-6 would therefore appear to be an ideal candidate molecule for the identification of a germinal center phenotype in lymphomas. Bcl-6 does appear to be expressed in almost all cases of follicular lymphoma to the extent that, if this is not present, the diagnosis should be regarded as highly questionable ***(14)***. Bcl-6 is also of value in identifying fragments of normal germinal centers in other types of lymphoma, including marginal zone and mantle cell lymphoma, with a nodular growth pattern. One of the most frequent errors in the diagnosis of follicular lymphoma arises in cases of B-CLL with an extensive follicular growth pattern. This is easily averted by demonstrating positive features of a B-CLL phenotype and by the absence of CD10 and bcl-6, although these can be expressed weakly in occasional cells in pseudofollicles. The interpretation of bcl-6 in diffuse large B-cell lymphomas is more difficult. Bcl-6 is expressed on a much larger group of tumors than CD10 and whereas CD10 probably underestimates the number of tumors with a germinal center phenotype, the reverse is probably the case with bcl-6. The reason for this is likely to be the result of abnormal expression of bcl-6 as a consequence of genetic abnormalities. Bcl-6 frequently is rearranged in a variety of types of B-cell lymphoma. Most commonly, this involves the immunoglobulin loci but many other translocation partners are described, and these may differ in the deregulation of the bcl-6 protein ***(34)*** and in their prognostic significance ***(35)***. *BCL*-6 is often mutated, and some mutations in the 5' regulatory sequences also may give rise to aberrant gene expression ***(36)***. For a further discussion and methodology *see also* Chapter 13.

From the point of view of assessing the prognosis of DLBCL, CD10 in combination with bcl-6 appears to give the optimum level of discrimination. DNA microarray studies have suggested that the t(14;18) is confined to tumors with a germinal center phenotype and this is also the case for tumors that co-express CD10 and bcl-6 by immunocytochemistry ***(38)***.

2.1.3. CD75

CD75 was widely used as an immunocytochemical reagent for germinal center cells before suitable antibodies to CD10 and bcl-6 became widely available. Despite being used for many years, the protein remains poorly characterized. Normal germinal center cells and most, if not all, follicular lymphomas express CD75; however, CDw75 also is known to react with non-GC cells, and in DLBCL a higher proportion of tumors express CD75 than express CD10. From the purely practical point of view, the presence of CD75 expression appears to add little to the expression of CD10 and bcl-6 in defining a germinal center phenotype. One practical use of this antibody is in the diagnosis of lymphocyte-predominant nodular Hodgkin lymphoma, in which very strong expression of CD75 by the tumor cells makes them easy to identify against a mixed B-cell background.

2.1.4. CD23

CD23 is expressed on virgin B-cells and a small proportion of germinal center cells. It also is found on the cells of the follicular mantle zone ***(39)***. CD23 also is a defining marker of typical B-CLL. When used as an immunocytochemical reagent, CD23 may be found on a small number of cases of follicular lymphoma. Interpretation of this antibody can be difficult because CD23 is expressed at much higher levels on follicular dendritic cells, which are found in both normal and neoplastic follicles. The proportion of cases of follicular lymphoma with CD23 expression is greater when flow cytometry is used. This may be caused by the greater sensitivity of detection on unfixed cells or better separation of the neoplastic population from normal B-cell and follicular dendritic cells. A small number of DLBCL are CD23+, bcl-6+, CD10–. This is likely to represent a subset of germinal center-type DLBCL, but the full significance of this phenotype is not yet known.

2.1.5. Bcl-2

Bcl-2 is not a marker for germinal center differentiation but is an essential component of the immunophenotypic assessment of all germinal center B-cell lymphomas. Using immunocytochemistry, normal germinal center cells do not express bcl-2, and its expression in this context is always significant. Bcl-2 expression is observed in approx 95% of follicular lymphomas, and its absence should lead to a re-evaluation of the diagnosis. Care must also be taken in interpreting the results of immunocytochemical studies because of the expression of bcl-2 by normal T-cells, which often are seen in considerable numbers in both normal and neoplastic follicles. Data on bcl-2 expression using flow cytometric methods that combine cell surface and cytoplasmic antigen detection have not yet been fully evaluated. In large cell lymphoma, interpretation of bcl-2 expression is more complex. Absence of bcl-2 is seen in both Burkitt lymphoma and in the best prognostic group of DLBCL. DLBCL with bcl-2 expression has a much poorer prognosis, but his group can be further subdivided according to the presence of a t(14;18). There is some evidence to suggest that the poor prognostic group is best defined by those that are bcl-2 and t(14;18) positive. This may reflect differences in the levels of expression of bcl-2 and hence the degree to which apoptosis is inhibited. The mechanism of expression of bcl-2 in tumors of germinal center type without rearrangement or amplification of *BCL*-2 is at present unknown.

2.1.6. Surface Immunoglobulin

The presence of surface immunoglobulin is a feature of all types of B-cell malignancy with the exception of acute lymphoblastic leukemia and myeloma. In tumors showing germinal center differentiation, there are a number of specific features that should be noted. A proportion of follicular lymphomas may have absence of surface immunoglobulin because of the disruption of the immunoglobulin genes by translocations. Surface immunoglobulin is also lost during plasma cell differentiation and, in the bone marrow, a substantial proportion of an infiltrate of follicular lymphoma may consist of plasma cells. Standard flow cytometry would underestimate the extent of infiltration in these circumstances. Immunoglobulin class switching is a feature of normal germinal center cells and it is, therefore, not surprising that follicular lymphomas expressing sIgG are found. In practice, this is very rare in other types of lymphomas and in the absence of obvious features of B-CLL the presence of sIgG is very strongly suggestive of a germinal center type tumor. This can be helpful in the bone marrow where CD10 expression can be weak or absent. The value of identification of sIgG in the assessment of DLBCL is not yet known.

2.1.7. P53 and p21

The role of p53 as a tumor-suppressor gene is well known. DNA damage leads to activation of p53 and, in normal cells, produces cell cycle arrest, induction of apoptosis, or cell senescence. Inactivation of the pathway by mutation of p53 or deletion of the gene is very frequent in malignant cells. Normal p53 induces the cyclin-dependent kinase p21, but this function is lost in cells with mutated p53. The use of these antibodies together is a simple screening test for mutated p53 ***(40)***. In germinal, center-derived B-cell lymphomas, in particular those with a t(14;18), p53 inactivation is a poor prognostic factor. p53 is induced indirectly by ARF in c-*MYC*-induced hyperproliferative states and, in most cases of Burkitt lymphoma, p53 is strongly expressed in the absence of p21. This is consistent with studies of the pathogenesis of Burkitt lymphoma in transgenic mice ***(41)***. In large cell lymphomas with a germinal center phenotype, expression of p53 but absence of p21 and bcl-2 and a Ki67 fraction of greater than 95% is a very useful screening test for Burkitt lymphoma.

2.2. Immunocytochemistry

2.2.1. Antigen Retrieval

1. Citrate buffer, pH 6.0: 10 m*M* citric acid, pH to 6.0 with 2 *N* sodium hydroxide.
2. Antigen Unmasking Fluid: Vector (cat. no. H-3300).

2.2.2. The Streptavidin/Biotin/Horseradish Peroxidase Technique

1. Primary Antisera: Use antibodies, as described previously, that have been optimally diluted in Tris-buffered saline or Dako ChemMate™ antibody Diluent (S-2022). Optimum dilutions and detection methods are given in the table below and are based on detection using the Dako ChemMate Kit (*see* **Note 1**).

Antigen	Source	Optimum dilution	Detection method
CD10	Novocastra	1/20 (1/50[a])	StrABC (TSA[a])
Bcl-6	Dako	1/20 (1/50[a])	StrABC (TSA[a])
CD75	Novocastra	1/20	StrABC
CD23[b]	Dako	1/200	TSA
Bcl-2	Dako	1/100	StrABC
P53	In House	1/350	StrABC
P21	Dako	1/15	StrABC
IgM	Dako	1/20	StrABC
IgD	Dako	1/200	StrABC
IgG	Dako	1/1000	StrABC
Kappa	Dako	1/800	StrABC
Lambda	Dako	1/6000	StrABC

[a]*See* **Note 2.**
[b]*See* **Note 3.**

2. StrABC/HRP Multispecies Immunocytochemistry Kit: The Dako ChemMate Kit (K-5001) consists of Reagent A, multilink biotinylated secondary (anti-mouse and anti-rabbit); reagent B, Streptavidin peroxidase; Reagent C, diaminobenzidene (DAB); and reagent D, HRP substrate. Other materials needed are as follows:
   - ChemMate Peroxidase Blocking solution (S-2022).
   - Tris-buffered saline (TBS).
   - 0.5 *M* Tris and 0.03 *M* NaCl, adjusted to pH 7.6 using 50% hydrochloric acid.
   - Tris buffer (Tris).
   - 0.5 *M* Tris-HCl, pH 7.6.

2.2.3. Signal Amplification: The Tyramide Signal Amplification Technique

1. 50 m*M* borate buffer.
2. 1.24 g of boric acid (molecular weight [MW] 62.0) dissolved in 100 mL of distilled water.
3. 1.9 g of sodium tetra borate (MW 381.4) dissolved in 100 mL of distilled water.
4. Sodium tetra borate solution added to 70 mL of boric acid until pH reaches 8.0.
5. Biotinylated tyramide.
6. Stock Solution:
   - 100 mg of sulfosuccinimidyl-6-(biotinamide) hexanoate (Sulfo-NHS-LC biotin).
   - 30 mg of tyramide hydrochloride.
   - 40 mL of 50 mM borate buffer, pH 8.0.

   Stir gently at room temperature until completely dissolved, then filtered through a 0.45-mm syringe filter.
7. Working Solution: Twenty microliters of stock solution and 1 mL of 0.05 *M* TBS stored at –20°C in 1-mL aliquots.

2.2.4. DAB

1. Stock Solution: Seven and a half grams of 3,3 diaminobenzidine tetrahydrochloride in 100 mL of Tris buffer, pH 7.6, stored at –20°C in 1-mL aliquots.
2. Working Solution: One milliliter of stock solution in 400 mL of Tris buffer, pH 7.6, with 0.15% hydrogen peroxide (30% w/v).

2.3. Flow Cytometry

1. Ammonium Chloride Lysing Solution: 0.86 g of ammonium chloride in 1 L of distilled water. Do not adjust pH. Stable for 1 wk.
2. Wash Buffer: FACSFlow (BD Biosciences, UK) containing 1% w/v bovine serum albumin (Sigma, Poole, UK).
3. Suggested Flow Cytometry Panel for Surface Antigens

FITC	PE[e]	PE[e]:Cy5
CD3[d]	CD3[d]	CD19[d]
CD20[b]	CD5[d]	CD19[d]
CD10[d]	CD38[a]	CD19[d]
Kappa[d]	Lambda[d]	CD19[d]
FMC7[c]	CD22[a]	CD19[d]
CD11a[d]	CD23[d]	CD19[d]
IgM[a]	IgD[a]	CD19[d]
IgG[a]	CD79b[b]	CD19[d]

[a]BD Biosciences.
[b]Coulter/Immunotech.
[c]Silenus.
[d]In-house reagent.
[e]PE, phycoerythrin.

3. Methods

3.1. Choice of Technique

In a diagnostic laboratory, the identification of neoplastic cells with a germinal center phenotype can be conducted using immunocytochemistry, flow cytometry, or a combination of both techniques. Immunocytochemistry has the advantage that the cells of interest are identified morphologically. The main disadvantage is that at the moment only single color staining is used in the routine setting; however, kits for dual-color immunocytochemistry are becoming increasingly available. Immunocytochemistry has the added advantage of being applicable retrospectively to fixed tissue, but there are limitations on the range of antibodies that can be used. Many antigens are altered or masked by fixation and where tissue preservation is less than optimal, inconsistency of staining occurs (*see* **Notes 4–6**). In particular, the reliable identification of monoclonality in a B-cell population using immunoglobulin light chain restriction can be extremely difficult. The sensitivity of detection of a number of antigens is reduced in comparison with unfixed cells. An additional major advantage of immunocytochemical methods is the ease of detection of cytoplasmic and nuclear antigens. In the context of the present discussion bcl-2 and Ki67 are of particular importance. However, in the absence of effective multicolor techniques, interpretation can be difficult where the infiltrate is a heterogeneous mixture of normal and neoplastic cells.

Flow cytometry can be readily conducted on samples of solid tissue that have been disaggregated and on bone marrow, peripheral blood, or effusion specimens. The cells of interest are identified by a combination of physical characteristics, such as size and granularity, and by the use of up to four antibodies labeled with different fluorochromes. The major advantages of using flow cytometry are that it allows the analysis of very large numbers of cells and the accurate definition of small populations of cells in heterogeneous mixtures of cells, such as bone marrow. Flow cytometry also is very fast, and results can be obtained within a few hours of the specimen being taken. Until recently, routine diagnostic flow cytometry was limited mainly to the detection of cell surface antigens. This is now changing with fixation and permeablization reagents, which allow the simultaneous detection of combinations of cell surface, cytoplasmic, and nuclear antigens. This is a significant extension of the technique that will have major implications for the effective investigation of many types of tumor and in particular of germinal center lymphomas.

3.2. Immunocytochemistry Methods

3.2.1. Specimen Handling

Lymph nodes should then be cut along the longitudinal axis into 1- to 2-mm slices (*see* **Note 5**). Fix representative slices for 24–48 h at room temperature and process to paraffin wax. The remainder of the tissue is used for flow cytometry and molecular studies as required.

3.2.2. Antigen Retrieval

One of the most important advances in immunocytochemistry in recent years has been the development of techniques designed to unmask antigen sites that have been obscured by tissue fixation. Traditionally, this was achieved by using proteolytic enzymes such as trypsin. However, proteolytic antigen retrieval has many limitations, principally that the digestion time is highly dependent on the extent and efficiency of fixation, which cannot be easily controlled. In recent years, the most popular and optimal methods of antigen retrieval have been heat-mediated methods. By heating the sections in a suitable buffer, the weak

Schiff bases formed during formalin fixation can be broken and the antigenic sites exposed, whereas the methylene bridges remain intact. Heating may be achieved using a microwave oven, pressure cooker, autoclave, or incubator (*see* **Note 7**).

1. Take 3-µm sections through xylene and graded alcohols to water.
2. a. *Microwave antigen retrieval*. Microwave the slides in 400 mL of citrate buffer, pH 6.0, on high power (800 W) for 15 min, rest for 5-min, top the buffer back up, then microwave for a further 5 min; or

   b. *Pressure cooking*. Heat 1500 mL of buffer in the pressure cooker and, when boiling, place slides into buffer and seal the cooker. Once full pressure (15 PSI) is reached, cook for 30 s.
3. After antigen-retrieval pretreatment, wash the sections in cold tap water and rinse in TBS, pH 7.6.

3.2.3. The Streptavidin/Biotin/Horseradish Peroxidase (StrABC/HRP) Technique

The most commonly used method for diagnostic immunocytochemistry is based on the StrABC/HRP technique, which exploits the binding capabilities of avidin and biotin. The technique involves four main stages (*see* **Fig. 1**).

1. Application and binding of primary antibody to specific antigenic sites in the tissue section for a minimum of 1 h, followed by blocking of endogenous peroxidase activity using ChemMate Peroxidase Blocking solution or 0.5% hydrogen peroxide.
2. Application of a multi-link biotinylated secondary antibody that will bind to the primary antibody for a minimum of 30 min.
3. Binding of StrABC/HRP complex to the biotinylated secondary antibody for a minimum of 30 min.
4. Visualization of HRP labeled sites using DAB working solution (*see* **Note 8**) for 10 min to give a brown final reaction product and counterstain with hematoxylin.

Washes between each incubation are for a minimum of 5 min in TBS.

The StrABC/HRP is prepared using streptavidin isolated from *Streptomyces avidinii* and horseradish peroxidase that has been optimally labeled with biotin using a 7-atom spacer arm. When streptavidin and biotinylated peroxidase are mixed as described in the procedure, the complex is stoichiometrically assembled to allow free streptavidin molecules to bind to the biotin of the secondary multi-link antibody, and optimal staining is achieved. The use of streptavidin in the complex ensures a particularly low background because the pH of streptavidin is close to neutral and, therefore, nonspecific ionic interactions with tissue components are avoided. The peroxidase enzyme present in the complex is used to localize the antigen by the production of a colored end product at the site of the reaction when the chromogen (DAB) is added in the presence of hydrogen peroxide, which catalyses the reaction (*see* **Note 8**).

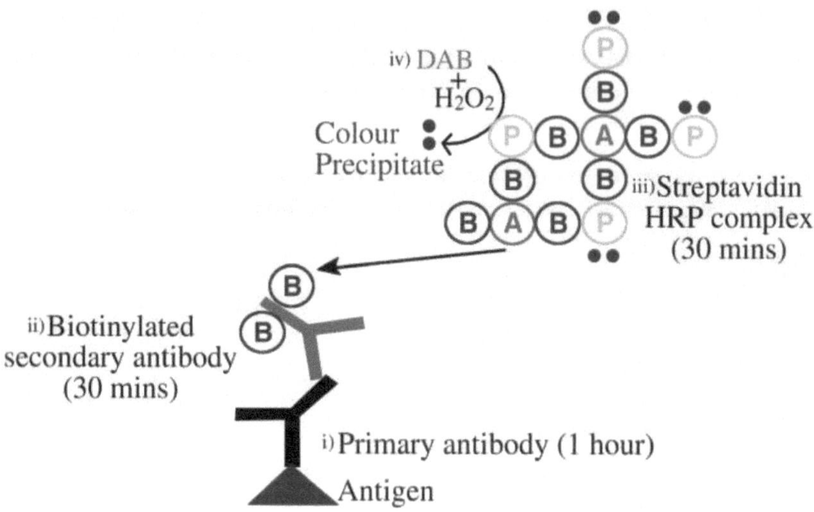

Fig. 1. Diagrammatic representation of the standard StrABC technique. (**i**) Application and binding of primary antibody to specific antigenic sites in the tissue section. (**ii**) Application of a multilink biotinylated secondary antibody that will bind to the primary antibody. (**iii**) Binding of StrABC/HRP comples. (**iv**) Visualisation of HRP labelled sites using Diaminobenzidene (DAB). Washes between each incubation are for a minimum of 5 min in TBS.

3.2.4. Signal Amplification: The Tyramide Signal Amplification Technique

The Tyramide Signal Amplification (TSA) technique ***(42)*** enables the detection of quantitatively small amounts of antigen that remain in tissues that have been fixed and processed and therefore allows the demonstration of antigens previously unreactive in formalin-fixed, paraffin-embedded, or resin-embedded tissue. This method requires a number of modifications of the standard StrABC/HRP method.

1. Antigen retrieval is conducted in Vector Antigen Unmasking Fluid (diluted 1/10 in distilled water).
2. Follow the standard StrABC protocol with 15-min incubations in primary and secondary antisera and StrABC (*see* **Fig. 2**).
3. After localization of the primary antibody with biotinylated secondary and StrABC, biotinyl tyramine is added to the sections, in the presence of hydrogen peroxidase (4 µL per 1.0-mL aliquot of biotinyl tyramine working solution) and incubated for 5 mins exactly (*see* **Fig. 2**).
4. After prolonged washing (at least 10 min), further StrABC/HRP is added in the final stage and incubated for a further 15 min before developing the reaction using DAB (*see* **Fig. 2**).

The use of antigen retrieval and signal amplification has greatly expanded the range of antigens that can be detected in fixed and routinely processed tissue specimens. These techniques can also be applied to methyl methacrylate embedded specimens of bone marrow (*see* **Note 3**). The combination of high-quality morphology and immunocytochemistry can allow even very low level infiltrates to be detected with confidence.

All the germinal center-related markers require the use antigen-retrieval techniques to achieve reliable results in fixed tissue specimens (*see* **Note 7**). In addition to heat-mediated antigen retrieval, to visualize these antigens in fixed tissue CD23 also requires additional signal amplification (*see* **Note 3**).

3.3. Flow Cytometry Methods

Flow cytometry is the method of choice for identifying germinal center B-cell lymphomas in which unfixed tissue specimens are available or for the detection of these tumors in the bone marrow, peripheral blood, or serous effusion specimens. As with immunocytochemistry, the quality of the specimen and its initial handling are crucial to obtaining satisfactory results. Tissue specimens must be fresh and ideally should be sent to the laboratory by the fastest route after being removed from the patient. Specimens of lymph node can be readily disaggregated into a single cell suspension by mechanical disruption and gentle perfusion with cell culture medium using a fine needle and syringe. Specially designed equipment is also available to carry out this function. A leucocyte suspension can also be readily prepared from peripheral blood or bone marrow.

The strategy used to identify the cells of interest is critical to the success of any flow cytometric method. Few of the antibodies used to define the germinal center phenotype are strictly lineage specific, for example, CD10 may be found on granulocytes, and CD38 is expressed on activated T-cells, granulocytes, and monocytes. Single-color techniques are therefore obsolete, and in all cases it is essential to identify the B-cells. This is especially important for the clear definition of monoclonality. Identification of B-cells is best achieved by a combination of a pan-B-cell marker, almost invariably CD19, in combination with the physical characteristics of the cells defined by light scatter. In a standard three-color technique using directly conjugated antibodies, this will allow the gated cells to be further defined by a number of paired combinations of antibodies selected from the list shown in **Subheading 2.2.2., item 1**.

Until recently, flow cytometry in routine diagnostic use was largely confined to the study of cell surface antigens. The development of reagents that fix cell suspensions and render the cell membrane permeable to conjugated antibodies while at the same time preserving cell surface antigens now are greatly expanding the scope of flow cytometry as a diagnostic technique. These reagents,

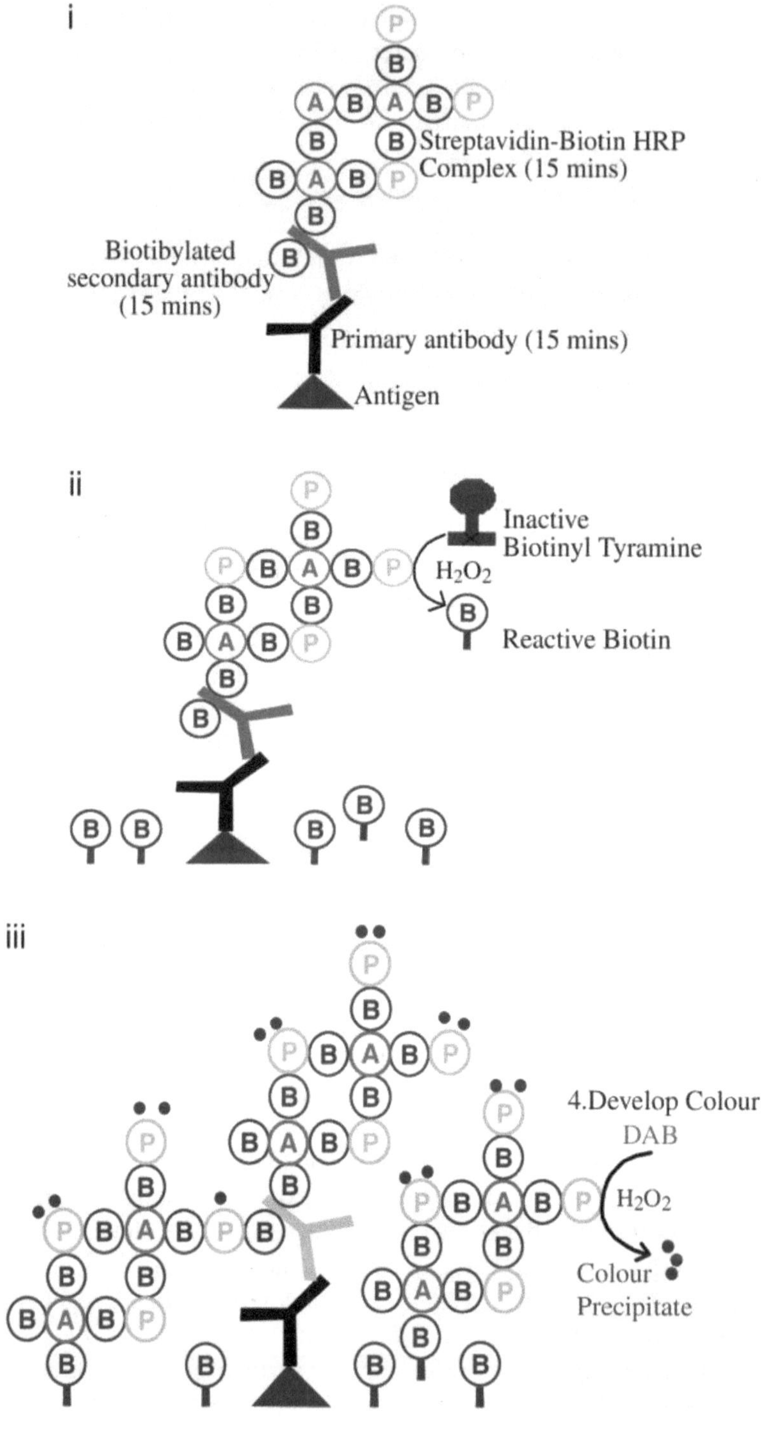
i
Streptavidin-Biotin HRP Complex (15 mins)
Biotibylated secondary antibody (15 mins)
Primary antibody (15 mins)
Antigen
ii
Inactive Biotinyl Tyramine
H_2O_2
Reactive Biotin
iii
4.Develop Colour
DAB
H_2O_2
Colour Precipitate

which usually involve a formaldehyde-based fixation step followed by a detergent-based permeabilization step, are available in several commercial formulations. This use of combined nuclear, cytoplasmic, and surface antigen demonstration is of particular relevance to the improved identification of normal and neoplastic germinal center cells because it will allow antibodies such as bcl-2, bcl-6, and Ki67 to be studied directly in relation to CD10 and surface immunoglobulin heavy chain. (Directly labeled antibodies to bcl-6 currently are unavailable commercially.)

Using these antibodies and techniques the identification and characterization of germinal center-type lymphomas in lymph nodes, effusions, or heavily involved bone marrow specimens is not usually a problem. If techniques to demonstrate only cell surface antigens are available, flow cytometric investigations can be supplemented by immunocytochemical analysis of bcl-2 and bcl-6. However, one of the main applications of flow cytometry is the ability to detect very small populations of tumor cells in a complex background of normal cells. If standard three-color cell surface flow cytometry is used, there are a number of problems in identifying small numbers of neoplastic germinal center cells in the bone marrow. Normal B-cell progenitors are CD19+, CD10+, and CD38+. These must be distinguished from neoplastic germinal center cells by the absence of surface immunoglobulin and by differences in the intensity of expression of CD19 and CD38. This problem is compounded by the apparent discordance in CD10 expression between germinal center-type lymphomas in lymph nodes and in bone marrow. This is well recognized in follicular lymphoma, but there are few data in DLBCL B-cell and Burkitt lymphoma. A small minority of germinal center lymphomas may lack surface immunoglobulin, possibly as a consequence of translocations into the immunoglobulin heavy chain locus. The ability to detect small numbers of any type of neoplastic B-cell in the bone marrow using light chain restriction is greatly limited by the dilutional effect of normal B-cells. To overcome these problems, more sophisticated flow cytometric techniques are required. The starting point for the development of these techniques is to identify a number of antigens that have a wide difference in expression between the neoplastic cells and any other population of B-cells, such as progenitor cells, which have an overlapping phenotype. This forms the

---

Fig. 2. *(opposite page)* TSA method. **(i)** Standard StrABC method with reduced incubation times. **(ii)** Biotinylated tyramine amplification. Horseradish peroxidase in the presence of hydrogen peroxidase catalyses the formation of reactive biotinylated tyramide and results in the deposition of biotin at the reaction site. **(iii)** Amplification of biotin sites. Subsequent reapplication of labeled streptavidin binds to the newly deposited biotin. The streptavidin is conjugated to horseradish peroxidase, which is used to develop the color of the chromogen.

basis for the development of an analytical technique, which will almost certainly involve four-color combinations of antibodies. Development of techniques of this type will have major implications for the diagnosis, bone marrow staging, and monitoring of patients with germinal center-type lymphomas. Experience with this type of approach in myeloma and B-CLL has shown that high specificity and sensitivity can be achieved ***(43,44)***.

3.3.1. Surface Antigen Detection

1. Tissue cell suspension: place into a 12-mL tube and centrifuge at 700*g* for 3 min, then discard supernatant. Resuspend in 12 mL of ammonium chloride lysis solution, and go to **step 3**.
2. Blood or marrow: aliquot up to 1 mL of whole blood or bone marrow into a 12-mL tube and make up to 12 mL with ammonium chloride lysis solution.
3. Incubate for 5 min at 37°C or until solution is transparent (*see* **Note 9**).
4. Centrifuge at 700*g* for 2 min and discard supernatant. Resuspend in 12 mL of wash buffer.
5. Repeat **step 4**.
6. Centrifuge at 700*g* for 2 min and discard supernatant. Resuspend in approx 1 mL of wash buffer.
7. Determine cell concentration.
8. Aliquot 5×10^5 cells into each of eight wells of a microtiter plate for standard panel. Centrifuge plate at 700*g* for 1 min and discard supernatant.
9. Add 15 µL of each antibody cocktail to the relevant well. Tap plate on bench to ensure that all antibody is at the bottom of the well. Resuspend the cells into the antibody suspension using a plateshaker.
10. Incubate cells with antibody at 4°C for 20 min.
11. Add 150 µL of wash buffer to each well. Centrifuge at 700*g* for 1 min, and then discard supernatant.
12. Repeat **step 11**, then resuspend in 250 µL of FACSFlow.

3.3.2. Surface and Intracellular Antigen Detection

There are various commercial reagents available. The manufacturer's instructions should be followed closely because small variations may have a dramatic impact on surface/intracellular staining quality. Surface staining will be compromised with most reagents, so analysis of surface antigens only is best performed without fixation. Analysis of surface immunoglobulin using standard manufacturer's instructions is generally not suitable.

3.3.3. Acquisition and Analysis

1. Ensure flow cytometer is adequately set-up for acquisition (*see* **Note 10**).
2. If necessary, transfer the contents of each microtiter plate well to a FACS tube.
3. Acquire a minimum of 20,000 cells (*see* **Note 11**). Acquire all leucocytes; do not

use a live gate because this may result in erroneous exclusion of B-lymphocytes, particularly DLBCL cells.

4. Assessing a CD19 vs side scatter plot is the first step (*see* **Fig. 3**). Gating strategies for B lymphoproliferative disorders are more straightforward than for other hematological malignancies. However, there is still considerable heterogeneity, particularly within germinal center neoplasias. As such, gating regions must be optimized for each case.
5. Set a wide region 1 on CD19 vs SSC plot. Normal B-cells are present in the upper left area of the plot (high CD19, low side scatter). In most B-cell neoplasias, the malignant B-cells fall within the same area. However, follicular lymphoma cells often show weak CD19. Diffuse large B-cell lymphoma cells frequently show a much higher level of side scatter. It is therefore necessary to set a wide region that may include other non-B-cell mononuclear cells. These are excluded at a later stage (*see* **Note 14**).
6. Set a wide region 2 on FSC vs SSC plot This is primarily used to exclude apoptotic cells and cellular debris but also may be used to identify neoplastic cells. A gating strategy combining these two regions is sufficient to identify the B-cell population with greater than 95% purity and usually greater than 99% purity. Optimizing the regions requires assessment of fluorescence characteristics for the surface antigens.
7. Assess the CD3 PE vs CD3 FITC plot to determine whether there is contamination by apoptotic cells/debris and/or T-cells (*see* **Notes 12** and **13**). Adjust region 1 and/or region 2 accordingly, taking care to ensure that follicular lymphoma cells are not excluded.
8. Assess kappa vs lambda plot. Identify lambda+/kappa– and lambda–/kappa+ populations. Cells lacking surface immunoglobulin should only be detected in bone marrow samples. Detection of more than two discrete populations (three on bone marrow) indicates the presence of aberrant B-cells or contamination.
9. If cells binding both kappa and lambda in equal proportions are present, this indicates contamination by monocytes or apoptotic cells/debris. Adjust region 1 and or region 2 to remove the contaminating events without excluding B-cells (*see* **Note 14**).
10. Once the B-lymphocyte population has been accurately identified, the analysis of other cell markers may be performed.

3.4. Future Developments

The antibodies described above allow B-cell lymphomas to be crudely divided into two groups: those with a germinal center phenotype and the remainder that are mainly postgerminal center tumors. As has been shown, this simple division has both prognostic significance and correlates with the presence of specific balanced translocations involving bcl-2 and c-myc. However, as knowledge of the normal biology of the germinal center develops, it will become possible to use immunophenotypic methods to more precisely classify

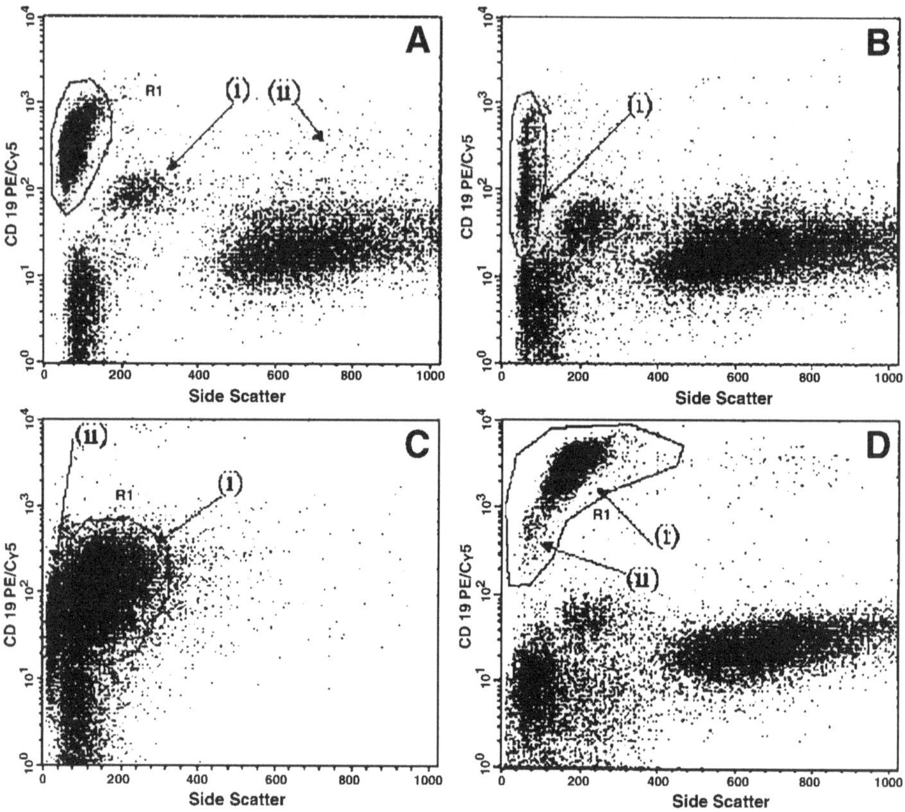

Fig. 3. Gating B-cells using CD19 and side scatter characteristics. In (**A**), a normal profile is shown that demonstrates the advantage of CD19/SSC gating to exclude monocytes (**i**) and nonviable granulocytes with high levels of nonspecific binding (**ii**). (**B**) shows a profile from a bone marrow involved with follicular lymphoma, demonstrating the low CD19 expression by the neoplastic cells (**i**) seen in many cases. (**C**) shows a profile from a disaggregated lymph node biopsy heavily involved with DLBCL, demonstrating the high side scatter of the neoplastic cells (**i**), which usually overlaps with monocytes in bone marrow/peripheral blood samples. Also shown are nonviable B-cells (**ii**), which frequently are seen in lymph node biopsies and should be excluded because they may show high levels of nonspecific binding to antibodies. (**D**) shows cells from a patient with hairy cell leukemia, showing the very high CD19 and high side scatter of the neoplastic cells (**i**) in comparison to the residual normal B-cells (**ii**).

DLBCL and, indeed, all types of mature B-cell malignancies. One approach may be to identify those tumors in which the process of somatic hypermutation remains active. Small studies using microarray techniques have already shown that tumors with a germinal center pattern of gene expression are likely to have evidence of intra-clonal heterogeneity with respect to immunoglobulin mutational pattern. Demonstrating clonal heterogeneity by cloning and sequencing immunoglobulin genes is unlikely to be a practical diagnostic method. However, antibodies to the AID protein, which appears to be a key element in the mutator mechanism, and, to some of the proteins involved in repair of double-stranded DNA breaks are becoming available, and these may allow tumors with active mutator mechanisms to be identified. Directly identifying tumors with active mutator mechanisms may be of value in assessing the risk of genetic progression. The presence of double-stranded DNA breaks may lead to balanced translocations. Alternatively, it has been shown that a wide range of nonimmunoglobulins genes, most notably bcl-6 but including other key regulatory genes, are mutated in malignant germinal center B-cells and that this may lead to tumor progression ***(45)***.

Cells that survive passage through a germinal center may become memory B-cells or plasma cells. This involves a complex switching mechanism in which a number of key transcription factors are regulated in response to signals through surface immunoglobulin and a number of cytokines including interleukin-4 and interleukin-10. Exit from the germinal center involves downregulation of bcl-6 and, in the case of cells destined to become plasma cells, induction of BLIMP-1 ***(46)***. Both of these proteins directly interact with IRF-4. BLIMP-1 represses BSAP and many other B-cell surface proteins ***(47,48)***. Less is known about the induction of memory B-cells. A second key pathway at this stage of B-cell development is the induction of NFkappa B, which is closely related to CD40 and CD30, both of which are tumor necrosis factor receptor family members. NFkappa B is has a powerful antiapoptotic effect and is able to induce a very wide diverse range of other molecules ***(49–52)***. Preliminary evidence exists to suggest that many DLBCL have an aberrant phenotype with respect to these molecules. These phenotype may give important clues to tumor pathogenesis and may be useful as surrogate markers of genetic abnormalities in the way that the expression of bcl-2 in germinal center cells strongly indicates the presence of a t(14;18).

4. Notes

1. When using the StrABC/HRP technique for each primary antibody, the pretreatment protocol and dilution required need to be established for each user, so that the best possible demonstration of antigen is achieved with minimal nonspecific binding, which is assessed using a negative control and by examination of internal cellular controls within the positive control and the test. Positive controls should be used for each antibody.
2. On paraffin sections, CD10 and Bcl-6 work optimally using the standard StrABC technique with the DAKO ChemMate Kit to detect the antigen; however,

tyramide signal amplification can be used to intensify the staining in resin-embedded samples or if weak staining is observed by routine methods.

3. With the TSA technique, the Dako CD23 clone (MHM6) requires tyramide signal amplification to optimize staining; however, the clone available from Novocastra and Serotec (1B12) produce optimal staining using the standard StrABC technique.
4. The reliability of immunocytochemistry methods is critically dependent on the initial handing of the tissue specimen. It is important that lymph node biopsies are sent to the laboratory unfixed and as quickly as possible.
5. Placing a whole specimen in formalin results in major artifacts, with wide variation in fixation between the center and edge of the node. As a result, the morphology and intensity of tinctorial and immunocytochemical staining are highly inconsistent across the tissue section. This is particularly apparent with many of the antibodies used for demonstrating a germinal center phenotype, and in extreme cases the diagnosis may be compromised if the specimen is poorly fixed. To avoid this, tissue should be thinly sliced into pieces of no more than 2- to 3-mm thick.
6. There has been a great deal written on methods of fixation of lymphoid tissue for the optimization of immunocytochemical staining. When modern immunocytochemistry is used, 10% formalin or neutral buffered formalin is adequate for all routine applications, and "special" fixatives are no longer required.
7. The advantage of pressure-cooking is that multiple 25-slide racks can be pressure-cooked at the same time and, therefore, it is less time-consuming than microwaving. Pressure-cooking also can result in superior demonstration of certain antigens. Pressure-cooking can, however, lead to poor morphology and inaccurate staining in suboptimally fixed specimens, particularly in very small biopsies in which fixation times are reduced. Microwaving is recommended in these situations.
8. If the Dako ChemMate kit is to be used, prepare ChemMate DAB solution by adding 20 µL of DAB concentrate (reagent C) per 1 mL of substrate (reagent D), allowing 200 µL of DAB solution per slide. Alternatively, use DAB working solution as described in the immunocytochemistry materials section.
9. When performing flow cytometry lysis also may be performed at room temperature, but this may be suboptimal if samples are older than 24 h. Complete lysis may take longer than 5 min, but leucocyte degradation begins to occur after 20 min.
10. For Becton Dickinson flow cytometers, initial calibration is best performed using FACSComp with CALIBrite beads, and then further calibrated using relevant reagents from the panel on cells. In particular, for CD19 PE/Cy5 reagents, an aliquot of cells should be stained with this reagent alone, and compensation optimized accordingly.
11. This number of cells will be adequate for immunophenotyping B-lymphocyte populations that represent more than 1% of leucocytes. For smaller populations, more accurate results may be obtained if 50,000 events are acquired. However, more specific antibody combinations may be required to detect minimal disease.

12. T-cell contamination: these cells are rarely a problem, and frequent contamination of a B-cell region by T-cells is usually indicative of a poor CD19 reagent. However, the expression of CD19 may be weak in follicular lymphoma/DLBCL, and in some very rare cases it may be necessary to repeat the analysis using a different B-cell gating reagent such as CD20. T-cell contamination is identifiable as a population of cells that bind both CD3 FITC and CD3 PE in equal proportions. In tissue biopsies, T-cells are often present in the B-cell gate at low level because of cell:cell adhesion of B-cells to T-cells that occurs in follicles.: these cannot be excluded by this gating strategy, but it is extremely rare that these represent more than 1% of events in the B-cell gate.
13. Apoptotic cell contamination: these are problematic because they show variable levels of nonspecific binding. Again, fluorescein isothiocyanate conjugates are most likely to bind nonspecifically. However, antibodies conjugated to other fluorochromes may also show very high levels of nonspecific binding to apoptotic cells, and there are also differences between identical antibodies conjugated by different companies. It is therefore necessary to exclude all apoptotic cells, including apoptotic B-cells, because their inclusion may lead to a false-positive result for certain antigens. Apoptotic cells frequently are present in bone marrow samples, particularly those in which normal B-cells also are present. In some tissue biopsies, virtually all of the B-cells may be apoptotic or necrotic, but this can be minimized by gentle disaggregation techniques and by analysis immediately after disaggregation. For definitive exclusion of apoptotic cells, a viability dye such as propidium iodide or preferably 7-AAD may be included, but this will limit the number of channels available to analyze antigen expression. In the panel used here, binding of CD3 FITC but not CD3 PE is indicative of contamination with apoptotic cells. In most case, they may be completely removed by adjusting the scatter region to gradually remove cells with the lowest forward scatter until there is no evidence of aberrant binding.
14. Monocyte contamination: these cells have high levels of nonspecific binding and as such may appear to have weak CD19 binding. The are readily separated from most B-LPDs by their high side scatter but often show overlapping characteristics with DLBCL cells. They also are present in bone marrow/peripheral blood samples or tissue samples with heavy blood contamination. Immunoglobulin is present on the surface of monocytes ligated to Fc receptors. Both normal and neoplastic B-cells express only one light chain or none at all, whereas monocytes will have both kappa and lambda bound to their cell surface. As such, assessment of kappa vs lambda binding will reveal a diagonal line if monocytes are present, with B-cells to the upper left, lower right, or lower left of the plot. In addition, monocytes tend to bind FITC antibodies nonspecifically to a greater extent than PE antibodies. Therefore, a population of cells with moderate side scatter, weak binding of several FITC reagents, and equivalent binding of both kappa and lambda antibodies should be excluded from analysis. This can be achieved by adjustment of gating regions allowing exclusion of monocytes without removal of any B-cells in the vast majority of cases.

References

1. Faili, A., Aoufouchi, S., Gueranger, Q., Zober, C., Leon, A., Bertocci, B.. et al. (2002) AID-dependent somatic hypermutation occurs as a DNA single-strand event in the BL2 cell line. *Nat. Immunol.* **3,** 815–821
2. Harris, R. S., Sale, J. E., Petersen-Mahrt, S. K., and Neuberger, M. S. (2002) AID is essential for immunoglobulin V gene conversion in a cultured B-cell line. *Curr. Biol.* **12,** 435–438.
3. Dunn-Walters, D., Thiede, C., Alpen, B., and Spencer, J. (2001) Somatic hypermutation and B-cell lymphoma. *Phil. Trans. R. Soc. Lond. B. Biol. Sci.* **356,** 73–82.
4. Klein, U., Goossens, T., Fischer, M., Kanzler, H., Braeuninger, A., Rajewsky, K., et al. (1998) Somatic hypermutation in normal and transformed human B-cells. *Immunol. Rev.* **162,** 261–280.
5. Nadel, B., Marculescu, R., Le, T., Rudnicki, M., Bocskor, S., and Jager, U. (2001) Novel insights into the mechanism of t(14;18)(q32;q21) translocation in follicular lymphoma. *Leuk. Lymphoma* **42,** 1181–1194.
6. Iida, S., Rao, P. H., Butler, M., Corradini, P., Boccadoro, M., Klein, B., et al. (1997) Deregulation of MUM1/IRF4 by chromosomal translocation in multiple myeloma. *Nat. Genet.* **17,** 226–230.
7. Bishop, P. C., Rao, V. K., and Wilson, W. H. (2000)Burkitt's lymphoma: molecular pathogenesis and treatment. *Cancer Invest.* **18,** 574–83.
8. Hecht, J. L., and Aster, J. C. (2000) Molecular biology of Burkitt's lymphoma. *J. Clin. Oncol.* **18,** 3707–3721.
9. Fenton, J. A., Pratt, G., Rawstron, A. C., and Morgan, G. J. (2002) Isotype class switching and the pathogenesis of multiple myeloma. *Hematol. Oncol.* **20,** 75–85.
10. Pasqualucci, L., Migliazza, A., Fracchiolla, N., William, C., Neri, A., Baldini, L., et al. (1998) BCL-6 mutations in normal germinal center B-cells: evidence of somatic hypermutation acting outside Ig loci. *Proc. Natl. Acad. Sci. USA* **95,** 11816–11821.
11. Pasqualucci, L., Neumeister, P., Goossens, T., Nanjangud, G., Chaganti, R. S., Kuppers, R., et al. (2001) Hypermutation of multiple proto-oncogenes in B-cell diffuse large-cell lymphomas. *Nature* **412,** 341–346.
12. Kuppers, R., Hansmann, M. L., and Rajewsky, K. Clonality and germinal center B-cell derivation of Hodgkin/Reed- Sternberg cells in Hodgkin's disease. *Ann. Oncol.* **9(Suppl 5),** S17–S20.
13. Kuppers, R., Schwering, I., Brauninger, A., Rajewsky, K., AND Hansmann, M. L. (2002) Biology of Hodgkin's lymphoma. *Ann. Oncol.* **13(Suppl 1),** 11–18.
14. Dunphy, C. H., Polski, J. M., Lance, Evans H., and Gardner, L. J. (2001) Paraffin immunoreactivity of CD10, CDw75, and Bcl-6 in follicle center cell lymphoma. *Leuk. Lymphoma* **41,** 585–592.
15. Abou-Elella, A., Shafer, M. T., Wan, X. Y., Velanker, M., Weisenburger, D. D., Nathwani, B. N., et al. (2000) Lymphomas with follicular and monocytoid B-cell components. Evidence for a common clonal origin from follicle center cells. *Am. J. Clin. Pathol.* **114,** 516–522.

16. Ott, G., Katzenberger, T., Lohr, A., Kindelberger, S., Rudiger, T., Wilhelm, M., et al. (2002) Cytomorphologic, immunohistochemical, and cytogenetic profiles of follicular lymphoma: 2 types of follicular lymphoma grade 3. *Blood* **99,** 3806–3812.
17. Alizadeh, A. A., Eisen, M. B., Davis, R. E., Ma, C., Lossos, I. S., Rosenwald, A., et al. (2000) Distinct types of diffuse large B-cell lymphoma identified by gene expression profiling. *Nature* **403,** 503–511.
18. Barrans, S. L., Carter, I., Owen, R. G., Davies, F. E., Patmore, R. D., Haynes, A. P., et al. (2002) Germinal center phenotype and bcl-2 expression combined with the International Prognostic Index improves patient risk stratification in diffuse large B-cell lymphoma. *Blood* **99,** 1136–1143.
19. King, B. E., Chen, C., Locker, J., Kant, J., Okuyama, K., Falini, B., et al. (2000) Immunophenotypic and genotypic markers of follicular center cell neoplasia in diffuse large B-cell lymphomas. *Mod. Pathol.* **13,** 1219–1231.
20. Kramer, M. H., Hermans, J., Wijburg, E., Philippo, K., Geelen, E., van Krieken, J. H., et al. (1998) Clinical relevance of BCL2, BCL6, and MYC rearrangements in diffuse large B-cell lymphoma. *Blood* **92,** 3152–3162.
21. Barrans, S. L., O'Connor, S. J., Evans, P. A., Davies, F. E., Owen, R. G., Haynes, A. P., et al. (2002) Rearrangement of the BCL6 locus at 3q27 is an independent poor prognostic factor in nodal diffuse large B-cell lymphoma. *Br. J. Haematol.* **117,** 322–332.
22. Chang, C. C., Liu, Y. C., Cleveland, R. P., and Perkins, S. L. (2000) Expression of c-Myc and p53 correlates with clinical outcome in diffuse large B-cell lymphomas. *Am. J. Clin. Pathol.* **113,** 512–518.
23. Leroy, K., Haioun, C., Lepage, E., Le Metayer, N., Berger, F., Labouyrie, E., et al. (2002) p53 gene mutations are associated with poor survival in low and low- intermediate risk diffuse large B-cell lymphomas. *Ann. Oncol.* **13,** 1108–1115.
24. Braziel, R. M., Arber, D. A., Slovak, M. L., Gulley, M. L., Spier, C., Kjeldsberg, C., et al. (2001) The Burkitt-like lymphomas: a Southwest Oncology Group study delineating phenotypic, genotypic, and clinical features. *Blood* **97,** 3713–3720.
25. Nakamura, N., Nakamine, H., Tamaru, J., Nakamura, S., Yoshino, T., Ohshima, K., et al. (2002) The distinction between Burkitt lymphoma and diffuse large B-cell lymphoma with c-myc rearrangement. *Mod. Pathol.* **15,** 771–776.
26. Macpherson, N., Lesack, D., Klasa, R., Horsman, D., Connors, J. M., Barnett, M. et al. (1999) Small noncleaved, non-Burkitt's (Burkit-Like) lymphoma: cytogenetics predict outcome and reflect clinical presentation. *J. Clin. Oncol.* **17,** 1558–1567.
27. Nagai, J., Kigasawa, H., Koga, N., Katoh, A., Nishihira, H., and Nagao, T. (1998) Clinical significance of detecting p53 protein in Burkitt lymphoma and B-cell acute lymphoblastic leukemia using immunocytochemistry. *Leuk. Lymphoma* **28,** 591–597.
28. Lindstrom, M., and Wiman, K. (2002) Role of genetic and epigenetic changes in Burkitt lymphoma. *Semin. Cancer Biol.* **12,** 381.
29. Sullivan, M. P., and Ramirez, I. (1985) Curability of Burkitt's lymphoma with high-dose cyclophosphamide-high- dose methotrexate therapy and intrathecal chemoprophylaxis. *J. Clin. Oncol.* **3,** 627–636.

30. Thomas, D. A., Cortes, J., O'Brien, S., Pierce, S., Faderl, S., Albitar, M., et al. (1999) Hyper-CVAD program in Burkitt's-type adult acute lymphoblastic leukemia. *J. Clin. Oncol.* **17,** 2461–2470.
31. Attygalle, A., Al Jehani, R., Diss, T. C., Munson, P., Liu, H., Du, M. Q., et al. (2002) Neoplastic T-cells in angioimmunoblastic T-cell lymphoma express CD10. *Blood* **99,** 627–633.
32. Ye, B. H., Cattoretti, G., Shen, Q., Zhang, J., Hawe, N., de Waard, R., et al. (1997) The BCL-6 proto-oncogene controls germinal-center formation and Th2-type inflammation. *Nat. Genet.* **16,** 161–170.
33. Ree, H. J., Kadin, M. E., Kikuchi, M., Ko, Y. H., Suzumiya, J., and Go, J. H. (1999) Bcl-6 expression in reactive follicular hyperplasia, follicular lymphoma, and angioimmunoblastic T-cell lymphoma with hyperplastic germinal centers: heterogeneity of intrafollicular T-cells and their altered distribution in the pathogenesis of angioimmunoblastic T-cell lymphoma. *Hum. Pathol.* **30,** 403–411.
34. Chaganti, S. R., Rao, P. H., Chen, W., Dyomin, V., Jhanwar, S. C., Parsa, N. Z., et al. (1998) Deregulation of BCL6 in non-Hodgkin lymphoma by insertion of IGH sequences in complex translocations involving band 3q27. *Genes Chromosomes Cancer* **23,** 328–336.
35. Akasaka, T., Ueda, C., Kurata, M., Akasaka, H., Yamabe, H., Uchiyama, T., and Ohno, H. (2000) Nonimmunoglobulin (non-Ig)/BCL6 gene fusion in diffuse large B-cell lymphoma results in worse prognosis than Ig/BCL6. *Blood* **96,** 2907–2909.
36. Artiga, M. J., Saez, A. I., Romero, C., Sanchez-Beato, M., Mateo, M. S., Navas, C., et al. (2002) A short mutational hot spot in the first intron of BCL-6 is associated with increased BCL-6 expression and with longer overall survival in large B-cell lymphomas. *Am. J. Pathol.* **160,** 1371–1380.
37. Vitolo, U., Botto, B., Capello, D., Vivenza, D., Zagonel, V., Gloghini, A., et al. (2002) Point mutations of the BCL-6 gene: clinical and prognostic correlation in B-diffuse large cell lymphoma. *Leukemia* **16,** 268–275.
38. Huang, J. Z., Sanger, W. G., Greiner, T. C., Staudt, L. M., Weisenburger, D. D., Pickering, D. L., et al. (2002) The t(14;18) defines a unique subset of diffuse large B-cell lymphoma with a germinal center B-cell gene expression profile. *Blood* **99,** 2285–2290.
39. Pallesen, G. (1987) The Distribution of CD23 in normal human tissues and in malignant lymphomas, in *Leucocyte Typing III. White Cell Differentiation Antigens* (McMichael A. J., ed), Oxford University Press, Oxford, pp. 383–386.
40. Aoyagi, K., Kohfuji, K., Yano, S., Murakami, N., Miyagi, M., Takeda, J., et al. (2002) The expression of proliferating cell nuclear antigen, p53, p21, and apoptosis in primary gastric lymphoma. *Surgery* **132,** 20–26.
41. Eischen, C. M., Weber, J. D., Roussel, M. F., Sherr, C. J., and Cleveland, J. L. (1999) Disruption of the ARF-Mdm2-p53 tumor suppressor pathway in Myc-induced lymphomagenesis. *Genes Dev.* **13,** 2658–2669.
42. Adams, J. (1992) Biotin amplification of biotin horseradish peroxidase signals in histochemical stains. *J. Histochem. Cytochem.* **40,** 1457–1463.
43. Rawstron, A. C., Kennedy, B., Evans, P. A., Davies, F. E., Richards, S. J., Haynes, A. P., et al. (2001) Quantitation of minimal disease levels in chronic lymphocytic

leukemia using a sensitive flow cytometric assay improves the prediction of outcome and can be used to optimize therapy. *Blood* **98,** 29–35.

44. Rawstron, A. C., Owen, R. G., Davies, F. E., Johnson, R. J., Jones, R. A., Richards, S. J., et al. (1997) Circulating plasma cells in multiple myeloma: characterization and correlation with disease stage. *Br. J. Haematol.* **97,** 46–55.
45. Pasqualucci, L., Neumeister, P., Goossens, T., Nanjangud, G., Chaganti, R. S., Kuppers, R., et al. (2001) Hypermutation of multiple proto-oncogenes in B-cell diffuse large-cell lymphomas. *Nature* **412,** 341–346.
46. Angelin-Duclos, C., Cattoretti, G., Lin, K. I., and Calame, K. (2000) Commitment of B lymphocytes to a plasma cell fate is associated with Blimp-1 expression in vivo. *J. Immunol.* **165,** 5462–5471.
47. Shaffer, A. L., Lin, K. I., Kuo, T. C., Yu, X., Hurt, E. M., Rosenwald, A., et al. (2002) Blimp-1 orchestrates plasma cell differentiation by extinguishing the mature B-cell gene expression program. *Immunity* **17,** 51–62.
48. Tsuboi, K., Iida, S., Inagaki, H., Kato, M., Hayami, Y., Hanamura, I., et al. (2000) MUM1/IRF4 expression as a frequent event in mature lymphoid malignancies. *Leukemia* **14,** 449–456.
49. Cerutti, A., Schaffer, A., Shah, S., Zan, H., Liou, H. C., Goodwin, R. G., et al. (1998) CD30 is a CD40-inducible molecule that negatively regulates CD40-mediated immunoglobulin class switching in non-antigen-selected human B-cells. *Immunity* **9,** 247–256.
50. Cerutti, A., Schaffer, A., Goodwin, R. G., Shah, S., Zan, H., Ely, S., et al. (2000) Engagement of CD153 (CD30 ligand) by CD30+ T-cells inhibits class switch DNA recombination and antibody production in human IgD+ IgM+ B-cells. *J. Immunol.* **165,** 786–794.
51. Aizawa, S., Nakano, H., Ishida, T., Horie, R., Nagai, M., Ito, K., et al. (1997) Tumor necrosis factor receptor-associated factor (TRAF) 5 and TRAF2 are involved in CD30-mediated NFkappaB activation. *J. Biol. Chem.* **272,** 2042–2045.
52. Clodi, K., Asgary, Z., Zhao, S., Kliche, K. O., Cabanillas, F., Andreeff, M., et al. Coexpression of CD40 and CD40 ligand in B-cell lymphoma cells. *Br. J. Haematol.* **103,** 270–275.

4

Karyotyping Lymph Node Biopsies in Non-Hodgkin's Lymphoma

Fiona M. Ross and Christine J. Harrison

Summary

Culture and transport methods are described that allow chromosomes to be obtained from lymph node biopsies with a high success rate, even when the biopsy is taken at a distant site from the cytogenetic laboratory. Optimal banding techniques for the identification of these chromosomes are given, along with hints on how to correct any problems encountered on initial staining. We also describe how to prepare this material for fluorescence *in situ* hybridization techniques, both for further delineation of complex chromosomal rearrangements and for interphase analysis in cases in which conventional cytogenetics has not been successful.

Key Words: Chromosomal abnormalities; cytogenetics; FISH; cell culture; chromosome preparations.

1. Introduction

Chromosomal analysis of non-Hodgkin's lymphoma (NHL) has clearly identified that several subtypes of lymphoma are associated with specific cytogenetic rearrangements *(1)*. In most of these abnormalities, the chromosomal breakpoints are widely scattered such that molecular analysis is not guaranteed to detect the rearrangement. Cytogenetic analysis of lymph node material is extremely effective with an expected abnormality rate of approx 90%. In contrast cytogenetic analysis of bone marrow and blood is much less informative except in the relatively rare instances of very high-level involvement.

To obtain chromosome preparations from lymph nodes, the cells must be cultured and then arrested in mitosis. A hypotonic solution is used to swell the mitoses and allow the resulting chromosomes to be spread flat on a slide after the cells are fixed. It is important to be aware that NHL encompasses a number of disease types, which behave differently in culture. This means that if the

From: *Methods in Molecular Medicine, Vol. 115: Lymphoma: Methods and Protocols*
Edited by: T. Illidge and P. W. M. Johnson © Humana Press Inc., Totowa, NJ

relevant cells are to be caught in division, a variety of cultures should be set up to ensure success. Minimizing the number of cultures while maximizing the success rate requires the use of all available information. Cell synchronization can improve mitotic indices and the quality of the resultant chromosomes *(2)*, and stimulation with a B-cell mitogen can be helpful for chronic lymphocytic leukemia (CLL)-like lymphomas *(3)*. Although the whole process is essentially straightforward, a number of stages are dependent on local conditions and, therefore, no methodology can detail precisely what to do in all locations. Consult the notes section and such local experience as is available to determine useful starting points. Also, no advice is given in this chapter on the interpretation of chromosome analysis in NHL. This is not something that should be attempted by anyone without either significant cytogenetic experience or access to someone with such experience.

Fluorescence *in situ* hybridization (FISH), in the context of this chapter, is considered as an extra banding technique. Therefore, we have only given the methodology relevant to material that has already been prepared for cytogenetics. Other uses of FISH, such as on paraffin-embedded sections, are rather different and are not considered here. A wide variety of FISH probes are available both from commercial companies and from individual laboratories worldwide. Individual probes require different hybridization and stringency washes. Probes obtained from research laboratories need to be grown up and labeled by the receiving laboratory. This chapter assumes that any laboratory capable of doing this will have their own protocols for hybridization and stringency washing. Therefore, the methodology presented here is confined to general preparation of the material to be tested. We recommend following your own FISH protocols, or those that are provided with commercial probes.

Because of the organizational difficulties in ensuring fresh lymph node material is available for chromosome analysis, the number of published lymphoma karyotypes is still relatively small, particularly in some of the rarer subtypes. Many of these karyotypes are complex, with rearrangements that cannot be fully described using conventional chromosome banding techniques. Recently a 24-color chromosome painting approach has been developed, which is highly successful as a complementary tool in the accurate characterization of complex karyotypes. As a result, new nonrandom chromosomal abnormalities have been identified and cryptic changes revealed. There are two main approaches, spectral karyotyping *(4)* and multiplex FISH (M-FISH) *(5)*, which use 24-color chromosome painting kits, sophisticated microscopes, and state-of-the-art computer software. By combining such modern FISH technologies with instituting chromosomal analysis of fresh lymph nodes as part of the routine diagnosis of lymphoma, it should be possible to generate much larger numbers of fully defined lymphoma karyotypes. It is likely that this will lead to the discovery of new recurring abnormalities of clinical or prognostic significance in NHL.

2. Materials

1. Culture and transport medium: RPMI 1640 Dutch modification (Sigma, Poole, UK). To each 100-mL bottle of medium add 25 mL of fetal calf serum (Sigma), 2 mL of 2% L-glutamine, and 1 mL of 1% penicillin and streptomycin (Sigma) by filtering through a MiniSart or equivalent 0.2-μm filter. The Dutch modification contains HEPES buffer. This is essential when using the medium as a transport medium and when culturing in an incubator without gassing. If the cells are to be cultured in a CO_2 incubator, then standard RPMI 1640 with bicarbonate buffering is adequate. The complete medium should be stored at 4°C and should not be used for culture if more than 3 d old. If only small amounts are likely to be needed, the medium can be frozen until required. Transport medium (if not frozen) should be replaced at least monthly.
2. Defibrinating sticks (BDH, UK cat. no. 402020300, applicators, wood): wrap pairs in aluminium foil and autoclave.
3. Red cell lysis solution for cell counting: Zap-oglobin® II lytic reagent (Coulter Corporation, Miami, FL). Dilute 1:1 with sterile water and store at room temperature protected from light.
4. Trypan blue solution 0.4% (Sigma).
5. Culture tubes: 10-mL flat-sided tube (Nunc 156758, Invitrogen Ltd, UK).
6. Phosphate-buffered saline (PBS; Sigma): one tablet dissolved in 200 mL of water and filter sterilized.
7. Fluorodeoxyuridine (FdU; Sigma): Working solution is 10^{-5} *M*. Make up stock solution of 10^{-3} *M* (24.6 mg in 100 mL of sterile PBS). Freeze this as 1-mL aliquots. Add 1 mL of stock solution to 99 mL of sterile PBS and refreeze in 2-mL aliquots. Solution in use should be kept in the fridge and changed weekly (although the shelf life is probably at least a month).
8. Uridine (Sigma). Working solution is 4×10^{-4} *M* (9.7 mg in 100 mL of sterile PBS). Freeze in 2-mL aliquots. Solution in use should be kept at 4°C and changed weekly (although the shelf life is probably at least a month).
9. Thymidine (Sigma, UK): Working solution is 10^{-3} *M* (24.2 mg in 100 mL of sterile PBS). Freeze in 2-mL aliquots. Solution in use should be kept at 4°C and changed weekly (although the shelf life is probably at least a month).
10. Colcemid (demecolcine solution) 10 μg/mL (Sigma).
11. Potassium chloride hypotonic solution (KCl): 0.075 *M* = 5.56 g/L in sterile water. Store at room temperature. Filter sterilization is only necessary if likely to be stored for more than a few days.
12. Fixative: 3:1 Analar methanol (BDH):Analar glacial acetic acid (BDH). It is essential for first fixation that this solution is prepared immediately before use. For later fix changes and slidemaking, it should also be fresh but can be up to approx 1 h old. (The mixture gradually esterifies and this destroys its air-drying effects.)
13. Tumor-promoting agent (TPA: phorbol 12-myristate 13-acetate; Sigma, UK). Dissolve the 1 mg as supplied in 1 mL of absolute ethanol and add to 9 mL of sterile distilled water. Freeze this stock in 0.5-mL aliquots. (Shelf life no more than 2 yr.) Working solution is made by adding 0.5 mL of stock solution to 19.5

mL of sterile distilled water. This should be dispensed into small quantities (e.g., 1 mL or less depending on use) and can be stored frozen for up to 3 mo. Solution in use should be kept at 4°C for no more than 4 d. Do not refreeze. Discarded TPA should be washed down the sink with methanol then lots of water.

14. Wright's stain (Sigma): Weigh out 1.5 g of Wright's stain and add this extremely slowly to 500 mL of Analar methanol that is already stirring in a 2-L flask (*see* **Note 1**). Leave to stir for 1 h with parafilm or aluminium foil over the top of the flask. Filter through a double thickness of Whatman No. 1 filter paper into a 500-mL brown glass bottle (i.e., requires some protection from light). Cap tightly and leave for at least 2 wk before use. Always cap tightly after each opening. As the stain is used up, transfer the remainder into smaller brown bottles to prevent the staining time increasing too far due to interaction with air in the bottle.
15. Wright's buffer: Sorensen's phosphate buffer pH 6.8 (Microgen Bioproducts Ltd, UK) diluted 1 in 10 with sterile distilled water to give a 0.06 *M* solution. Preferably make up at least 1 d before use. Keep tightly capped at room temperature.
16. Hydrogen peroxide: H_2O_2 solution (approx 30%; BDH). Dilute this approx 1 in 3 with tap water. This should be performed at least a few hours and preferably 1 d before use. Shelf life is somewhat variable but not more than a few days. If it does not fizz obviously when in contact with the slide replace it.
17. Histomount (Hughes & Hughes, UK).
18. 2X standard saline citrate (SSC): Make up 20X SSC (3 *M* NaCl, 0.3 *M* sodium citrate) by dissolving 175.3 g of NaCl and 88.2 g of sodium citrate in 1 L of distilled water. We prefer to use this at pH 6.2. Adjust with concentrated hydrochloric acid. Store at room temperature. Dilute 1 in 10 with distilled water to give 2X SSC, which should also be stored at room temperature.
19. RNase/pepsin: RNase A (Sigma; cat. no. R5503), 1 mg/mL in RNase buffer, which is 10 m*M* Tris/15 m*M* NaCl, pH 7.5. Boil for 30 min to destroy DNase and store as 50-μL aliquots at –20°C. Pepsin (Sigma; cat. no. P6887) 50 mg/mL in 0.01 *M* HCl. Store as 50-μL aliquots at –20°C. To make up RNase/pepsin solution, thaw one aliquot of each and add to 450 μL 2X SSC. Mix well and use immediately. Discard any excess.
20. Rubber solution: any quick drying clear sealant that can be easily peeled off will do. We use rubber solution intended for bicycle repair kits but other products are available. Clear nail varnish should only be used to seal the final coverslip once all FISH processing has been done, and not even then if there is any possibility that more rounds of detection may be necessary, as it is not easily removed.
21. Mountant for FISH slides: Vectashield containing DAPI (Vector Laboratories, UK).

3. Methods

3.1. Preparing the Tissue

Please note, tissue preparation is usually done at a distant site.

1. Cut out a section of the lymph node biopsy (as much as can be spared).

2. Trim off excess fat or connective tissue.
3. Place in sterile culture medium (usually provided by cytogenetics laboratory; **Subheading 2., step 1**) in a universal bottle or similar container as soon as possible after biopsy.
4. Transport to the appropriate laboratory as fast as is practicable (first class post in the UK in usually adequate; *see* **Note 2**).

3.2. Setting Up Cultures

1. Macerate the cut node between two sterile defibrinating sticks in a universal to make a cell suspension (*see* **Note 3**).
2. Remove any remaining pieces of tissue to a separate container and spin the cell suspension for 5 min at 200*g* in a bench centrifuge.
3. Replace the supernatant with fresh medium either at room temperature or 37°C but not still cold from the fridge.
4. Perform a total cell count and viability check. If you have access to an automated cell counter use this for the total cell count. Otherwise mix 50 µL of cell suspension with 50 µL of red cell lysis reagent such as Zap-oglobin and count the cells in a hemocytometer. Count the cells in the central square and multiply by 2 to allow for the dilution factor and by 10^4 to calculate the numbers of cells/milliliter in the original suspension. For the viable count mix with Trypan blue instead of Zap-oglobin. Dead cells will take up this vital dye and appear blue. Calculate the percentage viability, taking care to exclude any red cells (which can be identified by their small size) from the count.
5. Set up cultures at 10^6 viable cells/mL in 5 mL of culture medium, in flat-sided test tubes. *See* **Table 1** for optimal cultures to set up (*see* **Note 4**).
6. For TPA cultures, add 0.1mL TPA and wrap tube in aluminium foil to protect from light.
7. Incubate all cultures at 37°C.
8. For F1 cultures block the cells by adding 0.05 mL FdU and 0.05 mL of uridine sometime between 2 and 4 PM on day 1 or immediately if the cultures are set up later than this (*see* **Notes 4** and **5**).
9. For F2 cultures, carry out **step 8** between 2 and 4 PM the day after setting up the cultures.
10. For F1 and F2 cultures, release the block by adding 0.05 mL of thymidine between 9 and 11 AM the day after the cells were blocked.
11. For F1 and F2 cultures, start the harvest procedure at 5 h, 45 min after releasing the block.
12. For delayed direct cultures start the harvest procedure any time after the cells have warmed up to 37°C after having been set up (*see* **Note 6**).
13. For overnight cultures the harvest procedure can be done at any time the day after setting up.
14. For TPA-stimulated cultures, the harvest should be started as near to 72 h after the culture was set up as is practically possible.

Table 1
Optimum Culture Regimes for Different Types of Lymphoma

Known high grade or large cells and/or <80% viable	Low grade or small cells with >80% viability	Known/probable, CLL/SLVL or MCL
Deldir, ON, F1, (F2)	ON, F1, (F2)	ON, F1, (F2), TPA3

Deldir, delayed direct culture, harvested later the day it is set up; ON, overnight culture, harvested the day after it is set up; F1 or F2, FdU-synchronized culture harvested 1 (F1) or 2 (F2) after set-up; TPA3, TPA-stimulated culture harvested 3 d after set-up.

3.3. Harvesting

1. Add 50 µL of Colcemid to the culture, mix well and return to the incubator for 15 min.
2. Spin at 200*g* for 5 min.
3. Remove the supernatant (*see* **Note 7**) and gently resuspend the pellet (**Note 8**).
4. Add 5 mL of 0.075 *M* KCl prewarmed to 37°C.
5. Return to the incubator for an appropriate time. This is laboratory dependent. It will be of the order of 5–30 min (*see* **Note 9**).
6. Spin at 200*g* for 5 min.
7. Remove the supernatant and gently resuspend the pellet. Add freshly prepared fixative with the first 1 mL being added dropwise while gently but thoroughly mixing (*see* **Note 10**). Top up to at least 5 mL with fix and leave at –20°C for a minimum of 1 h (*see* **Note 11**).

3.4. Slide Making for Cytogenetics

1. Wash the cells in fixative four times by spinning at 200*g* for 10min and replacing the supernatant with freshly prepared fixative.
2. After the final spin, resuspend the pellet in enough fixative for the suspension to appear very slightly cloudy but not milky (*see* **Note 12**).
3. Take a fresh clean slide and drop a single drop of suspension (from either a glass or plastic narrow point pipet) on to the slide (*see* **Note 12**).
4. Examine under phase-contrast microscopy as the slide dries. Check for suitable cell density, quality of spreading of the chromosomes and phase darkness of chromosome appearance, and adjust the concentration of suspension and time to dry of the slide as necessary (**Notes 12** and **13**).
5. Make the number of slides required.
6. Age the slides in an oven at 60°C for 1 h (*see* **Note 14**).
7. Store spare suspensions at –20°C (*see* **Note 15**).

3.5. Banding Chromosomes (see *Note 16*)

1. Place slides horizontally on a rack over a sink.
2. Add enough H_2O_2 to cover the area with cells on, and leave for 1.5 min.
3. Rinse thoroughly with tap water and shake the slide to remove excess water.

4. Add 0.5 mL Wright's stain to 1.5 mL of Wright's buffer in a clean container. Mix rapidly and pour on to the slide (*see* **Note 17**).
5. Leave for 2–5 min depending on stain batch (*see* **Note 18**).
6. Rinse off gently in running tap water and dry with a hair drier.
7. Examine microscopically under a high dry lens (at least ×63).
8. Correct staining if necessary (*see* **Subheadings 3.4.1.** and **3.4.2.**).
9. Mount the slide using Histomount or similar and examine microscopically under a ×100 oil lens.

3.5.1. Correcting Understained Slides (Bloated, Pale Chromosomes With Only Landmark Bands)

1. Add 0.5 mL of Wright's stain to 1.5 mL of Wright's buffer in a clean container. Mix rapidly and pour on to the slide on a rack over the sink.
2. Leave for an amount of time estimated from the degree of underbanding and the length of the initial staining step.
3. Rinse in tap water and dry with the hair dryer
4. Re-examine with the high dry lens

3.5.2. Correcting Overstained Slides (Dark Chromosomes, Approaching Solid Staining)

1. Soak the slide for 2 min each in 70% ethanol, 95% ethanol containing 1% HCl and 100% ethanol ***OR***
2. Rinse the slide in 3:1 methanol:acetic acid fixative then soak in fresh fix for 5 min ***OR***
3. Rinse the slide in methanol, then water, then methanol again.
4. Leave to dry.
5. Add H_2O_2 to cover the area with cells on and leave for 1.5 min.
6. Wash off thoroughly with tap water and shake the slide to remove excess water.
7. Add 0.5 mL of Wright's stain to 1.5 mL of Wright's buffer in a clean container. Mix rapidly and pour on to the slide
8. Leave for an appropriate time less than the original staining time, estimated from the extent of overstaining and the length of time in the original stain.
9. Rinse off gently in running tap water and dry with a hair drier.

3.6. Making Slides for FISH

3.6.1. Making Slides for FISH From Fixed Cell Suspension of a Single Patient

1. Remove stored fixed cell suspension from the freezer.
2. If necessary, transfer to a centrifuge tube suitable for assessing the turbidity of the suspension.
3. Spin at 200*g* for 10 min.
4. Remove the supernatant and resuspend the pellet in a suitable quantity of fresh fix.

5. Drop a single drop of the suspension on to a slide and allow to air dry such that the appearance under phase contrast is as grey as possible (*see* **Note 13**).
6. When dry, run five or six further drops of fix down the slide and allow the slide to dry in a near vertical position.
7. Use within 8 h or store at –20°C in a sealed container containing desiccant until required (*see* **Note 19**).

3.6.2. Making a Slide From Two Patients for a Single Probe

1. Perform **steps 1–4** of **Subheading 3.5.1.** for both cell suspensions.
2. Drop a single drop of suspension 1 near the hatched end of the slide.
3. Air dry such as to give a pale grey appearance under phase contrast microscopy
4. Breathe gently on the slide to visualize the position of spot 1 and drop a spot of the second suspension at a suitable distance to allow only a small space between the two spots when both are spread.
5. Air dry as in **step 3.**
6. Examine under phase contrast microscopy to confirm a small but definite gap between the spots. If there is any suggestion of overlap discard the slide and start again.
7. Mark the back of the slide to be able to position a 22 × 22 coverslip evenly over part of both drops (*see* **Note 20**).

3.6.3. Making Slides for Simultaneous FISH Analysis of Multiple Patients (see **Note 21**)

1. Make a template for nine spots within a 22 × 22-mm square (*see* **Fig. 1**).
2. Store fresh slides in fixative in a Coplin jar at –20°C.
3. Remove fixed cell suspensions from the freezer but retain them in Eppendorf or similar tubes.
4. Mix well and count each suspension in an automated cell analyser (*see* **Note 22** if no automated analyzer available).
5. Adjust each suspension to approx 2500 cells/µL. These cells can be used immediately or stored for prolonged periods at –20°C.
6. Remove slides from cold fix and air dry.
7. Place slides on slide template and carefully mark the corners of the 22 × 22 mm square with an indelible marker pen keeping the marks small (*see* **Note 20**).
8. Turn the slides so that the marked side is underneath.
9. Use a Gilson pipet to take 0.2 µL of well-mixed cell suspension and place it carefully on the first spot of the template, taking care to press the pipet plunger only to the first stop.
10. Allow to air dry.
11. Repeat with the other suspensions for each of the spots.
12. Run five or six drops of fresh fix down the slide and allow to dry vertically.
13. Use within 8 h or store at –20°C in a sealed container that contains desiccant until required.

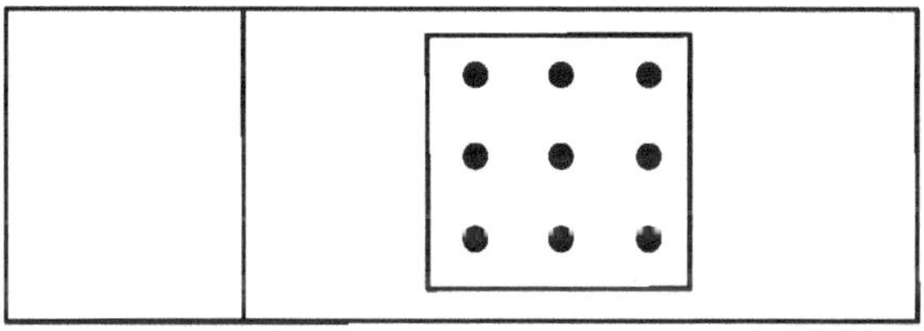

Fig. 1. Template for 9 spot FISH.

3.7. FISH Processing

1. Remove required probes from freezer and thaw at 37°C.
2. Set hotplate to correct temperature according to probe manufacturer's instructions and turn on.
3. Place 100 µL RNAse/pepsin solution on a 24 × 50-mm coverslip.
4. Invert slide to be FISHed, touch to coverslip, and carefully return to correct orientation.
5. Incubate for 2 min at room temperature.
6. Remove coverslip and place slide vertically in Coplin jar or equivalent containing 2X SSC for 2 min at room temperature.
7. Pour off 2X SSC and replace with 70% alcohol for 2 min at room temperature.
8. Pour off 70% alcohol and replace with 90% alcohol for 2 min at room temperature.
9. Pour off 90% alcohol and replace with 100% alcohol for 2 min at room temperature.
10. Air dry slides.
11. Vortex thawed probes or components of probe mixture and spin briefly in a Microfuge.
12. If necessary, make up probe mixture according to manufacturer's instructions.
13. Place probe mixture on a 22 × 22-mm coverslip taking care not to introduce air bubbles.
14. Invert slide to be FISHed over coverslip and touch to probe mixture taking care that the coverslip covers the appropriate cell area (*see* **Note 20**).
14. Carefully turn the slide right side up, adjust the coverslip position if necessary and use fine forceps to press the coverslip to remove air bubbles if necessary.
16. Seal the coverslip with rubber solution or equivalent and allow to dry completely
17. Place the slide on the hotplate for the time indicated by probe manufacturer or known local conditions.
18. Remove slide from hotplate and place in container where it can be held exactly horizontally at 37°C in a damp atmosphere for 1 to 60 h, depending on probe and convenience (*see* **Note 23**).
19. At the end of this time peel off the rubber solution and gently remove the coverslip taking care not to scrape the cell layer.
20. Stringency wash according to manufacturer's instructions or local protocol.
21. Detect if necessary according to manufacturer's instructions or local protocol, using 24 × 50-mm coverslips to cover the solutions on the slide.

22. Allow slide to dry (*see* **Note 24**).
23. Place one drop of mountant on a 22 × 50 coverslip and invert the slide onto it .
24. Return to correct orientation and carefully expel excess mountant by placing a double thickness of tissue over the slide and pressing firmly over the whole area of the coverslip.
25. Seal with rubber solution or nail varnish.
26. Examine under a fluorescence microscope with appropriate filters.

3.8. M-FISH

1. Make slides from fixed cell suspensions of a single patient as described in **Subheading 3.5.2.**
2. Before hybridization, examine the slide(s) for the presence of suitable metaphases; they need to be of good quality, and the chromosomes must be as separated as possible, with minimum touching and overlaps.
3. Localize an area with selected metaphases to which the probe can be applied under a 22 × 22-m coverslip.
4. Apply 24-color probe mixture to this area of the slide. Hybridize and detect adhering strictly to the manufacturer's recommendations (*see* **Note 25**).
5. Capture and analyze metaphases using an automated microscope, sensitive cooled coupled device camera and sophisticated specialized software

4. Notes

1. The original recipe for Wright's staining for G-banding chromosomes *(6)* was for 1.25 g of stain in 500 mL of methanol. However, a change in the late 1980s in the method that Sigma use to manufacture Wright's stain has meant that more stain has to be used to produce banding times in the 2- to 5-min range.
2. Rapid transport of the lymph node specimen to the cytogenetics laboratory is important, particularly for high-grade disease. However, most specimens will survive at least overnight and often longer so that in the UK first class post is adequate if the biopsy is taken at a distant hospital. Almost 90% of nodes should give an abnormal result according to our own results, where almost all samples are sent from distant hospitals. To achieve this success rate, it is essential to use an enriched medium for transport. The medium used for culture is recommended and this should be provided to referring laboratories monthly. It is preferable to transport lymph node samples as solid lumps of tissue. However, success rates are not markedly different when the cells are disaggregated into suspensions before being sent, although this may result in a slight reduction in mitotic index. If suspensions are to be sent they should contain adequate cells for at least two cultures (i.e., 10^7 viable cells) if possible. True-cut biopsies can also be used, but these rarely give enough cells for more than one culture. This means that, unless the precise diagnosis is known, the chance of choosing the optimal culture time and therefore obtaining analyzable mitoses, is reduced.
3. Scalpels should only be used to make a cut through the capsule if a whole node is received. They should never be used to make the cell suspension because the

sharp blade will damage too many cells. These damaged cells spill their DNA into the culture, which can agglutinate viable cells. The ease of obtaining a cell suspension can provide useful hints as to the diagnosis. Most NHL lymph nodes require minimal disruption to produce a smooth cell suspension once the capsule has been cut, but lymph nodes from reactive cases are much harder to disaggregate. Many Hodgkin's disease nodes are extremely rubbery, and most carcinomas produce an uneven suspension with lots of clumps of cells and tiny pieces of tissue remaining. These distinctions can be used as a guide but should never be taken as a guarantee of diagnosis. It is likely that a high proportion of lymph node biopsies considered suitable for lymphoma cytogenetic analysis will not have a diagnosis of NHL. Close liaison with the pathologists can reduce the amount of unnecessary culture, but there will always be a significant proportion of nodes in which all cultures have been harvested before the correct diagnosis is available. In the research setting, fixed cell suspensions can be stored and slides made only when the diagnosis of lymphoma has been confirmed or when cytogenetics is requested to help clarify the diagnosis. In a diagnostic setting, it is advisable to make slides as quickly as possible. However, because the expected abnormality rate in lymphoma is so high, a cursory examination of metaphases can identify those cases that only appear to have a normal karyotype. Full analysis can then be deferred. In most such instances, the pathology report makes it clear than the cytogenetic result is no longer necessary. An experienced cytogeneticist is also likely to be able to recognize on a cursory examination at least some instances where abnormalities are suggestive of a cancer other than lymphoma. The size and shape of the interphase nuclei can also be very suggestive. Large amounts of time should not be spent attempting full analyses on extremely complex karyotypes without obvious lymphoma-associated changes unless the pathologist has confirmed the diagnosis.

4. The choice of cultures depends on the likely diagnosis, the number of cells, and the amount of time available to maximize the results. A laboratory-dependent effect may also be evident, for example, the optimal time for synchronization may differ. Presently, we rarely find a 2-d synchronized culture to be superior to a 1-d culture, but in a previous laboratory the 2-d culture was frequently the best. If the subtype of lymphoma is known, then the choice of culture is easy but usually there is no information available at the time of establishing the cultures. As a general guide, cases with larger cells or low viability are more likely to be high grade, and therefore require shorter term culture, including a direct harvest on the day that the specimen is set up. This very short-term culture can usually be omitted on cases with smaller cells and a high viability. If the diagnosis is small cell lymphocytic lymphoma/CLL, then a culture stimulated with a B-cell mitogen, such as TPA, may be helpful. There is no reliable means of selecting these on appearance alone, but the age of the patient can be used as an indicator if immunophenotyping results are not readily available. CLL is rare in patients younger than the age of 50.
5. Optimal blocking times for FdU-synchronized cultures are between 17 and 22 h. We use a 6-h release time (with Colcemid added for the last 15 min). This seems

to give the best overall results, although it is likely that some types of NHL, with particularly slow or fast turnover rates, might be better with different times.

6. The timing of harvest of a delayed direct or overnight culture can be flexible. In general it is preferable to incubate for at least 1 h if possible. If only an overnight and a 1-day synchronized culture are set up on any sample, it is not advisable to harvest them together in case of subjecting both to the same mistake.
7. The speed of centrifugation recommended here results in a relatively loose cell pellet and therefore pouring off the supernatant is not advisable. A vacuum pump fitted with a glass pipet is practical. There is no need to change pipets between samples provided the supernatants are always sucked off from the top down and aspiration stops at least 3 mm above the pellet.
8. Suspensions must be thoroughly resuspended at each stage of the harvest procedure. Whirlimixing is too rough for lymph node cultures. We therefore simply tap the tube to resuspend the pellet. At the hypotonic stage final mixing can be ensured by inverting the tube several times after adding the KCl. However, for the first fixation step, it is essential that the pellet is completely resuspended before any fix is added.
9. The time of incubation of cells in hypotonic is laboratory dependent. In general lymph node cell suspensions seem to require slightly longer (usually approx 5 min) than would be used in the same laboratory for bone marrows.
10. The first fixation step is crucial to the eventual quality of chromosomes on the slide. Fixative should be made up immediately before use, and the cells must be thoroughly resuspended before the fix is added. It is essential that the first few drops are added slowly while gently tapping the tube to make sure that they mix thoroughly. If unable to tap the tube while adding the fix, add no more than three drops at a time before stopping to agitate the tube, until at least 0.5 mL of fix has been added.
11. If an urgent analysis is required it may be possible to omit the incubation at –20°C in first fix. However, this is likely to result in chromosomes of suboptimal quality and so only a minimal number of slides should be made. The suspension should be returned to the freezer after initial slide making and more slides made later if necessary. A minimum of 1 h in the first fixative in the freezer is recommended before routine slide making but this can be extended to several days or even weeks if more convenient. Longer periods in first fix are not recommended.
12. Judging the relationship between turbidity of the suspension and actual cell density on the slide comes with experience. A trial slide should always be made to assess both cell density and extent of chromosome spreading. For metaphase analysis in NHL, where the mitotic index is sometimes very low, a balance has to be struck between increasing the cell density to produce moderate numbers of mitoses on a single slide, and allowing those mitoses sufficient room to spread effectively. Trial slide(s) should be carefully scanned under phase contrast microscopy to find and assess the mitoses that are present, and modify the slide making technique if necessary. Time spent at this stage in ensuring good quality metaphases can reduce time spent searching for analyzable cells after G

banding. Chromosomes should be well spread and appear quite dark grey. Pale grey chromosomes result in "fuzzy" banding. Excessively black or gold chromosomes are smaller as they have not flattened out properly on the slide, and will produce only landmark bands. The major contributor to this appearance is the time taken for the fix to dry. This is related to the temperature, humidity and the quantity of fix on the slide. Temperatures in the range of 20–25°C and a humidity of 40–50% are usually best. If this cannot be controlled, the precise slide making technique will vary from day to day. The humidity in the immediate vicinity of the slide can be altered by gently breathing on the slide either before or after adding the drop of fix, by placing the slide on a pile of damp paper towels, by having a boiling kettle in the vicinity or by using something to absorb moisture if the humidity is too high. A slight increase in temperature can easily be achieved by drying the slide on the back of your hand or on your knee. Some laboratories favor freezing the slides, either dry or in fix. Spreading can be altered by changing the distance above the slide from which the cells are dropped or by adding an extra drop of fix. This can be done either before adding the cell suspension, or afterwards when the first drop has spread to its maximum. There are almost as many methods of making cytogenetic slides as there are cytogenetics laboratories.

13. For metaphase FISH, slides should be made to the same standard as for cytogenetics. However, for interphase FISH, it is important to ensure that the nuclei are as flat on the slide as possible. This means that they should have a pale grey appearance with as small a halo round each nucleus as possible. It also is preferable to have a slightly higher cell density to reduce the area of the slide that needs to be scanned when scoring the high numbers of cells needed in this type of analysis. A cell density that is too high will result in too many touching cells, in which case it can be difficult to interpret how many signals are in each cell.
14. Although artificial aging of slides is generally employed before banding, slides can be stored for weeks and continue to be suitable. As the slides age they tend to need slightly less time in Wright's stain. If analysis will not be carried out for many weeks or months it is advisable to band all slides shortly after they are made and store them in this state.
15. Cell suspensions can be stored in the freezer for years and still be suitable for FISH analysis. It is advisable to transfer them to small screw-cap Eppendorf tubes. They must be very tightly capped if the fix is not to evaporate and render the suspensions useless. It is beneficial to spin the cells down and replace the supernatant with freshly made up fix immediately prior to slide making.
16. Wright's banding is preferred to trypsin banding for lymph nodes because it is possible to adjust sub-optimal staining. This is crucial when there may be very few metaphases on the slide. The final G-banded appearance of Wright's banded chromosomes is similar to that of trypsin banded cells, except for the heterochromatin block on chromosome 9 which tends to be mid-grey on Wright's and white on trypsin. In general there is also less swelling of chromosomes with Wright's which is helpful if the spreading is poor. Note that underbanded Wright's stain is more equivalent to over-trypsinization and vice versa.

17. Batch banding with Wright's stain is possible, although it is limited by the time required for optimal staining. This is because banding is only successful with the slides in a horizontal position. Pairs of slides can be treated with peroxide at the same time, with the peroxide being added at 10-s intervals between each pair. Stain should be added with 30-s intervals between each pair to allow time for fresh stain to be made up for each pair of slides. Thus if the staining time is 3 min, 12 slides (6 pairs) can be banded in succession starting at point 0, then 30 s, 1 min, 1 min 30 s, 2 min, and 2 min 30 s before the first pair requires the stain to be rinsed off at 3 min. When banding pairs of slides together make up double the quantity of stain and divide it equally between the two slides.
18. One way to change the timing is to alter the buffer concentration as more dilute buffer results in shorter banding times. However, on the whole we think that crisper banding is achieved with the standard 0.06 *M* buffer and a stronger concentration of stain. Note that the time to produce optimal banding is also crucially dependent on the quantity of stain placed on the slide and the amount of time the water is in contact with the cells. It is therefore very important to ensure consistency of division of stain between two slides (*see* **Note 17**), even movement of the slide under the running tap water with a consistent flow rate, and placing of all slides in the fullest air flow from the hair dryer at least for the initial drying time.
19. If attempting metaphase FISH on suspensions with a low mitotic index, it is usually helpful to find the metaphases by examination of the slide under phase contrast microscopy before carrying out the FISH procedure. This is much simpler than trying to find DAPI-stained metaphases under a low magnification lens.
20. Various methods can be used to show where the coverslip and probe should be placed to ensure it covers the cells on the slide. The simplest is to breathe gently on the slide immediately before inverting it over the coverslip. This results in a thin layer of moisture on the surface of the slide, which evaporates rapidly but clearly indicates the area occupied by the cells. A more accurate alternative is to mark the area of the cells on the wrong side of the slide with a diamond pencil. However, this can weaken the slide and make it more prone to breakage. For the multi-spot method of **Subheading 3.5.3.**, it is essential to know exactly where to place the coverslip. This requires marking with an indelible marker, although the conditions used for FISH will probably cause the ink to run. Marks should therefore be kept to a minimum and should be on the underside of the slide to prevent ink running into the cells. For similar reasons, all slides for FISH should be labeled in pencil.
21. Using spots of many patients on a single slide reduces the problems of synchronizing timings and of possible excessive changes in temperature on the hotplate or in the stringency washes if large numbers of slides are used simultaneously. It also greatly reduces the cost of using commercial probes. It is only feasible if you have many patients requiring the same FISH test. The method described here is only suitable for interphase FISH. Metaphase FISH can be used successfully with more than one spot on a slide if the mitotic rate is high enough, but it is unlikely that more than three spots requiring metaphase FISH can be successfully placed under a 22 × 22-mm coverslip.

22. Even if no automated cell counter is available it is possible to count the cell number within fixed cell suspensions. The rapid evaporation of fixative makes counting in a hemocytometer problematical. Counts for these purposes do not have to be exact and therefore it is sufficient to estimate the number of cells in a 0.2-μL spot dried onto a slide and adjust accordingly.
23. Most hybridizations are performed overnight, although some large probes require less time. It is rarely detrimental if the time is increased, for example it may be more convenient to leave a hybridization over the weekend.
24. If indirect labeling is being used it is advisable to mount the slides before they have dried following the detection procedure. This allows the option of removing the mountant and adding an extra round of detection after initial examination if the probe signals are too weak.
25. There are a number of commercially available 24-color probe kits available. The delicate balance of probe concentrations and the complex combinatorial labeling with five different fluorochromes makes reproduction of these probes extremely difficult and labour intensive. Therefore, apart from specialist research laboratories, it is sensible to use the commercial kits, which, although expensive, are reliable and reproducible. The choice of probe is influenced by personal preference for both probe and image analysis system and advice is freely available from all companies. Notably the analytical approach is quite different between spectral karyotyping and M-FISH, which can be studied from the original references *(4,5)*. Experience is required in the interpretation of M-FISH results. Due to the complexity of the fluorochrome combinations the analyst must be aware that touching and overlapping chromosomes produce a false result from the interaction of the fluorochrome sets from the individual chromosomes involved. Several metaphases should be analyzed to confirm consistent chromosomal abnormalities. A complementary approach with G-banded analysis will improve the accuracy of analysis. Results from some small chromosomal rearrangements may need to be confirmed by the application of whole chromosome paints.

References

1. Heim, S. and Mitelman, F. (1995) *Cancer Cytogenetics.* Wiley Liss, New York.
2. Webber, L. M. and Garson, O. M. (1983) Fluorodeoxyuridine synchronization of bone marrow cultures. *Cancer Genet. Cytogenet.* **8,** 123–132.
3. Gahrton, G., Robert, K.-H., Friberg, K., Zech, L., and Bird, A. (1980) Nonrandom chromosomal aberrations in chronic lymphocytic leukemia revealed by polyclonal B-cell mitogen stimulation. *Blood* **56,** 640–647.
4. Schrock, E., du Manoir, S., Veldman, T., Schoell, B., Weinberg, J., Ferguson-Smith, M. A., et al. (1996) Multicolor spectral karyotyping of human chromosomes. *Science* **273,** 494–497.
5. Speicher, M. R., Gwyn Ballard, S., and Ward, D. C. (1996) Karyotyping human chromosomes by combinatorial multi-fluor FISH. *Nat. Genet.* **12,** 368–375.
6. Sanchez, O., Escobar, J. J., and Yunis, J. J. (1973) A simple G banding technique. *Lancet* **ii,** 279.

5

Identification of Lymphoma-Associated Antigens Using SEREX

Amanda P. Liggins, Barbara A. Guinn, and Alison H. Banham

Summary

Serological analysis of recombinant complementary deoxyribonucleic acid (cDNA) expression libraries (SEREX) is a powerful approach to identify immunogenic cancer-associated proteins using antibodies that are naturally present in the serum of cancer patients. This technique involves the screening of a relevant cDNA expression library with patient serum that has been cleaned to remove any antibodies that may recognize bacterial and/or viral proteins. Once antigens have been identified and their reactivity has been confirmed with a second round of screening, the gene encoding the protein can be sequenced and identified. Antigens can then be screened with a panel of allogenic sera from other patients and control individuals. This identifies disease-specific antigens, which may be useful diagnostic markers or, alternatively, targets for immunotherapy. This chapter describes the SEREX methodology in full.

Key Words: Serological analysis of recombinant cDNA expression libraries (SEREX), lymphoma; antigen; antibody; immune response; immunotherapy; expression cloning; serology; autologous serum; immunoscreening; cancer antigen.

1. Introduction

One approach to identify lymphoma-associated antigens is to exploit the circulating antibodies present in the serum of lymphoma patients. The presence of circulating antibodies against diagnostic lymphoma-associated proteins, such as the NPM-ALK protein in anaplastic large cell lymphoma patients, and the BCL-2 protein in follicular lymphoma patients, has been demonstrated previously *(1,2)*.

The SEREX technique (serological analysis of recombinant complementary deoxyribonucleic acid [cDNA] expression libraries) was first used to identify antigens in human melanoma, renal cancer, astrocytoma and Hodgkin's disease *(3)* and the technique subsequently has been modified to identify a wide range of tumor-associated antigens *(4–6)* reviewed by *(7)*. These antigens have

From: *Methods in Molecular Medicine, Vol. 115: Lymphoma: Methods and Protocols*
Edited by: T. Illidge and P. W. M. Johnson © Humana Press Inc., Totowa, NJ

included those previously identified by cloning cytotoxic T-lymphocyte (CTL)-recognized epitopes, such as MAGE-1 and tyrosinase ***(3,8,9)***, and novel antigens, such as NY-ESO-1 and SSX-2 ***(10,11)***. This technique therefore enables the detection of tumor antigens that elicit both cellular and humoral immunity ***(12)***, and as such is an excellent method for identifying potential targets for immunotherapy. As well as investigating Hodgkin's disease, the SEREX technique has been used to identify antigens in acute myeloid leukemia ***(13)***, chronic lymphocytic leukemia ***(14)***, and lymphoma-associated antigens in cutaneous T-cell lymphoma ***(15)***.

1.1. The SEREX Technique

The original SEREX technique relied on the detection of antigens expressed by a tumor-derived cDNA library screened with autologous serum (i.e., derived from the same patient as the tumor) ***(15)***. Subsequently, a number of variations of this technique have been developed and these are discussed where appropriate. There is a SEREX database (http://www.licr.org/SEREX.html) that is maintained by the "SEREX core group." This site provides information on sequences obtained using SEREX and links to other research groups using this technique. Both DNA and protein sequences can be searched through this database to investigate whether they represent a known antigen previously detected using the SEREX technique.

1.2. Obtaining Human Serum and/or Tumor Tissue

The original SEREX technique uses both tumor tissue and serum from the same patient. Therefore, the appropriate ethical permission for the project, and informed consent of the patient, must be obtained. Ideally, both tumor and serum should be obtained at the time of diagnosis as most treatments impair the patient's immune response; as such, if using serum from post-treatment patients, this should be tested for antibody reactivity before use. Additionally, because gene expression changes can occur after treatment, these patients may express a different repertoire of antigens. Although a large volume of serum is required for the primary library screening (20 mL maximum), tertiary screening requires smaller volumes (0.5–1 mL), thus, serum from residual routine blood samples is sufficient, reducing the inconvenience to patients.

1.3. cDNA Libraries

Screening a cDNA expression library with autologous serum requires the preparation of the library from mRNA extracted from tumor tissue derived from the same patient. This methodology is not within the scope of this chapter and adequate instructions are provided by the manufacturers of cDNA library synthesis kits, e.g., Stratagene (λ ZAP libraries). There are a number of variants of the original SEREX technique that do not rely on screening cDNA libraries with autologous serum, but instead use cDNA libraries derived from cancer cell lines, normal testis or germline cells ***(16–19)***. This enables cDNA expression libraries to be purchased commercially (e.g., Stratagene, Becton Dickinson), and subsequent screening can be performed with either single or pooled allogenic sera. However, these variants may not detect novel patient specific epitopes, e.g., those created by gene mutations.

1.4. Serum Cleaning

Before screening can commence, the human serum must be rigorously cleaned to remove any reactivity with either *Escherichia coli* or λ-phage proteins that might obscure a positive reaction with recombinant proteins expressed by the cDNA clones. This is an essential part of the technique that should not be bypassed and comprises the removal of antibodies from the serum that react with *E. coli* or λ-phage proteins by incubating it with columns to which the bacterial and λ-phage proteins have been coupled, and with membranes to which more of the same proteins have been transferred.

1.5. Library Screening

The λ-phage cDNA library is plated and the expression of recombinant proteins from the cDNA clones in the λ-phage is induced. The recombinant proteins are transferred onto nitrocellulose membranes, and are then screened with the cleaned human serum. The reactivity of the serum (or sera) with the primary plaques is confirmed with a round of secondary screening, which is also used to isolate individual positive phages.

1.6. Tertiary Screening/Clone Identification

To determine the biological significance of the SEREX antigens, their reactivity with serum from multiple lymphoma patients and with control individuals must be assessed. The identification of the cDNA clones encoding these antigens (by DNA sequencing) can be performed either before or after the tertiary screening. The advantages of identifying the clones first is that this significantly reduces the time spent on the tertiary screening as the number of clones can be reduced, i.e., where multiple cDNAs encoding the same gene have been identified. However, the disadvantages of this approach are that sequencing a large number of cDNA clones can be expensive (clones of no interest after tertiary screening need not be sequenced), and, if only partial sequencing is performed, then cDNAs that represent the same gene, but provide different epitopes through alternative splicing or mutation, may be inadvertently discarded.

1.7. Validation of Lymphoma Antigens

Further characterization of the expression of the SEREX antigens in normal tissues and in lymphomas is required to determine the expression pattern of the gene/protein and whether this has any diagnostic significance.

2. Materials

Unless stated, all chemicals are purchased from Merck BDH and/or Sigma Aldrich and are, where possible, of molecular biology grade. Where solutions are referred to as sterile, this should be achieved by autoclaving.

2.1. Serum Cleaning

1. *E. coli* XL1Blue MRF' bacteria.
2. *E. coli* XL1Blue MRF' cells in $MgSO_4$: Inoculate 50 mL LB (supplemented with 0.2% maltose and 10 m*M* $MgSO_4$) with a single *E. coli* XL1Blue MRF' colony from a freshly streaked LB/tetracycline plate, and grow overnight at 30°C and 250 rpm. The next morning, pellet the cells in a 50 mL Falcon tube by centrifuging 2000*g* for 10 min and resuspend in 25 mL 10 m*M* $MgSO_4$. Measure OD_{600} and dilute 10 mL cells to $OD_{600} = 0.5$ in 10 m*M* $MgSO_4$. *E. coli* cells in $MgSO_4$ can be stored at 4°C for up to 2 wk.
3. LB: 10g of NaCl, 5 g of tryptone, and 10 g of yeast extract per 1 L distilled water (dH_2O); pH 7.4); sterile.
4. LB agar (as LB with 1.5% bactoagar); sterile.
5. Tetracycline (Stock solution 10 mg/mL in 100% ethanol; store wrapped in foil at –20°C). The final concentration of tetracycline in LB/tetracycline plates should be 12.5 µg/mL.
6. Maltose (20%); sterile.
7. Magnesium sulfate (1 *M* and 10 m*M*); sterile.
8. Eluted blue phage in SM buffer/chloroform (*see* **Subheading 3.4.**)
9. CNBr-activated Sepharose 4B (Amersham Pharmacia Biotech).
10. 1 m*M* Hydrochloric acid. **Warning:** corrosive reagent.
11. Coupling buffer: 0.1 *M* $NaHCO_3$, pH 8.3, 0.5 *M* NaCl; sterile.
12. 0.1 *M* Tris-HCl, pH 8.0; sterile.
13. Wash buffer 1: 0.1 *M* NaOAc, pH 4.0, 0.5 *M* NaCl; sterile.
14. Wash buffer 2: 0.1 *M* Tris-HCl, pH 8.0, 0.5 *M* NaCl; sterile.
15. Sodium azide (10%). **Warning:** toxic reagent.
16. Tris-Buffered Saline (TBS) pH 8.0: 20 m*M* Tris-HCl, 137 m*M* NaCl.
17. TBS-Tween-20 pH 8.0: 20 m*M* Tris-HCl, 137 m*M* NaCl, 0.05% Tween-20.
18. Phosphate-Buffered Saline (PBS) pH 8.0: 137 m*M* NaCl, 3 m*M* KCl, 1.75 m*M* KH_2PO_4, 10 m*M* Na_2HPO_4.
19. NZY agar plates, 140 mm diameter. (NZY agar: 5 g of NaCl, 2 g of $MgSO_4 \cdot 7H_2O$, 5 g of yeast extract, 10 g of NZ amine, 15 g of agar per 1 L dH_2O; pH 7.5; sterile). Agar can be made in advance (400 mL in a 500 mL bottle) and stored at room temperature. It can be melted in a microwave, after loosening the bottle lid,

with frequent swirling to avoid the agar boiling over. Once the agar has cooled to between 55 and 60°C, it is poured into Petri dishes, and these agar plates should be stored, inverted and sealed (e.g., in a plastic sleeve), at 4°C for up to 3 mo.

20. NZY top agar (as NZY agar but use 7 g of agarose instead of 15 g of agar); sterile.
21. Isopropyl β-D-thiogalactiside (IPTG): 0.5 *M* in sterile dH_2O. Store in 1-mL aliquots at –20°C for 1 yr.
22. X-gal (250 g/mL in dimethylformamide [DMF]). Store in 1 mL aliquots, wrapped in foil, at –20°C for 3 mo.
23. Low-fat dried milk powder (Marvel is the only brand that seems to work).
24. Tween-20 (Polyoxyethylenesorbitan monolaurate).
25. Disinfectant suitable for viruses and bacteria (the authors use Virkon®).
26. 10- and 25-mL sterile pipets.
27. 15- and 50-mL sterile Falcon tubes.
28. Nitrocellulose membranes BioTrace™ NT membranes, (PALL Gelman Laboratory).
29. Parafilm.
30. Sintered glass filter.
31. Petri dishes (140 mm in diameter) for washing membranes.

2.2. Primary Screening

1. *E. coli* XL1Blue MRF' and growth media as in **Subheading 2.1., items 1–7**.
2. NZY agar plates as described in **Subheading 2.1., item 19**.
3. NZY top agar as described in **Subheading 2.1., item 20**.
4. SM buffer: 20 m*M* NaCl, 8 m*M* $MgSO_4$, 50 m*M* Tris-HCl, pH 7.5, 0.01% gelatin; sterile.
5. IPTG (0.5 *M* in sterile dH_2O).
6. Low-fat dried milk powder.
7. Tween-20.
8. TBS.
9. TBS-T.
10. Antibody: anti-human IgG, Fc fragment specific, conjugated to enzyme of choice (here Alkaline Phosphatase [AP]; Pierce). Follow the manufacturer's instructions for storage and reconstitution.
11. 15- and 50-mL sterile Falcon tubes.
12. 10- and 25-mL sterile pipets.
13. Nitrocellulose membranes.
14. Petri dishes (140 mm in diameter) for washing membranes.

2.3. Color Development

1. AP Color Development Buffer: 0.1 *M* Tris pH 9.5, 50 µ*M* $MgCl_2 \cdot 6H_2O$. Stable for up to 6 wk when stored at room temperature, wrapped in foil.
2. 5-Bromo-4-chloro-3-indoyl phosphate p-toluidene salt (BCIP; Bio-Rad; 30 mg/mL in 100% DMF). Light-sensitive; store wrapped in foil at 4°C; stable for up to 2 mo.

3. Nitroblue tetrazolium chloride (NBT; Bio-Rad; 60 mg/mL in 70% DMF). Light-sensitive; store wrapped in foil at 4°C; stable for up to 2 mo.
4. Petri dishes (140 mm in diameter).

2.4. Isolation of Positive Plaques

1. SM buffer.
2. Chloroform.
3. White light box.

2.5. Secondary Screening

1. As for primary screening (*see* **Subheading 2.2.**) except that Petri dishes for agar plates and washing membranes should be 90 mm in diameter.

2.6. Tertiary Screening

1. As for primary screening (*see* **Subheading 2.2.**).

In addition:

2. Eluted blue phage in SM buffer/chloroform (*see* **Subheading 3.4.**)
3. Eluted positive phage in SM buffer/chloroform (*see* **Subheading 3.5., step 8**).

3. Methods

The methods outlined below comprise (1) the cleaning of human serum, (2) the primary screening, (3) the color development reaction to identify positive plaques, (4) the isolation of the corresponding positive phages, (5) the secondary screening, and (6) the tertiary screening. A flow diagram of the entire SEREX technique is shown in **Fig. 1**.

3.1. Serum Cleaning

3.1.1. Lytic Column

1. Inoculate 50 mL LB (supplemented with 0.2% maltose and 10 m*M* $MgSO_4$) with a single *E. coli* XL1Blue MRF' colony from a freshly streaked LB/tetracycline plate, and grow overnight at 37°C and 225 rpm (*see* **Notes 1–3**).
2. Pellet the cells in a 50 mL Falcon tube by centrifuging at 2000*g* for 10 min. Resuspend the pellet in 2 mL LB containing 10 m*M* $MgSO_4$.
3. Introduce 200 µL of cells (store the remaining 1.8 mL at 4°C) into a 50 mL Falcon and add 5 mL LB, 50 µL 20% maltose, 50 µL 1 *M* $MgSO_4$ and 7.5 µL of a 12.5 µg/mL tetracycline solution.
4. Inoculate with the volume of one eluted blue phage (i.e., a blue phage that has been cored into SM buffer and allowed to elute into the buffer as described in **Subheading 3.4., steps 2–4**; spin the phage solution for 1 min at maximum speed and use the supernatant, leaving the chloroform behind).
5. Incubate the culture at 37°C and 250 rpm for 4 h.

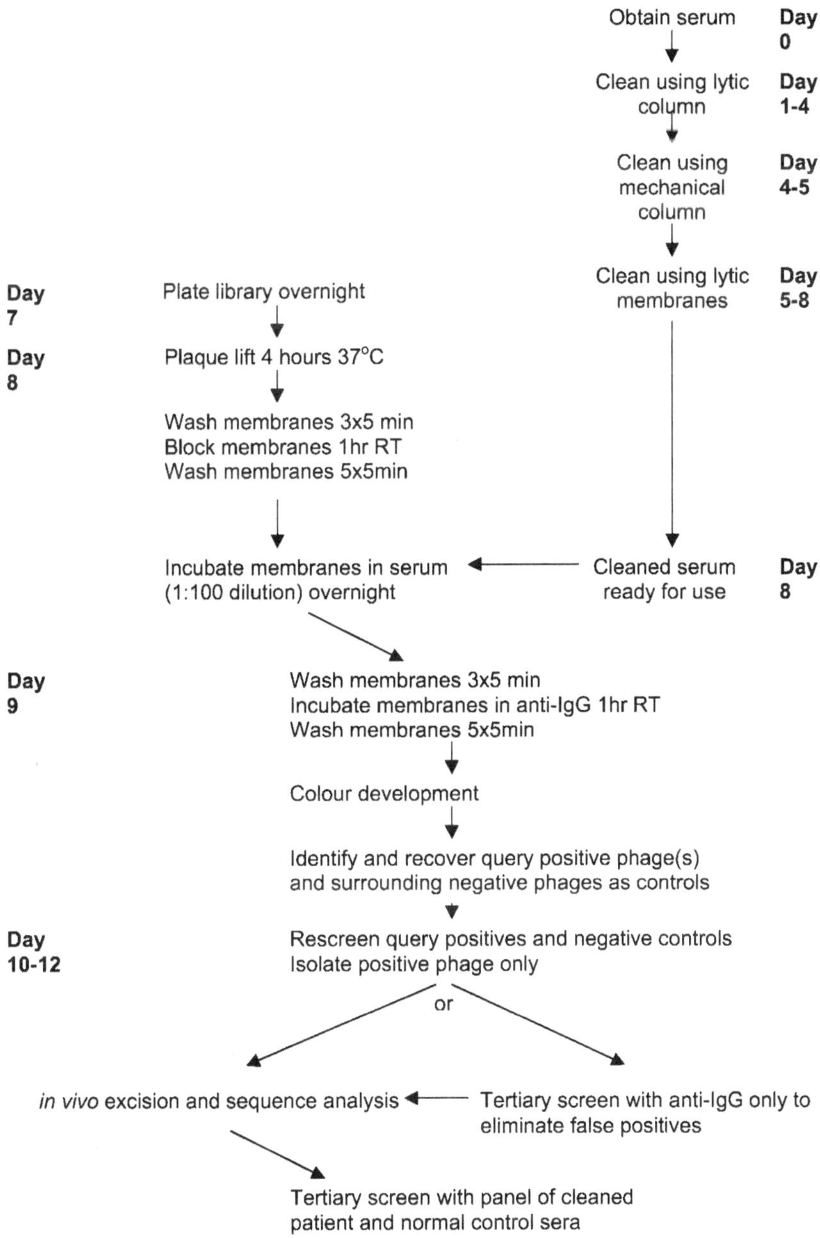

Fig. 1. Flow diagram, including an approximate time-scale, outlining the SEREX technique.

6. To the remaining 1.8 mL of culture from **step 3**, add 5 mL of LB, 50 µL of 20% maltose, 50 µL of 1 *M* $MgSO_4$, and 7.5 µL of a 12.5 µg/mL tetracycline solution. Mix this with the phage-inoculated culture from **step 5**.
7. Incubate the culture at 37°C and 250 rpm for 2 h.
8. Freeze-thaw the culture three times to lyse the bacterial cells, and then sonicate the cells, using eight 5-s pulses, to lyse the mitochondria.
9. Resuspend 1 g of CNBr-activated Sepharose in 10 mL of 1 m*M* HCl. Wash the beads with 200 mL of 1 m*M* HCl over a sintered glass filter to remove any additives (*see* **Note 4**).
10. Resuspend the beads in 7 mL (final volume) of 1 m*M* HCl (*see* **Notes 5** and **6**).
11. Add 5 mL of coupling buffer to the lysed bacteria from **step 8**. Add 4 mL (out of 7 mL final volume) washed Sepharose beads to the lysate. Seal the Falcon tube by wrapping parafilm around the lid/top of the tube, and rotate the mixture overnight at 4°C to couple the bacterial/phage proteins to the sepharose beads (*see* **Note 7**).
12. Pellet the matrix (Sepharose beads + proteins) by centrifuging at 2000*g* for 10 min and pour the supernatant into disinfectant solution. **Note:** Save the matrix.
13. Wash the matrix in 30 mL of coupling buffer by resuspending the matrix in the buffer, centrifuging at 2000*g*) for 10 min, and discarding the supernatant into disinfectant solution.
14. Block any remaining active groups by resuspending the matrix in 30 mL of 0.1 *M* Tris-HCl, pH 8.0, and leaving to stand at room temperature for 2 h (*see* **Note 8**).
15. Pellet the matrix and discard the supernatant.
16. Wash the matrix in 30 mL wash buffer 1 followed by 30 mL wash buffer 2.
17. Repeat **step 16** twice more.
18. Wash the matrix twice in 50 mL of 1X TBS/0.1% sodium azide. The matrix can be stored in 1X TBS/0.1% sodium azide at 4°C until required.
19. If using straight away, resuspend the matrix in a volume of 1X TBS/0.1% sodium azide that will yield a 1:10 dilution of serum after the serum is added (e.g., 18 mL 1X TBS/0.1% sodium azide + 2 mL serum) (*see* **Note 9**).
20. Add the serum to the resuspended matrix.
21. Seal the Falcon tube with parafilm (as in **step 11**) and rotate overnight at 4°C.
22. Pellet the matrix by centrifuging at 2000*g* for 10 min. Save the supernatant = serum. Discard the matrix. If not proceeding directly to the mechanical column method (**Subheading 3.1.2.**), store the serum at 4°C with the Falcon tube lid sealed with parafilm.

3.1.2. Mechanical Column

1. Inoculate 50 mL of LB (supplemented with 0.2% maltose and 10 m*M* $MgSO_4$) with a single *E. coli* XL1Blue MRF' colony from a freshly streaked LB/tetracycline plate, and grow overnight at 37°C and 225 rpm.
2. Pellet the cells in a 50 mL Falcon tube by centrifuging at 2000*g* for 10 min.
3. Resuspend the pellet in 5 mL PBS.
4. Freeze-thaw the culture three times, then sonicate the cells, using eight 5-s pulses.
5. Repeat **steps 9–18** from the lytic column method (**Subheading 3.1.1.**).

6. Do not resuspend the matrix in 1X TBS/0.1% sodium azide. Instead, add the serum (already at 1:10 dilution) from **Subheading 3.1.1., step 22**, directly to the matrix.
7. Seal the Falcon tube with parafilm (as in **Subheading 3.1.1., step 11**) and rotate overnight at 4°C.
8. Pellet the matrix by centrifuging at 2000*g* for 10 min. Save the supernatant = serum. Discard the matrix. If not proceeding directly to the lytic membrane method (**Subheading 3.1.3.**), store the serum at 4°C with the Falcon tube lid sealed with parafilm.

3.1.3. Lytic Membrane

1. Dry NZY agar plates (one per serum sample to be cleaned) inverted in an incubator at 37°C, or in a laminar flow-hood, and melt the top agar. Once melted, the agar should be placed in an incubator or waterbath set between 45–56°C to cool.
2. Prepare cells/phage mixture (one per plate): introduce 600 μL of *E. coli* XL1Blue MRF' cells (OD_{600} = 0.5; *see* **Subheading 2.1., item 2**), and 250 μL of eluted blue phage in SM buffer, into a 15 mL Falcon tube (spin the phage solution for 1 min at maximum speed and use the supernatant, leaving the chloroform behind). Mix the phage and the cells by inverting two to three times, then incubate at 37°C for 15 min.
3. Quickly add 10 mL of NZY top agar and 40 μL of IPTG to the phage/cells, mix gently by inversion, and pour onto the NZY agar plate. Leave to set at room temperature for 10 min and then incubate the plates, inverted, overnight at 37°C. If you wish to use blue/white color selection to distinguish recombinant from non-recombinant clones, X-gal (50 μL) should also be added to the cells/phage/IPTG mixture.
4. The next morning, perform a plaque lift. Using forceps, place a nitrocellulose membrane onto the plate, and lower it gently, eliminating any air bubbles. Incubate plate(s) and membrane(s), inverted, at 37°C for 4 h (*see* **Notes 10** and **11**).
5. Prepare the block solution, using 20 mL of solution per membrane. Boil approx 50 mL dH_2O in a 500 mL bottle to sterilize the bottle, and discard dH_2O. Boil the block solution (the appropriate volume of TBS with 5% [w/v]) low-fat dried milk powder) for 3 to 4 min to ensure sterilization. Leave to cool to room temperature; add Tween-20 to a final concentration of 0.05% just prior to use (*see* **Note 12**).
6. Remove membrane carefully, using forceps, into TBS. Gently brush off any excess agar, and place the membrane, protein-side down, into a clean Petri dish containing TBS-T. Repeat for any other membranes.
7. Place dishes on shaker and wash membranes for 5 min. Remove TBS-T and replace with fresh TBS-T. Wash for 5 min. Remove TBS-T and replace with TBS. Wash for 5 min.
8. Remove TBS and pipet 20 mL of block solution onto each membrane, ensuring full coverage. Incubate for 1 h at room temperature on the shaker.
9. Remove the block solution and wash the membranes four times for 5 min (each wash) in TBS-T, changing the Petri dish after the third wash (*see* **Note 13**). Finally, wash once with TBS for 5 min.

10. Pour the total volume of serum from **Subheading 3.1.2., step 8** onto the membrane and incubate overnight at room temperature on the shaker.
11. The next morning, remove the membrane from the serum using forceps. Allow excess serum to drip off and discard the membrane. Pipet the serum, using a 10-mL pipet, into a sterile 50-mL Falcon tube. Store at 4°C with the Falcon tube lid sealed with parafilm.
12. Repeat the lytic membrane method twice more. The serum should now be clean, and can be stored in 2-mL aliquots at 4°C for 6 mo or –80°C long term (*see* **Notes 14–17**).

3.2. Primary Screening

1. Dry the required number of NZY agar plates inverted in an incubator at 37°C, or in a laminar flow-hood, and melt the top agar. Once melted, the agar should be placed in an incubator or waterbath set to between 45–56°C to cool (*see* **Note 18**).
2. Introduce 600 µL *E. coli* XL1Blue MRF' cells (OD_{600} = 0.5), and the appropriate volume of phage in SM buffer, into a 15-mL Falcon tube (*see* **Note 19**). The standard density for library screening is 50000 pfu/140-mm plate, but the authors tend to use considerably lower densities (e.g., 10,000–20,000 pfu/140-mm plate) (*see* **Notes 20–22**). Mix the phage and the cells by inverting two to three times, then incubate, unshaken, at 37°C for 15 min.
3. Quickly add 10 mL of NZY top agar and 40 µL of IPTG to the phage/cells, mix gently by inversion, and pour onto the NZY agar plate. Leave to set at room temperature for 10 min and then incubate plates, inverted, overnight at 37°C (*see* **Note 23**).
4. Perform a plaque lift onto nitrocellulose membranes at 37°C as described in **Subheading 3.1.3., step 4**. Write the date and membrane number (or suitable annotation to identify the membrane at a later stage) on the membrane using a biro (*see* **Notes 24** and **25**).
5. Prepare the block solution, as described in **Subheading 3.1.3., step 5**.
6. Pierce the membrane and agar with a sterile needle, at three points approx 1 cm from the edge, to allow later orientation of the plaques and the membrane. Remove the membrane, using forceps, into TBS. Gently brush off any excess agar, and place the membrane, protein-side down, into clean Petri dishes containing TBS-T. Repeat for other membranes, and store the agar plates at 4°C as these are required for positive phage isolation.
7. Wash the membranes twice in TBS-T for 5 min each then once in TBS for 5 min, as described in **Subheading 3.1.3., step 7** (*see* **Notes 26** and **27**).
8. Remove the TBS and pipette 20 mL of block solution onto each membrane, ensuring full coverage. Incubate for 1 h at room temperature on the shaker (*see* **Note 28**).
9. Remove the block solution and wash the membranes four times for 5 min (each wash) in TBS-T, changing the Petri dish after the third wash. Finally, wash once with TBS for 5 min.
10. Remove the TBS and pipet 20 mL of serum onto each membrane as before. Incubate at room temperature on the shaker overnight (*see* **Note 29**).

11. The next morning, remove the membranes from the serum (*see* **Note 30**) and place into clean Petri dishes containing TBS-T. Pipet the serum into Falcon tubes and store the tubes, with the lid sealed with parafilm, at 4°C.
12. Wash the membranes as in **step 9**.
13. Remove the TBS and add 20 mL of antibody solution (Rabbit anti-human IgG, Fc fragment specific, alkaline phosphatase conjugated; 1:5000 dilution in 0.5% dried milk in TBS-T) (*see* **Note 31**). Incubate at room temperature on shaker for 1 h.
14. Remove the antibody solution and wash the membranes as in **step 9**.

3.3. Color Development

1. Introduce 20 mL of AP Color Development Reagent buffer into a clean Petri dish. Add 100 µL of BCIP and 100 µL of NBT. Mix thoroughly and cover with a light-protective box (e.g., cardboard) (*see* **Note 32**).
2. Using forceps, remove the membrane from the TBS (from **Subheading 3.2.**, **step 14**), draining excess TBS off onto tissue. Place the membrane, protein side up, into the development solution.
3. Allow the color reaction to develop for up to 30 min, keeping the reagents in the dark. Strongly-positive plaques will appear within 5 min, and background will appear within 10 min (*see* **Note 33**).
4. At the end of the reaction, place the membranes into dH_2O to stop the reaction.
5. Check the membranes when wet, and circle any positive plaques with a biro (*see* **Note 34**). Air-dry the membranes on filter paper and check again for any additional positive plaques, marking them in the same manner (*see* **Note 35**).

3.4. Isolation of Positive Plaques

1. Put the plate containing the positive plaques, upside down, next to the membrane on which the positives spots are marked. Use the needle marks to orientate the plate and membrane. Identify and mark the positive plaque(s) (*see* **Note 36**).
2. Turn the plate the right way up and place it on a light box. Using a sterile scalpel, cut out the positive plaque and its surrounding three to four negative neighbors as one piece, and place into a 1.5-mL eppendorf tube (labeled with the corresponding plaque number) containing 500 µL of SM buffer. Repeat for any other plaques.
3. Incubate the tubes on an end-over-end rotator overnight at 4°C to allow the phage to elute into the SM buffer.
4. The next morning, add 20 µL of chloroform to the eluted phage, vortex, microfuge at maximum speed for 1 min, and store at 4°C until ready to do secondary screening (*see* **Note 37**).

3.5. Secondary Screening

1. Dry the required number of NZY agar plates inverted in an incubator at 37°C, or in a laminar flow-hood, and melt the top agar. Once melted, the agar should be placed in an incubator or waterbath set to between 45–56°C to cool.

2. Dilute the phage from the primary screen (**Subheading 3.4., step 4**) 1:10 in SM buffer.
3. For each plate, introduce 200 µL *E. coli* XL1Blue MRF' cells (OD_{600} = 0.5), 96 µL of SM buffer and 4 µL of diluted phage from **step 2** into a 15-mL Falcon tube. Mix by inverting two to three times then incubate, unshaken, at 37°C for 15 min.
4. Quickly add 3 mL of NZY top agar and 18 µL of IPTG to the phage/cells. Mix gently by inversion, and pour onto the NZY agar plate. Leave to set at room temperature for 10 min and then incubate plates, inverted, overnight at 37°C.
5. Perform a plaque lift onto nitrocellulose membranes at 37°C, and prepare the block solution, as described in **Subheading 3.1.3., steps 4** and **5** respectively.
6. Perform the secondary screen as described for primary screening (**Subheading 3.2., steps 6–14**) but only 10 mL of block solution, antibody solution and serum are required for each membrane as the membranes used in this section are smaller than those used for primary screening.
7. Incubate the membranes in color development reagents as in **Subheading 3.3.**
8. Identify and isolate positive phages as in **Subheading 3.4.** except that in this second round of screening, the positive phage should be isolated alone (with no negatives), using the fine end of a sterile glass Pasteur pipet (*see* **Notes 38** and **39**). This method can also be used to isolate blue (or "empty") phage for use in serum cleaning and tertiary screening.

3.6. Tertiary Screening

Read **Notes 40–49** prior to this section.

1. Dry the required number of NZY agar plates inverted in an incubator at 37°C, or in a laminar flow-hood, and melt the top agar. Once melted, the agar should be placed in an incubator or waterbath set to between 45–56°C to cool.
2. For each plate, introduce 600 µL *E. coli* XL1Blue MRF' cells (OD_{600} = 0.5) into a 15-mL Falcon tube. Quickly add 10 mL of NZY top agar and 40 µL of IPTG, and pour onto NZY agar plates. Leave to set at room temperature for 15 min.
3. Spot 1 µL of positive phage (from **Subheading 3.5., step 8**) onto the plate, following the template suggested in **Fig. 2**, and spot 0.8 µL of blue phage as a negative control.
4. Once the phage has dried into the agar, incubate plates, inverted, overnight at 37°C.
5. Perform a 4-h plaque lift onto nitrocellulose membranes at 37°C, and prepare the block solution, as described in **Subheading 3.1.3., steps 4** and **5**, respectively.
6. Perform the tertiary screen as described for primary screening (**Subheading 3.2., steps 6–14**).
7. Incubate the membranes in color development reagents as described in **Subheading 3.3.**
8. Score the membranes, recording the reactivity of the plaques with the serum.

4. Notes

1. *E. coli* strains should be maintained on LB agar plates containing tetracycline (12.5 µg/mL; final concentration), and restreaked every 7–10 d. Plates can be stored, sealed with parafilm, at 4°C.

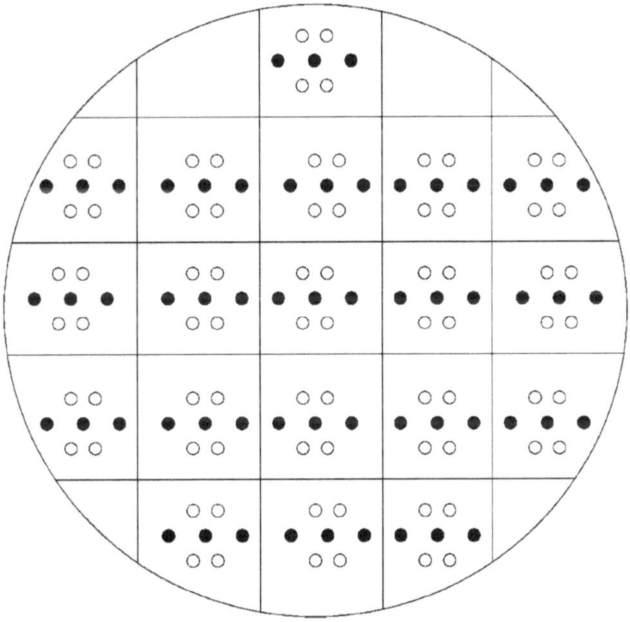

Fig. 2. Suggested template for tertiary screening. White circles represent blue phage negative control spots and black circles represent positive phage spots.

2. Bacterial cultures should always be grown in vessels of five times the volume of the culture.
3. Keep glycerol stocks of *E. coli* XL1Blue MRF' at –80°C.
4. The diameter of the Sepharose beads is 45–165 μm. Therefore, the pore size of the sintered glass filter should be less than 40 μm.
5. Remove the washed Sepharose beads from the columns using a 10 mL pipet; if the final volume of beads in 1 m*M* HCl is >7 mL, centrifuge at 200*g*) for 5 min to pellet the beads, and adjust the volume to 7 mL.
6. This protocol describes the preparation and use of one column; the authors tend to make batches of columns, which can be stored at –20°C for at least 6 mo after the freeze-thaw step, and clean multiple serum samples at one time.
7. Beads can be coupled to the lysate by rotating at room temperature for 4 h.
8. Blocking can also be achieved at 4°C for 16 h. An alternative chemical for blocking is 0.1 *M* ethanolamine.
9. For most efficient cleaning, use only 2–3 mL serum per column.
10. Label the nitrocellulose membrane with the plate name/number/ID and date, and lay it on the plate with the writing uppermost. Be careful not to touch the membranes with bare hands, as proteins from skin will stick to the nitrocellulose. Try to handle the membranes at the edges, with gloves on, preferably using flat-edged forceps, as these cause less damage to the membranes.

11. When placing the membrane on the agar plate, place it in a line down the centre of the dish and allow the membrane to wet. Slowly lower the outer edges, ensuring that no air bubbles are present, until there is complete and uniform contact between the membrane and the plate.
12. Boiling the block solution is of the utmost importance in order to destroy any micro-organism that might remain on the membrane, or in the dish, that could complicate results.
13. Changing the Petri dish after the third wash reduces any residual carry-over of reagents.
14. Serum cleaning is a vital step in the SEREX method — do not be tempted to cut corners.
15. The more times a serum is used, the less background there will be.
16. Serum cleaning takes approx 7–10 d.
17. Some serum will require more than one round of cleaning.
18. If plating the library late in the afternoon, melt the top agar mid-morning and allow to equilibrate to the recommended temperature. This temperature ranges from 45–56°C, and the authors have found no effect of different temperatures. Dry and/or warm NZY agar plates. Keep these at 37°C until ready to use (but replace the lids once the plates are dry).
19. *E. coli* cells in $MgSO_4$ (from **Subheading 2.1., item 2**) may be stored at 4°C for up to 2 wk. If this plating culture is used after this time, the bacterial lawn will be incomplete and appear grainy. The authors tend to switch to a fresh plating culture every 10–12 d.
20. Determine which plating density is best by titration—plaques that are too small to be seen are no good for future identification and isolation.
21. The number of plates to be screened in one batch may also help you to determine the optimum plating density. The authors have found that twenty large plates or twenty-four small plates is probably about the maximum that can be coped with in a screening protocol.
22. The number of clones included in the primary screening depends on the library complexity. Generally, 10^6 clones are screened from the amplified library if the number of primary clones is greater than 1 million, or the total number of primary clones is screened if this is less than one million. Libraries should be amplified to enhance stability, but only once to ensure that accurate representation of the cDNA population is not affected.
23. When plating the library, try to burst any bubbles in the top agar with a sterile pipette tip, as bubbles will leave marks on the membrane that may prevent a positive plaque being identified.
24. Some membranes can lift the top agar with them when performing a plaque lift, and removal of the agar will prevent you from being able to core a positive phage in this area. This was more common when plaque density was greater than 30% confluency. The authors use BioTrace™ NT nitrocellulose membranes (PALL Gelman Laboratory, MI) with no problems, but if problems do occur, putting the plates and membranes at 4°C for 30 min prior to performing the lift can help.

Alternatively, removing the lid for the last 10 min of the 4-h incubation, or briefly putting the plates and membranes in a laminar flow-hood, removes excess surface moisture, helping to dry off the membrane and prevent it sticking. However, care should be taken with these approaches as it is possible to over-dry the plates.

25. Following plaque lifts, plates can be stored at 4°C for 2–3 d.
26. Petri dishes used for washing membranes can be re-used, but should be washed in hot water with a small amount of detergent, and rinsed thoroughly.
27. Membranes being washed/blocked/incubated in dishes should be placed writing side up (protein side down). If anything should come into contact with the membrane, it will not damage the protein side and complicate/destroy interpretation of results. Membranes should only be placed protein side up during the colour development procedure.
28. Make fresh block solution each time it is required. Do not be tempted to store block solution at 4°C as micro-organisms can grow in it, which could lead to infection of the serum and increased nonspecific background staining of the membranes.
29. Dilutions of sera for screening vary from 1:100 to 1:1000. A lower dilution will allow detection of low titre antigens and is probably a good starting dilution.
30. When removing the serum from the petri dishes, using 10-mL pipets will ensure a greater recovery of the serum as they have smaller tips than larger pipets.
31. The optimum dilution of the secondary antibody should also be determined, although the manufacturer's advice regarding dilutions for Western blotting may be very useful.
32. 20 mL AP Colour Development Reagent buffer/100 µL each NBT and BCIP is sufficient to develop two large membranes or four small ones.
33. If positives take longer than 30 min to develop, the serum has reached the end of its life and should be discarded.
34. Positive plaques are identified as darker plaques, often donut-like in appearance, compared to their neighbors (*see* **Figs. 3–5**). Initially, it is better to select all possibles for follow-up rather than have missed one that may be groundbreaking. Experience leads to greater confidence in discerning true positives from false ones.
35. Once membranes are completely dry, store in plastic A4 clear wallets. Membranes should be kept dry to prevent any fungal growth. Some membranes are better kept in the dark as light can bleach the color and fade results.
36. To identify and isolate positive plaques, the authors tend to use the method described here. Using a pair of compasses, locate the positive phage from all needle-holes. Place the pointed compass on the first needle-hole on the membrane and extend the compasses until the pencil rests on the positive plaque. Transfer the compasses to the plate, putting the pointed compass onto the corresponding needle-hole mark. Use the pencil to draw a line through the positive plaque on the base of the plate. Repeat this process for the remaining holes; where the three lines cross is the location of the positive plaque. Circle the plaque and number it on the base of the plate. If there is more than one positive plaque, locate, mark and number the remainder in the same way.

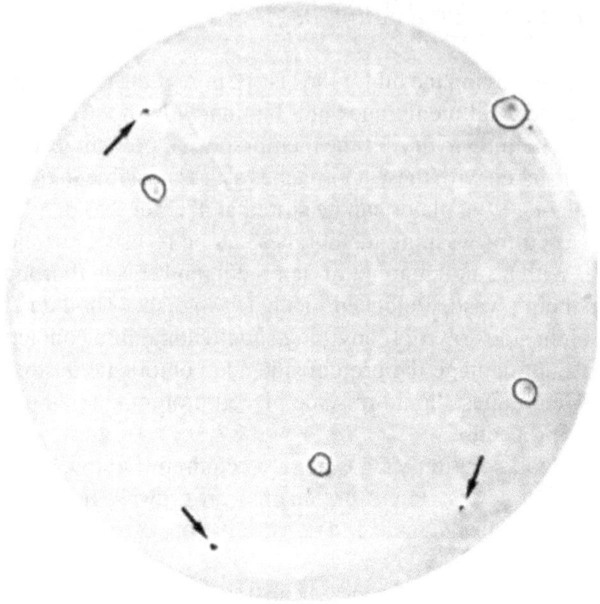

Fig. 3. Membrane following primary screening and color development. Query positive plaques, of differing size, shape and intensity, are circled. Orientation holes are indicated by arrows. *See* **Color Plate 2**, following page 270.

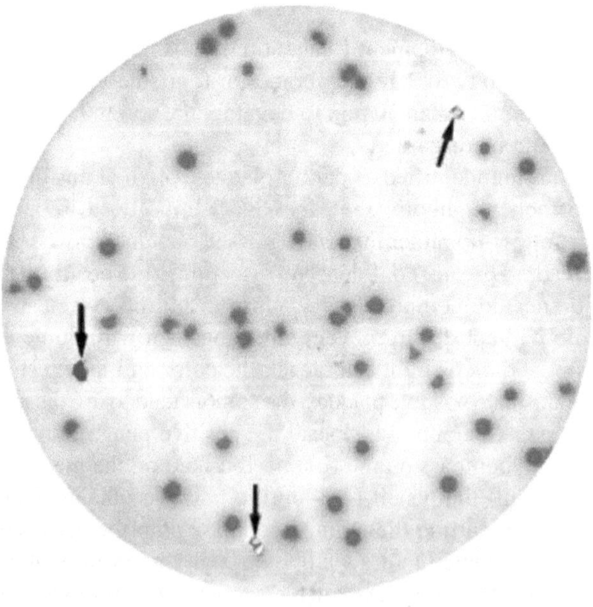

Fig. 4. Membrane following secondary screening and color development showing positive (darker circles) and negative (lighter circles) plaques. Orientation holes are indicated by arrows. *See* **Color Plate 3**, following page 270.

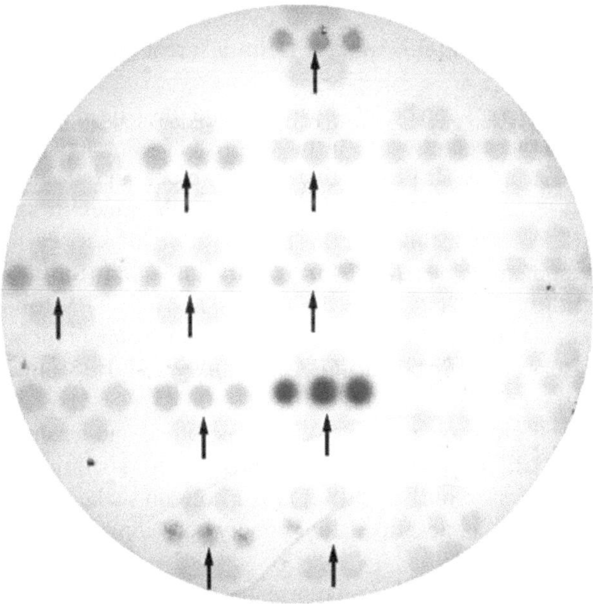

Fig. 5. Membrane following tertiary screening and color development. Examples of plaques that are positive, relative to the surrounding negative controls, are indicated by arrows. *See* **Color Plate 4**, following page 270.

37. Chloroform added to cored positive phage lyses the *E. coli* and prevents further bacterial growth. More chloroform may need to be added to the phage supernatant with time. The sample should then be vortexed and centrifuged briefly as in **Subheading 3.4., step 4**.
38. Select at least two plaques in the secondary screening to ensure that you get monoclonal positives. Choose a plaque that is isolated from neighbours to help attain monoclonality.
39. Clones are in vivo excised using standard protocols.
40. The tertiary screen of each antigen should be performed with each serum at least three times to ensure confidence of positivity.
41. Doing three separate screens can sometimes lead to conflicting results so doing duplicate lifts is an alternative, although it makes for a long day.
42. It should be remembered that antibodies are depleted from the serum with every screen so if a phage has been positive with a serum on one occasion, the chances are that this phage peptide/protein is recognised by the serum, even if the other subsequent results appear to be negative.
43. If the positive phage starts to produce small "speckly" plaques rather than a nice "circle" of plaques, more-recently cored phage (or phage that has been stored at –80°C) can often improve the situation.

44. Positive phage can be stored at –80°C (with 0.3% chloroform and 7% DMSO). The authors have found this to be a useful insurance against phage loss or contamination.
45. Some positive phages can be IgG positives, and these need to be eliminated. This can either be done as part of the primary screen, or as a separate tertiary screen.
46. Primary screen protocol: plaque lift, washes, block and washes as described in **Subheading 3.2., steps 4–9**; then incubate membranes in anti IgG antibody (1:5000 in 0.5% dried milk in TBS-T) for 1 h on shaker. Perform washes and color development as described for primary screening (**Subheading 3.2., step 14**; **Subheading 3.3.**) but place the membranes into TBS following the color development reaction. Wash the membranes and incubate them in serum overnight as described in **Subheading 3.2., steps 9** and **10**. Continue the primary screening protocol from **step 11** onwards.
47. Tertiary screen protocol: plaque lift, washes, block and washes as described in **Subheading 3.2., steps 4–9**; then incubate membranes in anti IgG antibody (1:5000 in 0.5% dried milk in TBS-T) for 1 hour on shaker. Perform washes and color development as described for primary screening (**Subheading 3.2., step 14**; **Subheading 3.3.**)
48. If this step is incorporated into the primary screen, it makes for a long day but means that the false positives can be eliminated before undertaking all the secondary screening. The IgG positives should be marked with a different-coloured pen, or in a different manner, so that they are not confused with true positives identified after incubation with serum.
49. Doing the IgG screen as a tertiary screen is a quicker protocol, but can result in some unnecessary secondary screening. Ultimately, the decision on when to incorporate this IgG screen may depend on whether the library is likely to have a high incidence of IgG cDNAs. If this is likely, an alternative approach to consider, especially when constructing a library, is the removal of IgG cDNAs by a subtraction technique prior to library construction *(5)*.

References

1. Pulford, K., Falini, B., Banham, A. H., Codrington, D., Roberton, D., Hatton, C., et al. (2000) Immune response to the ALK oncogenic tyrosine kinase in patients with anaplastic large-cell lymphoma. *Blood* **96,** 1605–1607.
2. Pulford, K., Roberton, H., Banham, A. H., Hatton, C. S. R., and Mason, D. Y. (2002) Immunochemical studies of antigenic lymphoma-associated proteins. *Br. J. Haematol.* **116,** 135–141.
3. Sahin, U., Türeci, Ö., Schmitt, H., Cochlovius, B., Johannes, T., Schmits, R., et al. (1995) Human neoplasms elicit multiple specific immune responses in the autologous host. *Proc. Natl. Acad. Sci. USA* **92,** 11810–11813.
4. Ling, M., Wen, Y.-J. and Lim, S. H. (1998) Prevalence of antibodies against proteins derived from leukemia cells in patients with chronic myeloid leukemia. *Blood* **92,** 4764–4770.

5. Scanlan, M. J., Chen, Y.-T., Williamson, B., Gure, A. O., Stockert, E., Gordan, J. D., Türeci, et al. (1998) Characterization of human colon cancer antigens recognized by autologous antibodies. *Int. J. Cancer* **76,** 652–658.
6. Itoh, M., Watanabe, M., Yamada, Y., Furukawa, K., Taniguchi, M., Hata, T., et al. (1999) HUB1 is an autoantigen frequently eliciting humoral immune response in patients with adult T-cell leukemia. *Int. J. Oncol.* **14,** 703–708.
7. Türeci, Ö., Sahin, U., Zwick, C., Neumann, F., and Pfreundschuh, M. (1999) Exploitation of the antibody repertoire of cancer patients for the identification of human tumor antigens. *Hybridoma* **18,** 23–28.
8. van der Bruggen, P., Traversari, C., Chomez, P., Lurquin, C., De Plaen, E., Van den Eynde, B., et al. (1991) A gene encoding an antigen recognized by cytolytic T lymphocytes on a human melanoma. *Science* **254,** 1643–1647.
9. Brichard, V., Van Pel, A., Wölfel, T., Wölfel, C., De Plaen, E., Lethé, B., et al. (1993) The tyrosinase gene codes for an antigen recognized by autologous cytolytic T lymphocytes on HLA-A2 melanomas. *J. Exp. Med.* **178,** 489–495.
10. Chen, Y. T., Scanlan, M. J., Sahin, U., Tureci, O., Gure, A. O., Tsang, S., et al. (1997) A testicular antigen aberrantly expressed in human cancers detected by autologous antibody screening. *Proc. Natl. Acad. Sci. USA* **94,** 1914–1918.
11. Gure, A. O., Tureci, O., Sahin, U., Tsang, S., Scanlan, M. J., Jager, E., et al. (1997) SSX: a multigene family with several members transcribed in normal testis and human cancer. *Int. J. Cancer* **72,** 965–971.
12. Jager, E., Chen, Y. T., Drijfhout, J. W., Karbach, J., Ringhoffer, M., Jager, D., et al. (1998) Simultaneous humoral and cellular immune response against cancer-testis antigen NY-ESO-1: definition of human histocompatibility leukocyte antigen (HLA)-A2-binding peptide epitopes. *J. Exp. Med.* **187,** 265–270.
13. Greiner, J., Ringhoffer, M., Simikoponkp, O., Szmaragowska, A., Huebsch, S., Maurer, U., et al. (2000) Simultaneous expression of different immunogenic antigens in acute myeloid leukemia. *Exp. Haematol.* **28,** 1413–1422.
14. Krackhardt, A. M., Witzens, M., Harig, S., Hodi, F. S., Zauls, A. J., Chessia, M., et al. (2002) Identification of tumor-associated antigens in chronic lymphocytic leukemia by SEREX. *Immunobiology* **100,** 2123–2131.
15. Eichmüller, S., Usener, D., Dummer, R., Stein, A., Thiel, D., and Schadendorf, D. (2001) Serological detection of cutaneous T-cell lymphoma-associated antigens. *Proc. Natl. Acad. Sci. USA* **98,** 629–634.
16. Huang, S., Preuss, K-D., Xie, X., Regitz, E., and Pfreundschuh, M. (2002). Analysis of the antibody repertoire of lymphoma patients. *Cancer Immunol. Immunother.* **51,** 655–662.
17. Türeci, O., Sahin, U., and Pfreundschuh, M. (1997) Serological analysis of human tumor antigens: molecular definition and implications. *Mol. Med. Today* **3,** 342–349.
18. Türeci, Ö., Sahin, U., Zwick, C., Koslowski, M., Seitz, G., and Pfreundschuh, M. (1998) Identification of a meiosis-specific protein as a member of the class of cancer/testis antigens. *Proc. Natl. Acad. Sci. USA* **95,** 5211–5216.

19. Güre, A., Stockert, E., Scanlan, M., Keresztes, R., Jäger, D., Altorlei, N., et al. (2000) Serological identification of embryonic neural proteins as highly immunogenic tumor antigens in small cell lung cancer. *Proc. Natl. Acad. Sci. USA* **97,** 4198–4203.

6

Determining Mutational Status of Immunoglobulin V Genes in Chronic Lymphocytic Leukemia

A Useful Prognostic Indicator

Surinder S. Sahota, Gavin Babbage, Niklas Zojer, Christian H. Ottensmeier, and Freda K. Stevenson

Summary

Determining the clonal origins of malignant B-cells will have an impact on disease understanding and management. In this regard, immunoglobulin variable (V) region gene analysis already is having a significant impact in delineating the tumor cell of origin. It can identify, among other features whether such a cell has undergone somatic mutation, which usually occurs within germinal centres. Remarkably, in chronic lymphocytic leukemia (CLL), the mutational status of V genes has allowed researchers to identify two subsets of disease, one originating from an unmutated B-cell with a markedly poorer disease outcome and the other from a mutated B-cell, which associates with long-term survival. The V gene status in CLL thus provides a robust indicator of disease outcome, which is beginning to shape clinical treatment. This chapter describes in detail the methodology for determining V gene usage in CLL, from acquisition of patient sample to generating the V-gene readout.

Key Words: Immunoglobulin; V gene; somatic mutation; prognosis; leukemia.

1. Introduction

The recognition of diverse antigens is critical to the humoral response and is mediated by the immunoglobulin (Ig) molecule expressed by B-cells. Specificity for antigen is determined by the variable (V) regions in the heavy (V_H) and light (V_L) chains, encoded by the corresponding V genes. Remarkably, affinity for antigen can be increased by the process of somatic mutation *(1)*. This process is activated after an encounter with the antigen in the T-cell-rich zones of secondary lymphoid organs and migration to follicular germinal centers (GCs). Once a GC reaction is initiated, somatic mutation can begin *(1,2)*.

From: *Methods in Molecular Medicine, Vol. 115: Lymphoma: Methods and Protocols*
Edited by: T. Illidge and P. W. M. Johnson © Humana Press Inc., Totowa, NJ

Although the precise details of this mechanism are as yet unclear, somatic mutation introduces nucleotide changes into the functionally rearranged V genes at a high rate, approaching 10^{-4} to 10^{-3} bp^{-1} per generation. Transitions are favored over transversions. Less frequently, these mutational events may include deletions or insertions *(3,4)*. Mutational changes lead to replacement of amino acids in the V regions, and B-cells expressing sIg of high affinity are selected *(1,2)*. A default pathway to apoptosis is in place for those cells failing affinity maturation *(2)*.

It is now possible to assess with confidence which B-cell has undergone somatic mutation because the germline genes used to encode V genes have been mapped. V region genes are assembled in early B-cell cells by deoxyribonucleic acid (DNA) recombination events to generate a functional transcriptional unit. For the V_H domain, this involves cutting and pasting of three germline elements, a V_H gene, a diversity (D_H) gene and a joining (J_H) gene, whereas for a functional V_L this involves V_LJ_L recombination. For the heavy chain, there are 51 potentially functional V_H genes, which can be grouped into seven families (V_H 1–7) on the basis of homology *(5)*; about 27 D_H genes *(6)*; and 6 J_H genes *(7)*, which map to chromosome 14q32. Polymorphism at the V_H locus involves insertions and deletions of gene segments, with the number of functional segments dependent on the haplotype. In addition, there is evidence of a low degree of allelic polymorphism *(5)*. Vκ light chains are encoded by 32 Vκ functional elements grouped into 6 families (VκI–VI) and 5 Jκ genes located on chromosome 2p11-12 *(8)*. Vλ assembly requires 37 Vλ genes, which can be grouped into 10 families (Vλ1–10) that are located upstream of 7 Jλ–Cλ pairs on chromosome 22q11.2 *(9)*.The recombinatorial processes that generate functional V(D)J units are imprecise, with nucleotide excision of coding exons and insertion of nontemplated (N) additions contributing to the unique third complementarity-determining region (CDR3) sequence in both V_H and V_L *(10)*. This mechanism contributes to generation of antibody diversity, and provides a unique CDR3 sequence that can be used to identify B-cell clones. Indeed, this forms the basis of analyzing V genes in neoplastic B-cells, because the CDR3 sequence is retained in the genome. Sequence analysis also provides an imprint of the clonal history of the cell of origin of a B-cell neoplasm and can indicate post-transformation events.

A number of important insights result from V gene analysis in B-cell tumors. The signature CDR3 identifies the tumor clone, and use of germline V gene elements can be assessed for any asymmetry of use. A striking bias is observed in the mandatory use of the V_H4 gene, $V_{4\text{-}34}$ in cold agglutinin disease *(11,12)*. In this disease, binding to the red cell surface carbohydrate I/i antigen is mediated by a framework region of the $V_{4\text{-}34}$ gene, resembling superantigen recognition in its unconventional binding site and accounting for the mandatory use

(13). Viral infections also can result in increased titers of $V_{4\text{-}34}$ Ig *(14)*, and its use in B-cell tumors has therefore created interest in a role for microbial agents in disease origins. The expansion of B-cells in response to a microbial superantigen carries a risk of neoplastic transformation. In CLL specifically, there appears to be overuse of the $V_{4\text{-}34}$ and $V_{1\text{-}69}$ genes in different disease subsets, suggesting a role for viral agents *(15,16)*.

Exposure of the tumor cell of origin to the somatic mutation mechanism can be readily assessed and, in fact, B-cell tumors can be classified in three categories: as having a pre-GC origin, as residing in the GC, and as having been exposed to the GC and exiting *(17)*. Tumor cells that occur in the GC environment bypass constraints of apoptosis in normal B-cells, with tumor progeny being continually targeted by somatic mutation in V genes, giving rise to intraclonal variation in V gene sequences. This feature of tumor V genes is seen in follicular lymphoma *(18)*.

In CLL, mutational status of tumor V genes has now delineated two important subsets that differ remarkably in clinical behavior. Tumors displaying unmutated V genes have a shorter median survival, in one study of 99 mo vs 293 mo in the mutated cases *(15)*. Here, a cut-off of ≥ 98% homology to donor germline gene has been used to define unmutated tumor V genes to allow for a low degree of polymorphic allelic variation (*see* **Note 1 [*5*]**). Because CDR3 assembly involves complex recombination events, it is not always possible to identify germline D gene use (*see* **Note 2 [*6*]**), and the use of J genes is similarly affected by these processes. As a result, analysis of a somatic mutational imprint on tumor V genes depends solely on characterizing deviation in homology to the donor germline V_H or V_L segment, as shown in **Figs. 1** and **2** (*see* **Notes 4–6**). It is likely that a significant clinical importance will be placed on accurately identifying the mutational status of V genes in CLL (*see* **Notes 7** and **8**) and the methodology to determine this is described below.

2. Materials

2.1. Extraction Reagents and Complimentary Deoxyribonucleic Acid Preparation

1. Ficoll-Hypaque (Amersham Pharmacia; Buckinghamshire, UK).
2. TRI reagent.
3. $CHCl_3$.
4. Ethanol.
5. Isopropanol, all molecular biology grade, (Sigma-Aldrich; Poole, Dorset, UK).
6. RPMI 1640 medium/bovine fetal calf serum (Gibco Invitrogen, Paisley, UK).
7. Dimethylsulfoxide (Sigma).
8. Wizard Genomic DNA Purification Kit (Promega, Southampton).
9. First-strand cDNA synthesis kit (Amersham Pharmacia).

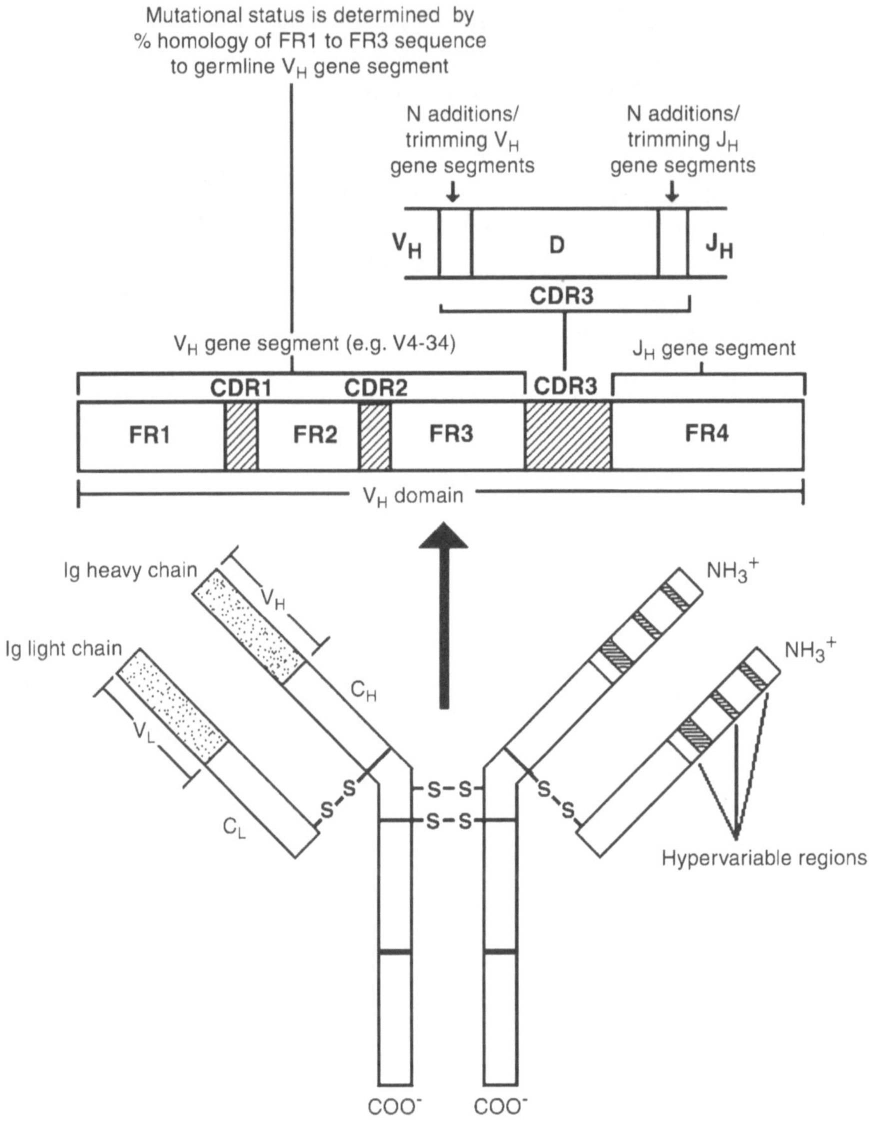

Fig. 1. A schematic representation of an immunoglobulin (Ig) molecule. Both the Ig variable (V) and constant (C) regions are shown for the heavy (V_H / C_H) and light (V_L / C_L) chains. The V_H region or domain has been further delineated to illustrate the contribution of germline V_H, D_H, and J_H gene segments in assembly of the functional V(D)J unit. Note that the mutational status is determined solely from the V_H gene segment as indicated.

```
CLL: Unmutated VH gene

          Q   V   Q   L   V   Q   S   G   A   E   V   K   K   P   G   A   S   V   K   V   S   C   K   A   S   G   Y   T   F   T
V1-02    CAG GTG CAG CTG GTG CAG TCT GGG GCT GAG GTG AAG AAG CCT GGG GCC TCA GTG AAG GTC TCC TGC AAG GCT TCT GGA TAC ACC TTC ACC
         ... ... ... ... ... ... ... ... ... ... ... ... ... ... ... ... ... ... ... ... ... ... ... ... ... ... ... ... ... ...
         |-------CDR1-------|                                                       |------------------------------CDR2-------
          G   Y   Y   M   H   W   V   R   Q   A   P   G   Q   G   L   E   W   M   G   W   I   N   P   N   S   G   G   T   N   Y
V1-02    GGC TAC TAT ATG CAC TGG GTG CGA CAG GCC CCT GGA CAA GGG CTT GAG TGG ATG GGA TGG ATC AAC CCT AAC AGT GGT GGC ACA AAC TAT
         ... ... ... ... ... ... ... ... ... ... ... ... ... ... ... ... ... ... ... ... ... ... ... ... ... ... ... ... ... ...
         -----------------------|
          A   Q   K   F   Q   G   W   V   T   M   T   R   D   T   S   I   S   T   A   Y   M   E   L   S   R   L   R   S   D   D
V1-02    GCA CAG AAG TTT CAG GGC TGG GTC ACC ATG ACC AGG GAC ACG TCC ATC AGC ACA GCC TAC ATG GAG CTG AGC AGG CTG AGA TCT GAC GAC
         ... ... ... ... ... ... ... ... ... ... ... ... ... ... ... ... ... ... ... ... ... ... ... ... ... ... ... ... ... ...
          T   A   V   Y   Y   C   A   R
V1-02    ACG GCC GTG TAT TAC TGT GCG AGA
         ... ... ... ... ... ... ... ...

CLL: mutated VH gene

          E   V   Q   L   V   E   S   G   G   G   L   V   Q   P   G   G   S   L   R   L   S   C   A   A   S   G   F   T   F   S
V3-7     GAG GTG CAG CTG GTG GAG TCT GGG GGA GGC TTG GTC CAG CCT GGG GGG TCC CTG AGA CTC TCC TGT GCA GCC TCT GGA TTC ACC TTT AGT
         ... ... ... ... ... ... ... ... ... .A. ... ... ... ... ... ... ... ... ... ... ... ... ... ... ... ... ... ..T ... ...
                                             *D                                                                        t
         |-------CDR1-------|                                                       |-------------------------------CDR2------
          S   Y   W   M   S   W   V   R   Q   A   P   G   K   G   L   E   W   V   A   N   I   K   Q   D   G   S   E   K   Y   Y
V3-7     AGC TAT TGG ATG AGC TGG GTC CGC CAG GCT CCA GGG AAG GGG CTG GAG TGG GTG GCC AAC ATA AAG CAA GAT GGA AGT GAG AAA TAC TAT
         CA. C.. ... ... ... ... ... ... ... A.. ... .AA ... ... ... ... .T. C.. ... ... ... ..T ACC ... ... .C. CTT GT. G.G ...
         *H  *H                              *T      *E                      *L  *L                  *N  *T          *T  *L  *V  *E
         ---------------------|
          V   D   S   V   K   G   R   F   T   I   S   R   D   N   A   K   N   S   L   Y   L   Q   M   N   S   L   R   A   E   D
V3-7     GTG GAC TCT GTG AAG GGC CGA TTC ACC ATC TCC AGA GAC AAC GCC AAG AAC TCA CTG TAT CTG CAA ATG AAC AGC CTG AGA GCC GAG GAC
         ... ... ... C.. ... ... ... ... ... ... ... C.. ... ... ... GC. C.. ... ..T ... ... ... ... ..T G.. ... ... ... ... ...
                     *L                              r                   *A  *H      l                       n   *G
          T   A   V   Y   Y   C   A   R
V3-7     ACG GCT GTG TAT TAC TGT GCG AGA
         ... ..C ... ... ... ... ..A ...
              a                   a
```

Fig. 2. Tumor-derived V_H genes from an unmutated and mutated CLL case. Each sequence is shown aligned at the nucleotide level with the germline V_H gene segment to determine mutational status. For the mutated CLL case shown, there is a 89.1% homology to the germline V3–7 gene, identified as donor by a best-fit homology match from the databases.

2.2. Primers

1. MWG Biotech; Milton Keynes (www.mwg-biotech.com).

2.3. PCR Reagents

1. Hotstart *Taq* DNA polymerase (QIAGEN; Crawley, West Sussex, UK).
2. dNTPs (BD Clontech, Oxford, UK).
3. Agarose (Gibco Invitrogen).
4. Ethidium bromide (Gibco Invitrogen).
5. Hybaid recovery DNA purification kit II (Hybaid; Ashford, Middlesex, UK).

2.4. Cloning Reagents

1. pGEM T vector kit (Promega; Southampton, UK).
2. *E. coli* strain JM109 competent cells (Promega).
3. Ampicillin (SmithKline Beecham Pharmaceuticals Ltd; Laoghaire, Co. Dublin).
4. LB (Millers Luria broth), agar (used at 1.5% w/v; Sigma-Aldrich).
5. X-Gal, 50 mg/mL (5-bromo-4-chloro-3-indolyl-β-D-galactopyranoside-Promega; Madison, WI).
6. Isopropyl-β-D-thio-galactopyranoside (IPTG; Calbiochem; Beeston, Nottingham, UK).
7. Spin Miniprep kit (QIAGEN).

2.5. DNA Sequence Analysis

1. Big dye version 1 (Applied Biosystems; Warrington, Cheshire, UK).
2. ABI 377 DNA sequencer (Applied Biosystems).
3. Sodium acetate, molecular biology grade (Sigma).

2.6. Software

1. MacVector (Oxford Molecular Group plc).
2. V base (MRC Centre for Protein Engineering; Cambridge, UK).

3. Methods

3.1. Patient Samples

1. Obtain 10–20 mL of peripheral blood (PB) by venepuncture and put into precoated heparinized or ethylenediamine tetraacetic acid tubes, for processing on the same day.
2. PB mononuclear cells (PBMCs) are obtained by standard Ficoll-hypaque density centrifugation.
3. PBMCs can be stored as pellets (approx 5×10^6) at –80°C or in dimethylsulfoxide (DMSO) containing storage medium (RPMI + 50% FCS + 10% DMSO) for ribonucleic acid (RNA).
4. For samples stored in DMSO, a wash step using sterile medium will be required before the extraction of RNA.

5. For DNA, cell pellets can be stored at 20°C. An aliquot of PB can be stored directly at –20°C for subsequent isolation of DNA. DNA may be isolated from transit samples within 48 h.

3.2. Extraction of RNA and DNA

1. Extract RNA from approx 5×10^6 PBMCs using the single phase phenol-based Tri reagent following the manufacturer's instructions.
2. Briefly, resuspend cells in 0.8 mL of RNAzol and lyse by multiple inversions.
3. To partition the phases, add $CHCl_3$ (160 µL) and mix suspension vigorously by inversion.
4. Place on ice for 5 min.
5. Centrifuge at 12,000*g* for 15 min.
6. Carefully remove top aqueous layer and precipitate RNA by addition of 0.7 vols isopropanol.
7. Store on ice approx 15 min and centrifuge at 12,000*g* for 15 min.
8. Decant supernatant and briefly spin again.
9. Remove traces of isopropanol.
10. Wash RNA pellet with 150 µL of 75% EtOH made with RNase-free H_2O.
11. Centrifuge for 5 min at 12,000*g*.
12. Remove wash supernatant carefully, and air dry pellet for approx 5 min.
13. Resuspend RNA in RNase-free H_2O (usually 100–150 µL). This must be stored at –80°C until required.
    Methods for extracting DNA will vary depending on which commercially available isolation kits are used, and protocols provided need to be followed precisely. For the kit used in our laboratory, DNA is eluted in 100 µL of DNase-free H_2O. Isolated DNA is stored at 4°C.

3.3. Preparation of cDNA

1. For the first-strand cDNA synthesis protocol (Pharmacia), mix 8 µL of RNA with 1 µL of oligo-dT (200 ng).
2. Heat 65°C for 10 min.
3. Place on ice for 2 min.
4. Add 1 µL of dithiothreitol and 5 µL of bulk mix (as supplied).
5. Incubate at 37°C for 1 h.
6. Store at –20°C. Alternative primers to prepare a specific cDNA pool for Cµ,δ,γ,α,ε are listed in **Table 1**.

3.4. Amplification of V Genes

For PCR amplification of V genes, a number of protocols can be used depending on the template source. For cDNA, the following primers can be used:

1. Mix of leader specific primers + constant region primer: for V_H genes, leader primers are for V_H families 1–6 (V_H7 is amplified by the V_H1 primer) and a C_H primer matching the tumor Ig isotype (**Table 1**). This mix of leader primers can

Table 1
Oligonucleotide PCR Primers

Primer	Location	Orientation	Sequence (5'–3')
V_H specific			
V_H1	LD	Sense	CTC ACC ATG GAC TGG ACC TGG AG
V_H2	LD	Sense	ATG GAC ACA CTT TGC TMC ACR CTC
V_H3	LD	Sense	CCA TGG AGT TTG GGC TGA GCT GG
V_H4	LD	Sense	ACA TGA AAC AYC TGT GGT TCT TCC
V_H5	LD	Sense	ATG GGG TCA ACC GCC ATC CTY G
V_H6	LD	Sense	ATG TCT GTC TCC TTC CTC ATC TTC
V_H1	FR1	Sense	TTG CGG CCG CCA GGT SCA GCT GGT RCA GTC
V_H2	FR1	Sense	TTG CGG CCG CCA GRT CAC CTT GAA GGA GTC
V_H3	FR1	Sense	TTG CGG CCG CSA GGT GCA GCT GGT GGA GTC
V_H4	FR1	Sense	TTG CGG CCG CCA GGT GCA GCT GCA GGA GTC
V_H5	FR1	Sense	TTG CGG CCG CGA RGT GCA GCT GGT GCA GTC
V_H6	FR1	Sense	TTG CGG CCG CCA GGT ACA GCT GCA GCA GTC
J_H1	FR4	Antisense	TGA GGA GAC GGT GAC CAG GGT GCC CTG
J_H2	FR4	Antisense	TGA GGA GAC AGT GAC CAG GGT GCC ACG
J_H3	FR4	Antisense	TGA AGA GAC GGT GAC CAT TGT CCC TTG
J_H4	FR4	Antisense	TGA GGA GAC GGT GAC CAG GGT TCC CTG
J_H5	FR4	Antisense	TGA GGA GAC GGT GAC CAG GGT TCC CTG
J_H6	FR4	Antisense	TGA GGA GAC GGT GAC CGT GGT CCC TTG
CH specific			
Cμ	CH1 (30–51)	Antisense	GGA ATT CTC ACA GGA GAC GAG G
Cμ16	CH1 (120–115)	Antisense	TTG GGG CGG ATG CAC T
Cδ1	CH1 (173–164)	Antisense	TTC TCT GGG GCT GTG TC
CγFF1	CH1 (192–184)	Antisense	GGT CAC CAC GCT GCT GAG GGA GTA GA
CαFF1	CH1 (187–179)	Antisense	CGT GGT GTA CAG GTC CCC GGA GGC A
Cα4	CH1 (125–118)	Antisense	GCT CAG CGG GAA GAC CTT GGG GCT

V_L specific			
Vκ1&4	FR1	Sense	GAC ATC SWG ATG ACC CAG TCT CC
Vκ2&6	FR1	Sense	GAW RTT GTG MTG ACT CAG TCT CC
Vκ3	FR1	Sense	GAA ATT GTG TTG ACG CAG TCT CC
Vκ5	FR1	Sense	GAA ACG ACA CTC ACG CAG TCT CC
Jκ1-4	FR4	Antisense	ACG TTT GAT HTC CAC YTT GGT CCC
Jκ5	FR4	Antisense	ACG TTT AAT CTC CAG TCG TGT CCC
$V_\lambda 1$	FR1	Sense	CAG TCT GTS BTG ACK CAG CCR CCY
$V_\lambda 2$	FR1	Sense	CAG TCT GCC CTG ACT CAG CCT SSY T
$V_\lambda 3$	FR1	Sense	TCY TMT GWG CTG ACT CAG SMM
$V_\lambda 7\&8$	FR1	Sense	CAG RCT GTG GTG ACY CAG GAG CCM TC
$V_\lambda 9$	FR1	Sense	CAG CCT GTG CTG ACT CAG CCA CCT TC
$J_\lambda C$	FR4	Antisense	ACC KAG GAC GGT SAS CTK GGT SCC
Sequencing			
T7	Vector	Sense	TAA TAC GAC TCA CTA TAG GG
SP6	Vector	AntiSense	ATT TAG GTG ACA CTA TAG AA

LD, leader; FR, framework

also be used with the J_H(1–6) mix of primers or the consensus J_H primer (cJ_H ; 5'-TGA GGA GAC GGT GAC CAG GAT CCC TTG GCC CCA G). Another strategy involves amplifying tumor cDNA with each individual leader primer and a downstream C_H or J_H mix(1–6) or cJ_H primer. In this case, each PCR product has to be analyzed separately or all products pooled prior to analysis. This procedure also minimizes 5'-primer competition.

2. Mix of framework (FR) 1 primers + downstream C_H or J_H mix / cJ_H primer.

For DNA, the same sense primer mix can be used as for cDNA PCR amplification, but use of leader-specific primers will also amplify up an approx 100 bp intron and increase the size of the PCR product for sequence analysis. For DNA though, only the J_H mix or cJ_H can be used as downstream primers.

Set up PCR mixture as follows using precautions described previously ***(19)***:

5 μL of 10X *Taq* polymerase buffer;
1 μL of dNTP mixture (20 m*M*);
6 μL of primer mix (leader-specific or FR1-specific; each at 20 pmol);
1 μL of C_H or J_H mix / cJ_H primer (each at 20 pmol);
3 μL of cDNA (or DNA);
1 μL of *Taq* polymerase enzyme (5 units); and
33 μL of H_2O.

1. PCR cycle conditions are: 94°C for 12 min (1X cycle; hot-start *Taq* polymerase); 30 cycles of 94°C for 1 min, 56°C for 1 min, and 72°C for 1 min; and 72°C for 5 min (1X cycle). For leader-specific primers, the annealing temperature can be increased to 65°C for 1 min.
2. Run out PCR products on a 1.2% agarose gel with ethidium bromide (5 μg/100 mL gel volume) and a 1-kb ladder for sizing and electrophoresis at 150v for 45 min.
3. Visualize PCR DNA under UV making sure there is no exposure to uncovered skin. Dispose ethidium bromide contaminated buffer as described ***(20)***.
4. Cut out the predicted size of V gene product (approx 360–480 bp).
5. Elute DNA from agarose slice using manufacturer's protocols for DNA recovery (Hybaid). This DNA can now be used for direct sequence analysis or cloned to assess intraclonal tumor variation in V gene sequence.

3.5. Analysis of Tumor Clonality

PCR DNA from amplified tumor V genes can be cloned using basic, standard procedures to examine clonal variation in tumor-derived V gene sequences. Because tumor cells represent a specific, clonal expansion of B-cells, it follows that the predominant cDNA species in the oligo dT primed pool is derived from tumor cells. By cloning PCR DNA and analyzing multiple colonies, the predominant sequence is readily identified by a common CDR3 sequence and represents the tumor V gene. This is now an established procedure, confirmed by evidence from idiotypic antibody phenotype and from analysis of expressed recombinant V genes in a ScFv format ***(21,22)***.

1. Set up a ligation reaction: 10X ligase buffer (1 µL) + PCR DNA (7.5 µL) + pGEM-T vector (0.5 µL) + T4 DNA ligase (1 µL).
2. Incubate at 14°C for 3–4 h or overnight.
3. For transformation, remove an aliquot of *E. coli* JM109 competent cells from –80°C storage and thaw on ice for 10 min.
4. Add ligated product (5 µL) to cells (50 µL) on ice.
5. Gently mix by shaking tube on ice, and leave for 15–30 min.
6. Heat shock cells at 42°C for 45 min; place on ice for an additional 2 min.
7. Add LB broth (0.8 mL) and shake for 1 h at 37°C.
8. Centrifuge cells briefly (1200*g*).
9. Remove most of the supernatant.
10. Resuspend cells for plating on LB-agar + ampicillin (100 µg/mL) + IPTG (0.1 *M*; 100 µL per plate) + X-gal (25 µL per plate).
11. Incubate overnight at 37°C.
12. Place cultured agar plates at 4°C for approx 1 h to maximize blue/white color selection.
13. Pick 12–15 white colonies representing inserts and culture in LB + ampicillin (50 µg/mL or 2 mL) overnight at 37°C.
14. Prepare plasmids from approx 1.5 mL of culture broth using manufacturer's instructions for column-based purification (QIAGEN).
15. Elute plasmid preparation in 50–75 µL of sterile H_2O.
16. Confirm cloned PCR DNA insert by restriction enzyme digests flanking cloning site or by resolving an aliquot (3 µL) of plasmid in agarose (0.7%) and comparing migration pattern with control plasmids lacking inserts (blue colonies).
17. Plasmids verified with inserts can then be sequenced (bidirectionally).

3.6. DNA Sequence Analysis

The protocol described here is for the automated central DNA sequence analysis facility available in our laboratory. If manual sequencing is required, standard molecular biology methods are available ***(20)***. The protocol below is adapted for the ABI 377 DNA automated sequence analyzer.

1. Set up sequencing reactions: Dye master mix (2 µL) + 5X reaction buffer (2 µL) + H_2O (3 µL) + plasmid or eluted PCR DNA (3 mL).
2. PCR amplification is as follows: 96°C for 10 s (x1 cycle), 25 cycles of 50°C for 5 s and 60°C for 4 min.
3. Precipitate sequencing products: PCR sequence reaction mixture (10 µL) + 3 *M* sodium acetate, pH 5.2 (2 µL) + H_2O (10 µL). Mix and add ethanol (85µL).
4. Place on ice 30 min.
5. Centrifuge 12,000*g* for 30 min.
6. Decant and wash pellet with 75% ethanol (150 µL).
7. Centrifuge 12000*g* for 5 min.
8. Decant and air dry pellet.

9. Resuspend DNA in loading dye:formamide (1:5; 2 µL) for fractionation in a sequencing gel.
10. Resuspended samples can also be stored at –20°C for a approx 3 d.

3.7. Analysis and Interpretation of Data

The complete V-BASE directory can be downloaded as a reference database and is available on request (**ref. *5***; Dr. I. Tomlinson, MRC Centre for Protein Engineering, University of Cambridge, UK). Alternatively, V gene sequences can be aligned to web directories at http://www.mrc-cpe.cam.ac.uk/imt-doc/vbase-home-page.html and http://www.ncbi.nlm.nih.gov/igblast. The web alignments are particularly useful because they also define each functional V gene by FR and CDR domains. For analysis, each donor germline V(D)J gene element used in tumor V gene rearrangement is first identified. Next, the mutational status of the tumor V gene is determined by analysis of % homology to the donor germline V_H or V_L gene segment (*see* **Notes 1** and **3**) and by the exclusion of the (D)J genes, as discussed in **Subheading 1**.

Word data files from the automated sequencer can be opened directly as MacVector files (or other sequence analysis software files) for further analysis:

1. Each file is aligned to the V base directory, and donor germline genes (V, D, and J) are identified as those with the closest match to test sequence. The sequence is next trimmed to read from the first codon of FR1 to J or constant region depending on use of primers, and translated into an amino acid sequence with MacVector software. If the derived Ig sequence isolated is in-frame and potentially functional, it can then be subjected to further evaluation. Amino acid sequences of germline V genes are available from the web directories or the literature for comparison ***(5–9)***.
2. Assessing the presence of somatic mutation: a cut-off of greater than or equal to 98% homology at the nucleotide level to donor germline V_H or V_L gene segment defines the mutational status of tumor V gene as unmutated. For this, the nucleotide sequence from FR1–FR3 inclusive from the in-frame V gene sequence (encompassing the complete FR1-CDR1-FR2-CDR2-FR3 sequence) but avoiding the primer sequence (*see* **Note 1**), is used for comparison. Because extensive trimming can occur at the FR3-CDR3 boundary, the last remaining nucleotides in FR3 need to be assessed with care (*see* **Note 3**).
3. The web-based alignment will give a direct readout of the germline gene used and percent homology.
4. Determining intraclonal variation: each tumor-derived clonal V gene sequence is placed in a software folder and compared for homology. An estimate of the *Taq* error rate, made by amplification of reference genes ***(23)***, will enable background variation to be eliminated. Evidence for intraclonal variation in tumor-derived V gene sequences rests on identical base changes or other mutational events being detected in two or more clones in separate PCRs. These generally occur in addition to shared common mutational events in tumor V genes.

4. Notes

1. When a mixture of FR1 primers are used to amplify and identify the tumor V gene, this sequence must be excluded from comparisons of homology to the germline V gene segment. Ideally, the tumor V gene sequence should be re-assessed using a leader-specific primer.
2. The most stringent criteria for identifying D-gene use in tumor V_H genes relies on a consecutive 10 nucleotide match with the donor D-gene segment *(6)*.
3. During V(D)J recombination, nucleotides are often removed from the coding exons of the rearranging V(D)J segments, and there may be N additions catalyzed by TdT, as observed in naive B-cells. Consequently, nucleotide differences at the very end of V gene segments, that is, the last codon of FR3, should not be regarded as somatic mutations unless followed by an at least 2 bp homology to the germline V gene. This then excludes junctional diversity generated in the V gene recombination process at an antigen-independent stage.
4. Analysis of mutational base changes leading to replacement (R) amino acids or are silent (S) in this respect can be informative as to the nature of underlying selection, assumed to be driven by the antigen. From a comprehensive analysis of normal memory B-cells, an overall R:S ratio of less than 1.7 in the overall FRs (FR1, 2, and 3 combined) is indicative of selection to maintain structural integrity *(24)*. Two or three nucleotide changes in a single codon (e.g., TTA to CTT) is overall silent because both codons encode Leu, but the two distinct nucleotide exchanges, TTA to CTA and TTA to TTT, represent 1S and 1R mutations. These determinations will influence the overall assessment.
5. Polymorphism of germline V genes mainly has been addressed in the V_H locus. The exact number of functional segments depends on two types of polymorphism in different haplotypes: the insertion or deletion of V_H segments and the occurrence of different alleles of the same segment (reviewed in **ref. *5***). Insertional polymorphism can vary. In 73% of individuals, an approx 50-kb insertion introduces five functional segments, including V30.3, with V3–30 and V4–31 duplicated. Another insertion event in 50% of cases, at the telomeric or 5' region of the V_H locus, introduces at least four segments. Other insertions introduce single V_H segments, and these have been mapped. Analysis of allelic variation between different haplotypes suggests that this is very low, and variation in available repertoire between individuals is most likely to involve insertion or deletional polymorphism. As further haplotypes are mapped, this finding may need to be modified. Consequently, in assessing mutational status in CLL, a 98% or greater homology cut-off is used to define the unmutated status. **Figure 2** shows examples of aligned tumor-derived V_H genes in CLL with germline donor V_H gene segments at the nucleotide level. Both unmutated CLL and mutated CLL cases are shown.
6. To assess mutational status of V genes in CLL, it is preferable to analyze V_H genes because they will, in general, have a higher amount of mutations than V_L *(24)*, enabling a more ready determination of deviation from germline.
7. In those CLL cases displaying somatically mutated V genes, extensive analysis is required to verify absence of intraclonal variation *(15)*. Replicate PCRs

(between 2 and 4) are performed to verify tumor V gene usage. The presence of stop codons in tumor V gene sequences generally is caused by amplification of the nonfunctional allele in CLL. However, CLL tumor cells can in rare cases express multiple functional V_H and V_L rearrangements, which occur by allelic inclusion *(25)*.

8. Somatically mutated $V_{3\text{-}21}$ genes define a further, specific subset in CLL associated with a significantly shorter survival than other mutated cases *(26)*. Analysis of V gene usage in CLL, therefore, is clearly important in defining important features of disease behavior.

Acknowledgments

This work was funded by The Leukaemia Research Fund UK, Tenovus UK, Cancer Research UK, and a European Society for Medical Oncology Fellowship (to N.Z.).

References

1. Berek, C. (1992) The development of B-cells and the B-cell repertoire in the microenvironment of the germinal center. *Immunol. Rev.* **126,** 5–19.
2. MacLennan, I. C. (1994) Germinal centers. *Ann. Rev. Immunol.* **12,** 117–139.
3. Goossens, T., Klein, U., and Kuppers, R. (1998) Frequent occurrence of deletions and duplications during somatic hypermutation: implications for oncogene translocations and heavy chain disease. *Proc. Natl. Acad. Sci. USA* **95,** 2463–2468.
4. Wilson, P. C., de Bouteiller, O., Liu, Y. J., Potter, K., Banchereau, J., Capra, J. D., et al. (1998) Somatic hypermutation introduces insertions and deletions into immunoglobulin V genes. *J. Exp. Med.* **187,** 59–70.
5. Cook, G. P., and Tomlinson, I. M. (1995) The human immunoglobulin V_H repertoire. *Immunol. Today.* **16,** 237–242.
6. Corbett, S. J., Tomlinson, I. M., Sonnhammer, E. L. L., Buck, D., and Winter, G. (1997) Sequence of the human immunoglobulin diversity (D) segment locus: a systematic analysis provides no evidence for the use of DIR segment, inverted D segments, "minor" D segments or D-D recombination. *J. Mol. Biol.* **270,** 587–597.
7. Ravetch, J.V., Siebenlist, U., Korsmeyer, S., Waldmann, T. and Leder, P. (1981) Structure of the human immunoglobulin mu locus: characteristics of embryonic and rearranged J and D genes. *Cell.* **27,** 583–591.
8. Zachau, H. G. (1995) The human immunoglobulin κ genes, in *Immunoglobulin Genes* (Honjo, T., and Alt, F. W., eds.), Academic, San Diego, CA, pp 173–191.
9. Williams, S. C., Frippiat, J.-P., TomLinson, I. M., Ignatovich, O., Lefranc, M.-P. and Winter, G. (1996) Sequence and evolution of the human germLine Vλ repertoire. *J. Mol. Biol.* **264,** 220–232.
10. Kirkham, P. M., and Schroeder, H. W. Jr (1994) Antibody structure and the evolution of immunoglobulin V gene segments. *Semin. Immunol.* **6,** 347–360.
11. Silberstein, L. E., Jefferies, L. C., Goldman, J., Friedman, D., Moore, J. S., Nowell, P. C., et al. (1991) Variable region gene analysis of pathologic human autoantibodies to the related i and I red blood cell antigens. *Blood.* **78,** 2372–2386.

12. Pascual, V., Victor, K., Spellerberg, M., Hamblin, T.J., Stevenson, F.K., and Capra, J. D. (1992) VH restriction among human cold agglutinins. The VH4–21 gene segment is required to encode anti-I and anti-i specificities. *J. Immunol.* **149,** 2337–2344.
13. Li, Y., Spellerberg, M. B., Stevenson, F. K., Capra, D., and Potter, K. N. (1996) The I binding specificity of human VH4–34 (VH4–21) encoded antibodies is determined by both VH framework region 1 and complementarity determining region 3. *J. Mol. Biol.* **256,** 577–589.
14. Chapman, C. J., Spellerberg, M. B., Smith, G. A., Carter, S. J., Hamblin, T. J., and Stevenson, F. K. (1993) Autoanti-red cell antibodies synthesized by patients with infectious mononucleosis utilize the VH4–21 gene segment. *J. Immunol.* **151,** 1051–1061.
15. Hamblin, T. J., Davis, Z., Gardiner, A., Oscier, D. G., and Stevenson, F. K. (1999) Unmutated Ig V(H) genes are associated with a more aggressive form of chronic lymphocytic leukemia. *Blood.* **94,** 1848–1854.
16. Damle, R. N., Wasil, T., Fais, F., Ghiotto, F., Valetto, A., Allen, S. L., et al. (1999) Ig V gene mutation status and CD38 expression as novel prognostic indicators in chronic lymphocytic leukemia. *Blood.* **94,** 1840–1847.
17. Stevenson, F., Sahota, S., Zhu, D., Ottensmeier, C., Chapman, C., Oscier, D., and Hamblin, T. (1998) Insight into the origin and clonal history of B-cell tumors as revealed by analysis of immunoglobulin variable region genes. *Immunol. Rev.* **162,** 247–259.
18. Zhu, D., Hawkins, R. E., Hamblin, T. J., and Stevenson, F. K. (1994) Clonal history of a human follicular lymphoma as revealed in the immunoglobulin variable region genes. *Br. J. Haematol.* **86,** 505–512.
19. Kwok, S., and Higuchi, R. (1989) Avoiding false positives with PCR. *Nature.* **339,** 237–238.
20. Sambrook, J., Fritsch, E. F., and Maniatis, T. (1989) *Molecular Cloning.* Cold Spring Harbor Laboratory Press, Plainview, NY.
21. Stevenson, F. K., Spellerberg, M. B., Treasure, J., Chapman, C. J., Silberstein, L. E., Hamblin, T. J., and Jones, D. B. (1993) Differential usage of an Ig heavy chain variable region gene by human B-cell tumors. *J. Immunol.* **82,** 224–230.
22. Forconi, F., King, C. A., Sahota, S. S., Kennaway, C. K., Russell, N. H., and Stevenson, F. K. (2002) Insight into the potential for DNA idiotypic fusion vaccines designed for patients by analysing xenogeneic anti-idiotypic antibody responses. *Immunology.* **107,** 39–45.
23. Sahota S. S., Davis, Z., Hamblin, T. J., and Stevenson, F. K. (2000) Somatic mutation of *bcl-6* genes can occur in the absence of V_H mutations in chronic lymphocytic leukemia. *Blood* **95,** 3534–3540.
24. Dorner, T., Foster, S. J., Brezinschek, H. P., and Lipsky, P. E. (1998) Analysis of the targeting of the hypermutational machinery and the impact of subsequent selection on the distribution of nucleotide changes in human VHDJH rearrangements. *Immunol Rev.* **162,** 161–171.

25. Rassenti, L. Z., and Kipps, T. J. (1997) Lack of allelic exclusion in B-cell chronic lymphocytic leukemia. *J. Exp. Med.* **185,** 1435–1445.
26. Tobin, G., Thunberg, U., Johnson, A., Thorn, I., Soderberg, O., Hultdin, M., et al. (2002) Somatically mutated Ig V(H) 3–21 genes characterize a new subset of chronic lymphocytic leukemia. *Blood* **99,** 2262–2264.

7

Idiotype Gene Rescue in Follicular Lymphoma

Katy McCann, Surinder S. Sahota, Freda K. Stevenson, and Christian H. Ottensmeier

Summary

Beyond the morphological, immunophenotypic, and genetic information used for the diagnosis of lymphoid malignancies, molecular analyses have deepened our insights into the development of B-cell lymphomas. We have learned that B-cell tumors can be grouped according to the mutational status of their immunoglobulin variable (V) region genes, and this has become an important prognostic tool in chronic lymphocytic leukemia. The analysis of V genes also has allowed us to more precisely place B-cell lymphomas relative to their normal B-cell counterparts and to the germinal center where somatic hypermutation takes place. It has become evident that many of the common B-cell tumors arise at this site and are able to respond to stimuli, which govern normal B-cells. In this chapter, we focus on the analysis of V genes in follicular lymphomas based on the experience in our laboratory and provide a detailed guide for this analysis.

Key Words: Follicular lymphoma; non-Hodgkin's lymphoma; immunoglobulin; V-gene analysis; immunogenetics; PCR; sequencing; cloning.

1. Introduction

Follicular lymphomas (FLs) account for approx 30 to 40% of all newly diagnosed cases of non-Hodgkin's lymphoma (NHL) *(1)* and display a wide spectrum of clinical presentations. Although rare in patients younger than the age of 25, the frequency of these lymphomas increases steadily with age, with a median presentation at 50–60 yr. They occur as frequently in men as in women, in contrast to many other NHLs, and their incidence is increasing. FL typically follows an indolent course, with waxing and waning of the disease. In most cases, standard treatments cannot secure a prolonged remission or cure, and the median survival is 7–8 yr *(2–4)*.

From: *Methods in Molecular Medicine, Vol. 115: Lymphoma: Methods and Protocols*
Edited by: T. Illidge and P. W. M. Johnson © Humana Press Inc., Totowa, NJ

1.1. Morphology

FL is defined as a tumor in which the normal architecture of the lymph node has been destroyed and is replaced by malignant cells, which grow, at least in part, in patterns reminiscent of lymphoid follicles. The tumor cell population consists of variable mixtures of cells, although centrocytes predominate and, by definition, centroblasts form only a minority in the population.

FL is believed to be of a germinal center (GC) origin with the $CD5^{-}$ $CD23^{-}$ peripheral B-cell of the inner follicle mantle being the presumed normal counterpart. More than 90% of FLs express surface immunoglobulins (Ig)—in the absence of cytoplasmic Ig—and typically are surface IgM^{+} but also are $sIgD^{+}$, $sIgG^{+}$, or $sIgA^{+}$, albeit less frequently ***(5–8)*** Characteristically, tumor cells are CD5 and CD43 negative, and CD10 and CD23 are variably expressed ***(9)***. Genetic analysis reveals a t(14;18)(q32;q21) translocation in the most cases ***(10–12)***.

1.2. Immunoglobulin Gene Rearrangement

Ig gene rearrangement is the defining molecular event in the development of a B-cell. In the early stages of B-cell development, the Ig heavy chain locus on chromosome 14 brings together a variable (V_H), a diversity (D), and a joining segment (J_H) in a process of somatic deoxyribonucleic acid (DNA) rearrangement known as V(D)J recombination. If successful, rearrangement of the light chain at the kappa locus on chromosome 2 and the lambda locus on chromosome 22 follows, respectively, until a functional light chain terminates the recombination process. Subsequent somatic hypermutation (SHM) and class switch recombination provide mechanisms by which Ig is further diversified and constitute central events in the life of a B-cell tightly associated with developmental stages. Scrutiny of the evidence these processes leave in the Ig gene sequence reveals the stage of development that the cells have reached at a particular time point compared with normal B-cells.

With the exception of Hodgkin's disease, B-cell malignancies typically have functional Ig genes, which may reflect the requirement for Ig expression in normal B-cells ***(13)***. As is the case with normal B-cells, SHM and class switch recombination events will leave a lasting imprint in the genome, which will be present in each cell of a tumor clone. Therefore, V genes can serve as specific markers for B-cell lymphomas. With the development of modern molecular techniques, this genetic information has become accessible and now analysis of Ig genes can provide details of the molecular events that a malignant B-cell has been exposed to, revealing information about the clonal history of the neoplastic cell ***(14,15)***.

V gene analysis also provides an independent marker for the presence of a clonal population. This markers permits one the ability to distinguish neoplasms from reactive processes and, therefore, it contributes to the interpretation of clinical and histological findings in difficult situations.

Genetic analysis also may reveal information related to pathogenesis. Preferential usage of individual V_H gene segments suggest the role of classical antigens (Ag) or superantigens (SAg) in the initial proliferation of B-cells, leading to overt neoplasia, because it has been shown that SAgs can bind to the (unmutated) framework (FR) regions of an antibody molecule ***(16–18)***. Because the human V gene repertoire is known, it is now possible to confidently identify somatic mutations in individual B-cells, which in turn allows assessment of whether a tumor cell, or its parent, has undergone SHM and affinity maturation. In tumors thought to be of GC origin, heterogeneity of the somatic mutations in the V genes within the tumor cell population indicates that SHM is still ongoing. Interestingly, in some cases, a narrowing of this heterogeneity has been found after treatment, implying selection of treatment resistant cells ***(14,19–21)***. More recently, isotype-switching events have been analyzed and reveal the presence of multiple isotypes in some tumors ***(22–24)***. The presence of these isotypes provides more evidence that the tumor cells can to some degree respond to stimuli that govern the life of the normal cellular counterparts.

The findings of these studies contribute to the understanding of differentiation and development of malignant B-cells and to the classification of these malignancies relative to normal B-cell development ***(9,14,15,25)***. Within some disease entities individual subgroups exist, which might arise at different time points in B-cell development ***(26,27)***.

1.3. Tumors of the Germinal Center

Most B-cell lymphomas, that is, FL, diffuse large B-cell lymphomas (DLBCL), MALT lymphomas, and Burkitt lymphoma, arise from cells that have undergone SHM. In combination with the morphological and immunophenotypic evidence, this progress is suggestive of a GC origin.

Normal cells undergo SHM of their V_H and V_L genes and may additionally class switch. They then leave the GC ***(28)***. Some cells re-enter the GC dark zone for further rounds of mutation, or alternatively become plasma cells. Although V gene analysis shows that many B-cell tumors have undergone, and in some cases can continue to undergo SHM, it is possible that prolonged cell survival and residence in the GC may blur the information that V gene analysis generates. Factors that are known to increase cell survival, such as deregulation of bcl-2, are in fact observed in the vast majority of FL with a t(14;18), and p53 mutations commonly are observed. Although the initial t(14;18) rearrangement likely occurs in the bone marrow ***(29)***, it may exert its influence only after the tumor cell has arrived in the GC and has additionally undergone some yet undefined additional transforming event.

In mouse models, it has been shown that the RAG1 and RAG2 genes can be reactivated in the GC, opening a new window for susceptibility to (abnormal) rearrangements (***30***; reviewed in **ref. *31***). It appears likely that such mechanisms can be active in humans too, because the salvage of cells from death by receptor editing in the GC requires reactivation of the recombinase machinery ***(32–34)***. An open question remains whether lymphomas, like normal B-cells, need the presence of Ag or of SAgs for ongoing somatic hypermutation.

1.4. V Gene Analysis in FL

Several studies have addressed V gene usage in FL and have reported a high degree of somatic mutations in the V genes of these lymphomas ***(20,21,35–40)***. V_H gene usage appears to be similar to that of the normal B-cell repertoire, with the possibility of a small excess of V_H4 genes. A well-documented feature is the presence of intraclonal heterogeneity, implying that the cells of this lymphoma remain under the influence of the somatic mutator in the GC, and it often is possible to deduce genealogical trees depicting the relationship between individual cell clones ***(41)***. In these lymphomas, the presence of antigen-presenting cells in the form of follicular dendritic cells is well recognized ***(8)*** and T-cells are invariably present. The presence of the third key component antigen, which drives somatic mutation in normal B-cells, has not been functionally demonstrated in FL. Nonetheless, in some cases, the evaluation of the patterns of somatic mutations has shown preferential sequence maintenance in FRs vs clustering of mutations in the complementarity-determining regions (CDRs) and this has been interpreted as evidence for antigen-driven clonal selection ***(19,21,38,42,43)***. Model systems are being established in which somatic mutations occur without external antigen (***44***), and it may be that for lymphomas arising in the GC, antigen is no longer an absolute requirement for SHM.

Most studies have assessed V_H genes only. However, light chain gene analysis has been reported in two studies ***(21,38)***. The latter study investigated light chain V_κ genes and V_H genes in 10 FL cases and found that the V_κ genes fell into two groups: one that demonstrated extensively mutated V_κ genes (6/10 cases) and a second with a very low degree of V_κ mutations (4/10 cases). To date this observation has not been confirmed and its relevance remains to be assessed.

More recently, it has become appreciated that disease progression or treatment may have an impact on V_H gene sequences, and loss of intraclonal heterogeneity has been observed ***(20,21)***.

As part of our clinical trial of anti-idiotypic DNA vaccination against FL, we have sequenced 36 cases, identifying both the V_H and V_L sequences from the tumor clone. All cases demonstrated mutated V genes, with higher levels of

SHM in V_H genes as compared with V_L. We could consistently identify J_H segments. However, if the stringent criteria of Corbett et al. ***(45)*** are applied, which require at least 10 nucleotides identity to a germline D segment,the identification of D region segments was ambiguous in most cases.

To measure the immune responses of the patients in our study, it was necessary to express idiotypic protein for use in immunological assays ***(40)***. Analysis of the recombinant proteins showed that they had undergone glycosylation. This observation prompted the systematic analysis of the V_H and V_L sequences for potential *N*-linked glycosylation sites ***(40)***. The motif for *N*-glycosylation is AsnXSer/Thr, for which X can be any amino acid except Pro, Glu, or Asp. Natural sites occur in three V_H germline segments (V1-08, V4-34, and VH5a) and in three V_L germline segments (VKV21(1), VL514115e, and 1173e). Sequence analysis of our own data show that 34/36 FL acquired one or more new glycosylation sites in either V_H, V_L, or both. In contrast, normal B-cell V gene rearrangements, nonfunctional V gene sequences, and sequences from multiple myeloma and the mutated subset of chronic lymphocytic leukemia have a low incidence of approx 10% glycosylation sites ***(40)***. Other germinal center lymphomas, such as DLBCL or sporadic Burkitt lymphoma, show an intermediate frequency of approx 40%; 90% of sites were located in the CDRs, particularly CDR2. FR2 and FR4 had no sites. Novel sites are limited to a few positions in the CDRs and focussed on codon 33-35 in CDR1 (14/14) and codon 50 at the N-terminus of CDR2 (20/36). In addition, replacement Asn residues commonly were acquired at or near the N-terminus of the CDR3 sequence. These may be derived from N-addition or from D-segment genes. Naturally occurring sites showed no preference as to retention or loss.

Together, these data suggest that the V gene sequences in FL are unusual in the acquisition of glycosylation sites and that these sites may be functional. The high incidence in these tumors suggests a positive selection and that glycosylation of V genes in these tumors may play an important role in the pathogenesis of FL and it is possible that they functionally take on the role of the "missing antigen" in the germinal center.

1.5. Technical Aspects of V-Gene Analysis From FL Cells

Ribonucleic acid (RNA) is extracted from tumor cells and followed by complimentary DNA (cDNA) synthesis using oligo (dT) primers. For this purpose, single-cell suspensions or frozen tissue can be used. For the analysis of heavy chain V genes, initial PCR reactions use individual family specific leader primers (1–6), and a mix thereof, together with an appropriate constant region primer (*see* **Table 1** and **Fig. 1**). If dealing with a tumor of unknown Ig isotype, it is judicious to begin investigation with a FR2 consensus primer to constant regions Cμ, Cγ, and Cα. The outcome of these initial PCRs will indicate which

Table 1
Primers for V_H and V_L PCR

Primer Name	Sequence
V_H primers	
V_H Leader 1/7	CTC ACC ATG GAC TGG ACC TGG AG
V_H Leader 2	ATG GAC ATA CTT TGT TCC AGG CTC
V_H Leader 3	CCA TGG AGT TTG GGC TGA GCT GG
V_H Leader 4	ACA TGA AAC AYC TGT GGT TCT TCC
V_H Leader 5	AGT GGG TCA ACC GCC ATC CTC G
V_H Leader 6	ATG TCT GTC TCC TTC CTC ATC TTC
V_H 1/7 FR1 consensus	CAG GTG CAG CTG GTG CAR YCT G
V_H 2 FR1 consensus	CAG RTC ACC TTG AAG GAG TCT G
V_H 3 FR1 consensus	GAG GTG CAG CTG GTG SAG TCY G
V_H 4a FR1 consensus	CAG STG CAG CTG CAG GAG TCS G
V_H 4b FR1 consensus	CAG GTG CAG CTA CAR CAG TGG G
V_H 5 FR1 consensus	GAG GTG CAG CTG KTG CAG TCT G
V_H 6 FR1 consensus	CAG GTA CAG CTG CAG CAG TCA G
FR2 a consensus	TGG RTC CGM CAG SCY YCN GG
FR2 b consensus	GTC CTG CAG GCY YCC GGR AAR RGT CTG GAG TGG
FR3 consensus	ACA CGG CYG TRT ATT ACT GT
Constant μ	GGA ATT CTC ACA GGA GAC GAG G
Constant γ	CTG AGT TCC ACG ACA CCG TCA
Constant α	ATC TGG CTG GGT GCT GCA GAG GCT
J_Ha consensus	ACC TGA GGA GAC GGT GAC C
J_Hb consensus	GTG ACC AGG GTN CCT TGG CCC CAG
J_Hc consensus	TGA GGA GAC GGT GAC CAG GAT CCC TTG GCC CCA G
J_H1	CAG GGC ACC CTG GTC ACC GTC TCC TCA
J_H2	CGT GGC ACC CTG GTC ACT GTC TCC TCA
J_H3	CAA GGG ACA ATG GTC ACC GTC TCT TCA
J_H4/5	CAG GGA ACC CTG GTC ACC GTC TCC TCA
J_H6	CAA GGG ACC ACG GTC ACC GTC TCC TCA
V_κ primers	
Leader 1 consensus	ATR GAC ATG AGR GTS CYY GCT CAG CKC
Leader 2 consensus	ATG AGG CTC CYT GCT CAG CTY CTG GGG
Leader 3 consensus	ATG GAA ACC CCA GCG CAG CTT CTC TTC
Leader 4	ATG GTG TTG CAG ACC CAG GTC TTC ATT
Leader 5	ATG GGG TCC CAG GTT CAC CTC CTC AGC
Leader 6a	ATG TTG CCA TCA CAA CTC ATT GGG TTT
Leader 6b	ATG GTG TCC CCG TTG CAA TTC CTG CGG
Constant κ27	CAA CTG CTC ATC AGA TGG CGG GAA
Constant κ69	AGT TAT TCA GCA GGC ACA CAA C

(continued)

Table 1 (Continued)

Primer Name	Sequence
V_λ primers	
Leader 1 consensus	ATG RCC DGS TYY CCT CTC YTC CTC
Leader 2 consensus	ATG GCC TGG GCT CTG CTS CTC CTC
Leader 3 consensus	ATG GCM TGG RYC VYW CTM YKB CTS
Leader 4a	ATG GCC TGG ACC CAA CTC CTC CTC
Leader 4b	ATG GCT TGG ACC CCA CTC CTC CTC
Leader 4c	ATG GCC TGG GTC TCC TTC TAC
Leader 5 consensus	AGT GCC TGG ACT CYT CTY CTY CTC
Leader 6	ATG GCC TGG GCT CCA CTA CTT CTC
Leader 7	ATG GCC TGG ACT CCT CTC TTT CTG
Leader 8	ATG GCC TGG ATG ATG CTT CTC CTC
Leader 9	ATG GCC TGG GCT CCT CTG CTC CTG
Leader 10	ATG CCC TGG GCT CTG CTC CTC CTG
V_λ FR1-1a	CAG TCT GTG CTG ACT CAG
V_λ FR1-1b	CAG TCT GTG YTG ACG CAG
V_λ FR1-1c	CAG TCT GTC GTG ACG CAG
V_λ FR1-2	CAG TCT GCC CTG ACT CAG
V_λ FR1-3a	TCC TAT GWG CTG ACT CAG
V_λ FR1-3b	TCC TAT GAG CTG ACA CAG
V_λ FR1-3c	TCT TCT GAG CTG ACT CAG
V_λ FR1-3d	TCC TAT GAG CTG ATG CAG
V_λ FR1-4	CAG CYT GTG CTG ACT CAA
V_λ FR1-5	CAG SCT GTG CTG ACT CAG
V_λ FR1-6	AAT TTT ATG CTG ACT CAG
V_λ FR1-7	CAG TCT GTG GTG ACT CAG
V_λ FR1-8	CAG ACT GTG GTG ACC CAG
V_λ FR1-9	CWG CCT GTG CTG ACT CAG
V_λ FR1-10	CAG GCA GGG CTG ACT CAG
Constant λ33	GTT GGC TTG AAG CTC CTC AGA GGA
Constant λ85	CAC RGC TCC CGG GTA GAA GTC ACT
Cloning	
T7	TAA TAC GAC TCA CTA TAG GG
SP6	ATT TAG GTG ACA CTA TAG AA
β actin	
β actin F	TCA TGT TTG AGA CCT TCA A
β actin R	GTC TTT GCG GAT GTC CAC G

R = A+G; Y = C +T; K = G+T; S = C+G; N = A+C+G+T, M = A+C, W = A+T

Where primers have more than 1 consensus sequence, for example. JH a, b and c, an equal mix is prepared.

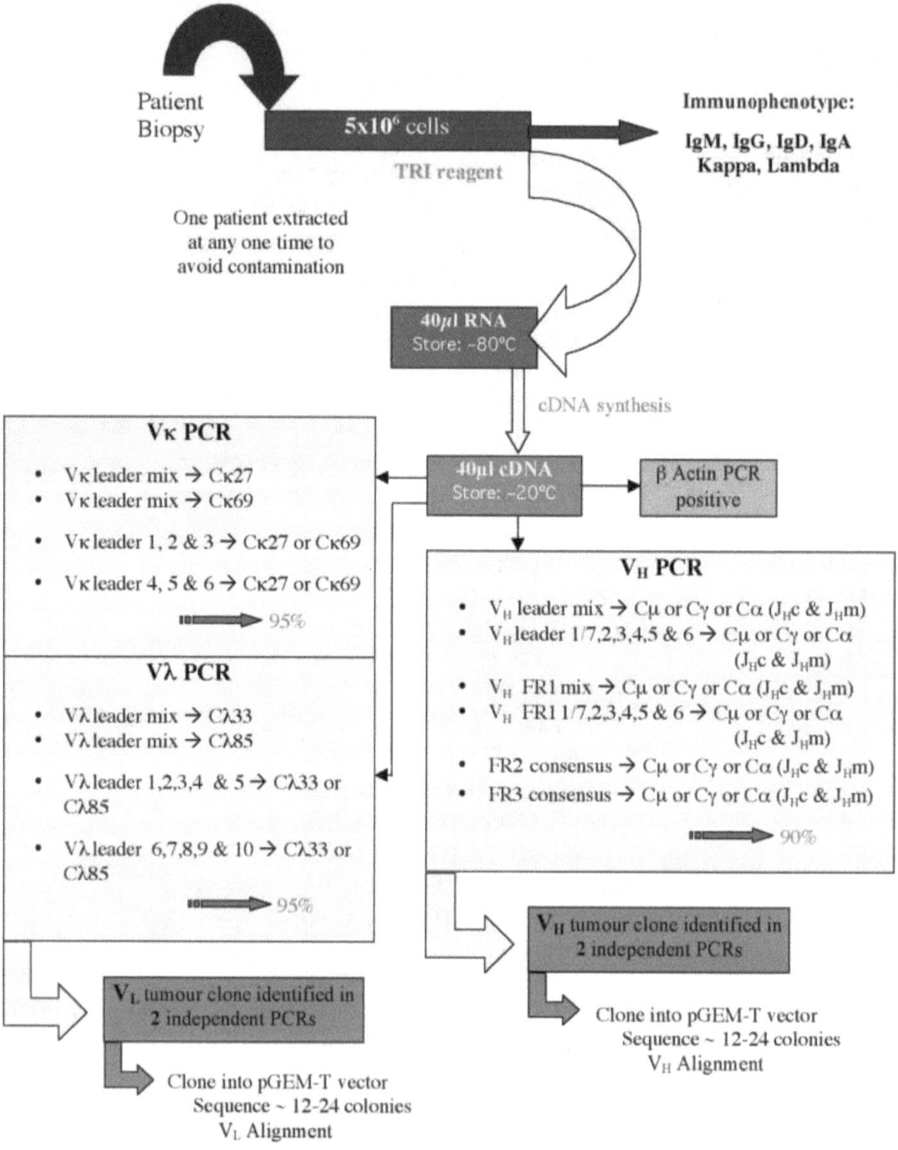

Fig. 1. Flowchart of V gene analysis. *See* **Color Plate 5**, following page 270.

heavy chain constant region is used by the tumor clone and will focus subsequent efforts with individual leader primers. It also is possible to use a J_H consensus primer as the 3' primer, but this is more likely to fail due to the presence of mutations in J_H.

For the amplification of the light chain, PCRs using family specific leader primers (Vκ1-6 or Vλ1-10), either individually or as a mix, together with a constant region primer is usually sufficient to identify the tumor clone (*see* **Fig. 1**). In general, we find that the V_L gene of a tumor clone is identified more easily than the V_H gene. This is most likely caused by the intrinsically lower mutational rates found in these genes.

Ideally, we seek to obtain a single product produced from any particular primer pair, although multiple products occur. Amplified products are gel extracted, directly sequenced, and aligned to the V Base database. For those sequences that align cleanly to V and J segments, a proposed germ line can be constructed.

PCR products that are polyclonal, either across the entire sequence or over the CDR3 alone as identified through analysis of the electropherogram (EPG), are not pursued. Accordingly, and for cases in which the initial PCR fails, revised cycling conditions for the PCR with a touch-down protocol or using existing primer pairs or with different primer combinations are likely to give a PCR product. For V_H genes, "reserve primers" are designed to anneal to FR1, FR2 and FR3 regions and the individual J_H segments (*see* **Fig. 1**).

Potentially clonal sequences are always confirmed by a second independent PCR. After two PCR products with identical sequence have been identified, one or both PCR products are cloned and 12–24 colonies sequenced. 10 tumor derived sequences are sufficient to assess the intraclonal variation of the tumor clone.

Although this approach is successful in the majority of cases, there are instances when it is not possible to define the V_H and/or V_L clone. This may be either because there are not enough tumor cells in the population or perhaps because the mutation in the leader or framework regions is too extensive to permit binding of the primers. In such cases, it can be useful to employ gene scan of FR3-$J_H$consensus PCR products to confirm a clonal population is present. Polyclonality, as revealed by gene scan, makes it less likely that the clonal signature of a tumor sample will be determined and therefore gene-scanning can avoid extensive and unsuccessful PCR and cloning.

Very occasionally, cloning reveals more than one sequence, suggesting the presence of multiple clones. We have observed this phenomenon in the light chains of a small number of FL cases, which can be explained by dual light chain rearrangement or receptor editing. In these cases, we have increased our cloning to determine and select the dominant clone. However, we have not experienced this when rescuing heavy chain variable regions in FL. We think this is related to the use of cDNA rather than genomic DNA, which avoids amplification of the second allelically excluded and nonfunctional rearranged V_H genes. In the single instance during which we observed two sequences in multiple clones identified from a single patient, it proved to be the result of contamination with material from a different patient and was resolved, but highlighted the potential risk of working with samples from multiple patients at one time. Theoretically, it is possible that a small minority of tumors express two V_H sequences in the same tumor cell population or that tumors may be truly biclonal. In other B-cell malignancies, this has been reported, and we have observed this occasionally in DLBCL, but in germinal center type B-cell lymphomas we would expect to find this in less than 5% of cases. In practical terms such a result is highly suspicious of contamination.

2. Materials

2.1. Cell Storage and Freezing

2.1.1. Preparing the Cell Suspension

All work should be conducted in a laminar flow tissue culture hood.

1. Patient biopsy.
2. Sterile tissue plates (10 cm in diameter).
3. Sterile scalpel.
4. Sterile tweezers.
5. Sterile metal tea strainer.
6. Sterile RMPI, store at 4°C.
7. Sterile 10- or 20-mL syringes.
8. 50-mL Falcon tubes.

2.1.2. Cell Counting

1. A hemocytometer, light microscope, and counter.
2. Trypan blue stain 0.4% (0.85% saline, Sigma).

2.1.3. Culture Media

1. RPMI 1640 Medium + 25 mM HEPES + L-glutamine (Gibco, Paisley, UK). Complete RPMI:
   - 500 mL of RPMI 1640 Medium + 25 m*M* HEPES + L-glutamine.
   - 5 mL of PSG, 100X (penicillin, 10,000 U/mL, streptomycin sulfate, 10,000 U/mL; L-glutamine, 29.2 mg/mL; sodium citrate, 10 m*M*; Gibco)
   - 5 mL of sodium pyruvate, 100 m*M* (Gibco).

2.1.4. Freezing of Cells

1. 1.6-mL Sterile cryovials and a cryo 1°C freezing container.
2. Freezing medium: 50% human Ab serum, complement free, batch tested (Sigma); 40% complete RPMI (*see* **Subheading 2.1.3.**); and 10% dimethylsulfoxide (DMSO).
3. Isopropanol (warning: flammable).

2.2. Preparation of cDNA

2.2.1. RNA Extraction

TRI Reagent (Sigma). In addition to the items listed below, a tabletop temperature-controlled microcentrifuge, a vortex, and 1.6-mL polypropylene Eppendorf (RNase-free) tubes are required.

NOTE: Phenol and TRI reagent are toxic carcinogens and irritant. Meticulous handling and adherence to laboratory safety and good laboratory practice is essential; *see* also **Note 1.**

1. TRI Reagent™; store at 4°C.
2. Chloroform.
3. Isopropanol (warning: flammable).
4. Ethanol (warning: flammable).
5. RNase-free water (as a cheap and easy alternative we use standard water for injection, available in 5-mL or 10-mL aliquots from NHS hospital supplies).

2.2.2. cDNA Synthesis

Superscript™ First-Strand Synthesis system for RT-PCR (Invitrogen, Paisley, UK). In addition to the items listed below, a tabletop microcentrifuge, wet ice, a thermocycler and the appropriate thin-walled polypropylene tubes are also required.

1. Diethylpyrocarbonate-treated water/water for injection.
2. 10 m*M* dNTP mix: 10 m*M* each of dATP, dCTP, dGTP, and dTTP.
3. Oligo$(dT)_{12-18}$, 0.5 µg/µL.
4. 10X RT buffer: 200 m*M* Tris-HCl, pH 8.4, 500 n*M* KCl.
5. 25 m*M* $MgCl_2$.
6. 0.1 *M* dithiothreitol (DTT).
7. RNaseOUT™ Recombinant RNase Inhibitor (40 U/mL).
8. Superscript™ II Reverse Transcriptase (50 U/µL).
9. *Escherichia coli* RNase H (2 U/µL).
10. 1 µL of control GSP.
11. 1–5 µg of total RNA from the sample.
12. 1 µL of control RNA.

2.3. PCR and Related Procedures

2.3.1. PCR

HotStartTaq™ (QIAGEN, Crawley, UK). The PCR is performed using a thermocycler with the corresponding thin-walled polypropylene tubes. Additional items required are wet ice, a laminar flow cabinet, and a tabletop microcentrifuge.

1. 10X PCR buffer: 15 m*M* $MgCl_2$, Tris-HCl, KCl, $(NH_4)SO_4$.
2. HotStartTaq DNA Polymerase (2.5 U/µL).
3. 2.5 m*M* dNTP mix: 2.5 m*M* each dATP, dCTP, dGTP, dTTP.
4. 1–5 µL template cDNA.
5. 1 µL 5' Primer(20 pmol/µL).
6. 1 µL 3' Primer(20 pmol/µL).
7. Diethylpyrocarbonate-treated water.

Primers are diluted to working concentration from stocks solutions and stored as aliquots at –20°C to minimize the possibility of contamination.

2.3.2. Agarose gel Electrophoresis

Items required are a gel tray and comb, a microwave, a gel tank, a power source and a UV light source, sterile scalpels, gloves, and face shield.

NOTE: Ethidium bromide is a carcinogen. Meticulous handling and adherence to laboratory safety and good laboratory practice is essential.

1. Agarose (Sigma).
2. Ethidium bromide, 10 mg/mL (Sigma).
3. 1X TAE buffer (40 m*M* Tris-acetate, 10 m*M* ethylenediamine tetraacetic acid).
4. 2µL of 1 kb + DNA ladder, 1 µg/µL (Invitrogen).

2.3.3. PCR Purification

Purification requires the use of the QIAquick Gel Extraction kit (QIAGEN). Other items required are 1.6-mL polypropylene Eppendorf tubes, a sterile scalpel, a precision scale, a heat block at 50°C, and a tabletop microcentrifuge.

1. Gel solubilization buffer QG.
2. Isopropanol (warning: flammable).
3. QIAquick spin column and 2-mL collection tube.
4. Ethanol (warning: flammable).
5. Wash buffer PE.
6. Elution buffer (EB) = 10 m*M* Tris-Cl, pH 8.5.

2.4. Sequencing

2.4.1. Sequencing Reaction

BigDye® Terminator v1.1 Cycle Sequencing Kit and ABI 377 automatic DNA sequencer (Applied Biosystems, Warrington, UK). The sequencing reaction is performed using a thermocycler with the corresponding thin-walled polypropylene tubes.

1. BigDye Terminator Ready Reaction Mix (A-dye terminator labeled with dichloro [R6G], C-dye terminator labeled with dichloro [R0X], G-dye terminator labeled with dichloro [R110], T-dye terminator labeled with dichloro [TAMRA], dNTP [dATP, dCTP, dITP, dUTP], and AmpliTaq DNA polymerase).
2. 5X sequencing buffer: 400 m*M* Tris-HCl, 10 m*M* $MgCl_2$, pH 9.0.
3. 1 µL of 5' or 3' primer, 1.6 pmol.
4. 5 µL of template DNA (PCR product or purified plasmid).

Additional items required for precipitation of sequencing reactions after cycling include 1.6-mL polypropylene Eppendorf tubes, wet ice, and a temperature-controlled tabletop microcentrifuge.

1. 3 *M* sodium acetate (pH 4.2).
2. Ethanol, 100% and 75% (warning: flammable).
3. Loading buffer = Loading dye: 25 m*M* EDTA, pH 8.0, 50 mg/mL Blue Dextran, Formamide at 1:5.

2.4.2. Sequencing Analysis

MacVector software (Oxford Molecular, Oxford, UK) and Entrez and V-Base databases (Center for Protein Engineering, MRC Center, Cambridge, UK; http://www.mrc-cpe.cam.ac.uk/vbase-ok) are required for analysis.

2.5. Cloning

2.5.1. Ligation

pGEM®-T Vector System I (Promega, Southampton, UK). Additional items required are 1.6-mL polypropylene Eppendorf tubes and a fridge at 4°C.

1. pGEM-T empty vector (50 ng/µL).
2. T4 DNA Ligase (3 Weiss U/µL).
3. 2X rapid ligation buffer: 60 m*M* Tris-HCl, pH 7.8, 20 m*M* $MgCl_2$, 20 m*M* DTT, 2 m*M* ATP 10% polyethylene glycol. Store 2X buffer in single use aliquots at –20°C. Avoid multiple freeze-thaw cycles.
4. 3 µL of purified PCR product.

2.5.2. Transformation

JM109 Competent cells (Promega). Additional items required are 20-mL universal tubes, 1.6-mL polypropylene Eppendorf tubes, wet ice, a waterbath set at 42°C, an orbital shaker set at 37°C, a tabletop microcentrifuge, spreaders, and a warm room set at 37°C.

1. 50 µL of JM109 competent cells.
2. 5 µL of ligate.

3. 1 mL of LB.
4. LB/Agar Amp, 100 plates.

2.5.2.1. LB

Millers LB broth (Sigma) is used. Additional items required include glassware, weighing scales, a flea and stirring plate, and an autoclave.

1. 25 g/L LB.
2. Autoclave and cool.

LB Amp 100 contains: Penbritin® Ampicillin, 100 mg/mL; add at 1 µL/mL to cool LB.

2.5.2.2. LB/Agar

Millers LB broth (Sigma.) and Bacto®-Agar (BD Biosciences, Oxford, UK) should be used. Additional items required include glassware, weighing scales, a flea and stirring plate, and an autoclave.

1. 25g/L LB.
2. 15g/L Agar.
3. Autoclave and cool.

LB/Agar Amp 100 contains: Penbritin® ampicillin, 100 mg/mL; add at 1 µL/mL to LB/Agar cooled to less than 50°C.

2.5.2.3. LB/Agar Amp100 Plates

Additional items required include a microwave, sterile Petri dishes, and a spreader.

1. LB/Agar Amp100 plates.
2. X-Gal (5-bromo-4-chloro-3 indolyl-β-D-galactoside), 50 mg/mL; use 20 µL/plate.
3. Isopropyl β-D-thiogalactopyranoside, 100 m*M*; use 100 µL/plate.

2.5.3. Plasmid Purification

QIAprep® Miniprep (QIAGEN) is needed, as well as 1.6-mL polypropylene Eppendorf tubes, a tabletop microcentrifuge, a vortex, and a QIAvac vacuum manifold (optional).

1. Resuspension buffer P1.
2. Lysis buffer P2.
3. Neutralization buffer N3.
4. QIAprep spin column and 2-mL collection tube.
5. Binding buffer PB.
6. Ethanol, flammable.
7. Wash buffer PE.
8. Elution buffer: 10 m*M* Tris-HCl, pH 8.5.

3. Methods

3.1. Technical Comments

The immunophenotype of the tumor provides a useful starting point for analysis. Expression of IgM, IgD, IgG, and IgA is evaluated and can be used to determine which constant region primer is most likely to identify the tumor clone. Knowledge of kappa and lambda expression can identify the light chain used by the tumor clone and, thus, the appropriate primers can be selected. In conjunction with other B-cell markers, including CD20 and CD19, immunophenotypic information can give an indication as to the percentage of tumor cells in the cell population. A low percentage can be a reason for failure to identify a tumor-derived clone.

3.2. Cell Storage and Freezing

Diagnostic lymph node biopsies are received fresh on the day of surgery and processed on the same day. An aliquot of cells is used for immunophenotyping by fluorescence-activated cell sorting analysis for IgM, IgD, IgG, and IgA and kappa and lambda expression.

1. Using a sterile scalpel, lymph nodes are cut into small pieces and the cells dispersed by forcing through a fine sieve (e.g., a sterile metal tea strainer) into sterile RPMI medium.
2. Cells are collected, centrifuged, and washed once in RPMI.
3. After resuspension, cell viability is assessed with 0.4% trypan blue stain and aliquots of 1×10^7 cells/mL are resuspended in freezing medium.
4. Freezing follows a step-wise drop in temperature to –80°C using cryopreservation protocols.
5. Cells are transferred to Liquid N_2 after 24 h.

Alternatively, material from frozen tissue blocks can be used. 5- to 10-μm sections are cut using a cryostat and transferred directly into 1mL TRI Reagent with a sterile needle. Five to 20 sections per milliliter of TRI reagent should be sufficient to obtain enough RNA for analysis, but the number of sections needed ultimately is dependent on the size of the tissue block. Care should be taken to avoid thawing of the tissue block prior to, during and after cutting.

3.3. Preparation of cDNA

3.3.1. RNA Extraction

RNA is extracted from 5×10^6 to 1×10^7 cells using 1 mL of TRI reagent (Sigma) and following the manufacturers instructions in a triphasic separation (*see* **Note 1** regarding RNA handling).

1. Rapidly thaw one aliquot of cells at 37°C and pellet by touch spin.
2. Resuspend cells in approx 100 µL of RPMI medium before adding 1 mL of TRI reagent; Mix thoroughly and allow the sample to stand for 5 min at room temperature.
3. Add 0.2 mL of chloroform, shake vigorously, and allow to stand for 15 min.
4. Centrifuge at 12000*g* for 15 min at 4°C.
5. Transfer the colorless upper aqueous phase containing the RNA into a fresh tube with 0.5 mL isopropanol and allow to stand for 5–10 min.
6. Centrifuge at 12000*g* for 10 min at 4°C.
7. Remove the supernatant and wash once with 75% ethanol.
8. After a final centrifugation step at 12,000*g* for 5 min, air dry the resulting RNA pellet for a few minutes and resuspend into an appropriate volume of RNase-free sterile water (approx 40–80 µL).
9. Quantitative analysis of the RNA is performed using a spectrophotometer (A_{260}) and the RNA is then stored at –80°C.

3.3.2. cDNA Synthesis

First-strand cDNA is synthesized from total RNA using the Superscript II system (Invitrogen) with an oligo-dT primer according to the manufacturer's instructions (*see* **Note 1**).

1. Up to 5 µg of total RNA is transferred to an RNase-free sterile tube, mixed with 2 µg of oligo-dT primer and incubated at 65°C for 5 min.
2. A mix of 10X RT buffer, 25 m*M* $MgCl_2$, 0.1 *M* DTT, and RNaseOUT-RNase inhibitor is added and incubated at 42°C for 2 min.
3. 50 units of Superscript II reverse transcriptase is then added and incubated for a further 50 min at 42°C.
4. The reaction is terminated by heating to 70°C for 15 min and placed on ice.
5. After a final addition of 1 µL of RNaseH and incubation at 37°C for 20 min, the synthesized cDNA can be immediately amplified or stored at –20°C.

3.4. Heavy-Chain PCR

3.4.1. V_H PCR: Set-Up and Cycling Conditions

V_H genes are amplified from the cDNA by PCR with HotStart Taq (QIAGEN) using 5' and 3' oligonucleotide primers designed specifically (*see* **Subheading 3.4.2.**). It is advisable to check the quality of the cDNA before attempting V gene rescue using primers designed to amplify a standard house-keeping gene, such as β actin.

1. 1–5 µL of cDNA template.
2. 1 µL of 5' primer, 20 pmol.
3. 1µL of 3' primer, 20 pmol.
4. 10 µL of dNTPs, 2.5 m*M*.
5. 1 µL (2.5U) HotStart Taq DNA polymerase.

6. 10 µL of 10X PCR buffer.
7. Up to 50 µL of total volume with sterile water.

All PCRs are set up in a laminar flow cabinet to avoid contamination. Negative controls, in which the cDNA is absent from the reaction, are run in parallel for every primer pair. Thus contamination of any component of the PCR reaction with cDNA or DNA can be identified immediately (*see* also **Notes 2–6**).

"Touchdown" PCR cycling conditions for the amplification of V_H genes and β actin (with the exception of FR3-constant region primer combinations; see below) consists of the following:

1. Initial denaturing step at 94°C for 15 min.
2. A single cycle of 94°C for 30 s, 60°C for 45 s, and 72°C for 45 s followed by a single cycle of 94°C for 30 s, 59.5°C for 45 s, and 72°C for 45 s followed by a single cycle of 94°C for 30 s, 59°C for 45 s, and 72°C for 45 s. In the touchdown PCR, the primer annealing temperature is reduced from 60°C by 0.5°C per cycle, to 54°C.
3. 30 cycles of 94°C for 30 s, 54°C for 45 s, and 72°C for 45 s.
4. A final extension step is performed for 10 min at 72°C.

Standard PCR cycling conditions for the amplification of FR3-constant region are as follows:

1. Initial denaturing step at 94°C for 15 min.
2. 55 cycles of 94°C for 10 s, 57°C for 10 s, and 72°C for 25 s.
3. Final extension step of 10 min at 72°C.

3.4.2. Primer Combinations

3.4.2.1. If the Constant Region Phenotype Is Known

Begin V_H gene rescue with the following:

1. V_H leader mix: constant (Cµ or Cγ or Cα , as indicated by immunophenotype).
2. Individual V_H leader 1/7 and 2 and 3 and 4 and 5 and 6: constant.

3.4.2.2. If the Constant Region Phenotype Is NOT Known

In this situation, it is beneficial to perform a small number of preliminary PCRs to identify the constant region using a 5' primer designed to anneal to the FR2 region together with all available 3' constant region and J_H primers:

FR2 consensus—Cµ and Cγ and Cα and J_H consensus and J_H mix

FR2 is selected because it is less likely to be mutated than the leader and FR1 regions. Therefore, the chance of mismatches between the V_H gene and the primers designed to hybridize to this region is lower resulting in a greater chance of amplification.

3.4.3. Outcome of First PCR (see also 3.6. Gel Analysis and 3.7. Sequencing)

See also **Notes 2** to **6.**

3.4.3.1. If the Constant Region Phenotype Is Known

1. If two or more PCR products have similar or repeated sequences with a clonally related CDR3, then the tumor-related V_H gene has been identified and confirmed; proceed to clone one PCR product.
2. If one PCR product has a clonal sequence through V_H, CDR3 ,and J_H that can be aligned successfully to VBase, attempt to confirm this sequence by repeating the PCR using the same primer pair and/or set up a second PCR using the family specific leader primer for the identified germ line donor together with the constant region primer. One or both of these PCR products should confirm the sequence and clonally related CDR3. Proceed to cloning.
3. If multiple PCR products have clonal sequence through V_H, CDR3 to J_H, but the sequences are not similar and do not share a clonally related CDR3, then attempt to identify the "true" tumor-related V_H gene by repeating all the relevant PCRs. If more than one sequence is repeated, pursue both sequences via cloning. It is rare to find true V_H biclonality in FL; therefore, rigorous checks for contamination need to be performed at this point to eliminate this possibility.
4. If the V_H leader PCRs failed to recover an unambiguous sequence, then, in this case, the primer pairs used for the PCR need to be revised. It is useful to perform FR2 to all possible constant region primers and to J_H consensus and J_H mix primers as a next step, since we have found that these primer combinations have a high hit rate for identification of V_H (for outcome, *see* **Subheading 3.4.3.2.**).

3.4.3.2. If the Constant Region Phenotype Is Not Known

In this instance, the preliminary PCR serves to identify the heavy chain constant region used by the tumor clone and to determine which constant region primers to use in later PCRs.

1. If one FR2 PCR product has a clonal sequence through the end of V_H, CDR3 and J_H that can be aligned successfully to VBase, then a partial sequence for the tumor-related V_H gene (FR2-constant) and the constant region it uses has been identified. Proceed to perform PCRs using the appropriate individual family-specific V_H leader primers to the identified constant primer as in **Subheading 3.4.2.1.** Once confirmed, the leader PCR product (full-length V_H gene) can be cloned.
2. Two or more FR2 PCR products amplified from different constant region primers have similar or repeated sequences with a clonally related CDR3: A partial sequence for the tumor-related V_H gene (FR2-constant) is identified and is shown to express multiple isotypes. Proceed to perform PCRs using the appropriate individual family specific V_H leader primers to one or all of the identified constant primer, as in 3.4.2.1. Once confirmed a single leader PCR product (full-length V_H gene) can be cloned.
3. If multiple FR2 PCR products have clonal sequence through the end of V_H, CDR3 to J_H but the sequences are not similar and do not share a clonally related CDR3,

attempt to identify the "true" tumor-related V_H gene by performing PCRs using the appropriate individual family specific V_H leader primers to the identified constant primer, as in **Subheading 3.4.2.1.** If more than one sequence is repeated, pursue both sequences via cloning if contamination has been ruled out.

4. If the FR2 PCRs failed to recover an unambiguous sequence, then experience has shown that FR2 and constant primer pairs for PCR usually will lead to the identification of the tumor-related V_H if it is there to be found, but this is not always the case and, therefore, further primer combinations should be investigated (*see* **Subheading 3.4.4.**). However, if failure to detect a clonal V_H sequence from a FR2 PCR is accompanied by failure to identify the partner V_L, it is likely that further investigation will be fruitless and may indicate problems with the tumor load. Genescan of FR3-$J_H$consensus PCR products can be employed the confirm polyclonality of the sample (*see* **Subheading 3.7.3.**).

3.4.4. If V_H Leader PCRs Yield Polyclonal Sequences

It is possible that extensive mutation of the tumor-related V_H gene within the leader region causes failure of V_H leader primers to hybridize to this region and results in a lower amplification efficiency. This is masked by the amplification of normal B-cell V_H rearrangements and leads to polyclonal products. The next step is to use primers designed to anneal to the framework regions, where sequence is inherently conserved. The following primer pairs are used until the clone is identified or the primer combinations are exhausted. In our laboratory the failure rate for the identification of tumor-related V_H genes using these primer sets is approx 10%.

3.4.4.1. Framework 1 Region Primers

1. V_H FR1 mix: Cμ and Cγ and Cα and J_H consensus and J_H mix.
2. V_H FR1 1/7and 2, 3, 4, 5, and 6: Cμ and Cγ and Cα and J_H consensus and J_H mix.

3.4.4.2. Framework 2 Region Primers

V_H FR2 consensus: Cμ and Cγ and Cα and J_H consensus and J_H mix.

3.4.4.3. Framework 3 Region Primers

V_H FR3 consensus: Cμ and Cγ and Cα and J_H consensus and J_H mix.

3.5. Light-Chain PCR

3.5.1. V_L PCR: Set-Up and Cycling Conditions

V_L genes are amplified by PCR in the same way as for V_H genes (refer to **Subheading 3.4.1.**) with the exception of the "Touchdown" PCR cycling conditions, which are listed below.

1. Initial denaturing step at 94°C for 15 min.
2. A single cycle of 94°C for 30 s, 56°C for 45 s, and 72°C for 45 s followed by a single cycle of 94°C for 30 s, 55.5°C for 45 s, and 72°C for 45 s followed by a

single cycle of 94°C for 30 s, 55°C for 45 s. and 72°C for 45 s. In the touchdown PCR, the primer annealing temperature is reduced from 56°C by 0.5°C per cycle to 50°C.

3. 30 cycles of 94°C for 30 s, 50°C for 45 s, and 72°C for 45 s.
4. Final extension step at 72°C for 10 min.

3.5.2. Primer Combinations

3.5.2.1. If the Light-Chain Restriction Is Known

Begin Vκ gene rescue with, Vκ leader mix constant (constant κ27 and constant κ69).

Begin Vλ gene rescue with, Vλ leader mix constant (constant λ33 and constant λ85).

Duplicating PCRs with two different constant region primers increases the likelihood of identifying and confirming the V_L tumor clone in a single PCR.

3.5.2.2. If the Light-Chain Restriction Is NOT Known

For an unknown light-chain restriction, both Vκ and Vλ leader mix to constant PCRs (as listed above) are performed.

3.5.3. Outcome of First PCR (see also 3.6. Gel Analysis and 3.7. Sequencing)

For more information, also *See* **Notes 2–6.**

1. If both light-chain PCR products have similar or repeated sequences with a clonally related CDR3, then Tumor-related V_L gene has been identified and confirmed; proceed to clone one PCR product.
2. If only one PCR product has a clonal sequence through V_L, CDR3 to J_L that can be aligned successfully to VBase, then attempt to confirm this sequence by repeating the PCR using the same primer combination and/or set up a second PCR using the family-specific leader primer for the identified germ line donor. It is likely that one or both of these PCRs will confirm the sequence and clonally related CDR3. Proceed to cloning.
3. If both PCR products have clonal sequence through V_L, CDR3 to J_L but the sequences are not similar and do not share a clonally related CDR3, then attempt to confirm both the V_L gene sequences by repeating the relevant PCRs and in addition set up a second PCR using the family-specific leader primer for each of the identified germ line donors. If both sequences are validated by a second independent PCR, pursue both via cloning. In our experience, dual light chain rearrangements occur in about 8% of FL; however, be sure to rule out possible PCR contamination.
4. If both PCR products fail to recover an unambiguous sequence then, in this case, the primer pairs used for the PCR need to be revised (*see* **Subheading 3.5.4.**)

The outcomes listed above also apply in cases where the light chain restriction is not known. Both Vκ and Vλ PCRs are performed and the products analyzed independently. In the majority of cases, either one or both of the Vκ or Vλ PCR products will have a clonal sequence that can be aligned to VBase, with polyclonal products for the second light chain. However, it is possible that both Vκ and Vλ PCR products yield polyclonal sequences and, therefore, it is necessary to use individual family-specific primers for both Vκ and Vλ, sequentially until the tumor-related V_L is identified. Because Vκ rearrangements are found more frequently than Vλ (60:40, for normal B-cells), it is logical to start with the investigation of Vκ followed by Vλ. For more information, *see* **Notes 2–6**.

3.5.4. If V_L Leader Mix PCRs Yield Polyclonal Sequences

In many cases, the tumor-related V_L gene can be readily identified using a leader mix together with a constant region primer. However, if this primer pair yields only polyclonal sequences, individual family-specific leader primers can be used. Because Vκ and Vλ have numerous families, each with a disproportionate number of germ line donors, we begin investigation with the largest families first before moving on to those families with fewer germ line donors until the clone is identified or the primer combinations are exhausted. In our laboratory the failure rate for the identification of tumor-related V_L using these primer sets is less than 5%. This is lower than for the V_H genes and is likely a consequence of an intrinsically lower level of somatic mutation in V_L genes.

3.5.4.1. Individual Family-Specific Vκ Leader Primers

Vκ Leader 1 and 2 and 3 (constant κ27 or constant κ69) followed by Vκ Leader 4 and 5 and 6 (constant κ27 or constant κ69).

3.5.4.2. Individual Family-Specific Vλ Leader Primers

Vλ leader 1 and 2 and 3 and 4 and 5: constant (constant λ33 or constant λ85), followed by Vλ leader 6 and 7 and 8 and 9 and 10: contstant (constant λ33 or constant λ85).

3.6. Agarose Gel Electrophoresis

PCR products are separated by 1% agarose gel electrophoresis against 1 kb+ DNA ladder (Life Technologies, Paisley, UK) and visualized with ethidium bromide under UV light. Bands of the appropriate size (350–400 bp) were excised and purified using the QIAquick Gel Extraction Kit (QIAGEN). Remember to take a photograph for documentation!

1. Excise band and weigh.
2. Add 3 volumes of buffer QG to 1 volume gel (100 mg~100 µL) and incubate at 50°C for 10 min.

3. Add 1 volume of isopropanol, mix, and apply to the column.
4. Centrifuge at 20,000*g* for 1 min.
5. Wash once with buffer QG (optional) followed by one wash with buffer PE.
6. Elute DNA in an appropriate volume of buffer EB.

3.7. Sequencing

3.7.1. Sequencing Reaction

Direct DNA sequencing of PCR products is performed on an ABI 377 automatic DNA sequencer (Applied Biosystems, Warrington, UK) using ABI Prism BigDye Terminator Kit (Applied Biosystems) in a final volume of 10 µL.

1. 5 µL of PCR product.
2. 1 µL 5' primer, 1.6 pmol.
3. 2 µL Big Dye.
4. 2 µL 5X sequencing buffer.

Sequencing PCR cycling conditions consist of 25 cycles of 96°C for 10 s, 50°C for 50 s, and 60°C for 4 min. This is followed by Sodium Acetate and ethanol precipitation.

1. 10 µL of sequencing reaction is added to 1 µL of 3 *M* sodium acetate (pH 5.2) and 25 µL 100% ethanol and placed on ice for 15 min.
2. Samples are centrifuged at 20,000*g* for 30 min at 4°C.
3. Samples are washed once with 75% ethanol.
4. After air drying, pellets are resuspended in 1 µL of loading buffer (1:5 of loading dye:formamide) for immediate analysis or storage at –20°C.

3.7.2. Sequence Analysis

For sequence alignment analysis, use MacVector software (Oxford Molecular, Oxford, UK) aligned to Entrez and V-BASE databases (Center for Protein Engineering, MRC Center, Cambridge, UK; http://www.mrc-cpe.cam.ac.uk./vbase-ok), which contain all known human germ line Ig V region genes.

Tumor-related V genes were defined by the presence of repeated sequences with a clonally related CDR3. Somatic hypermutation is determined by comparison of the sequence to the germline V genes with the greatest homology. The percentage of somatic mutation is calculated from the aligned sequences from the beginning of FR1 to the end of FR3 (*see* **Notes 7–9**).

3.7.2. Genescan Analysis

In the event that all PCR attempts using the available primer sets fail to identify the tumor-related V_H and V_L clones, GeneScan™ can be used to assess the polyclonality of a sample. This technique uses a simple V_H PCR from FR3 to a 6-FAM-labeled J_H consensus primer according to the set up and cycling conditions listed in **Subheading 3.4.1.** The resulting approx 100 bp PCR product is run directly on an ABI 377 automatic DNA sequencer (Applied Biosystems) incorporating the GeneScan™ Analysis software. If the product is polyclonal, it is very unlikely that the clonal signature of the tumor will be identified with further investigation. Alternatively, GeneScan™ may reveal a clonal population. The FR3-J_H PCR can then be sequenced to identify the clonal CDR3 and subsequent PCR using a CDR3-specific reverse primer. This, together with individual leader and FR1 primers, may resolve the full-length V_H gene sequence.

3.8. Cloning

3.8.1. Ligation

Clonal PCR products are ligated into pGEM-T vector system I (Promega).

1. 3 µL of PCR product.
2. 1 µL of Empty pGEM-T vector.
3. 1 µL of T4 DNA ligase.
4. 5 µL of 2X buffer.

Ligations reactions are incubated at 4°C overnight.

3.8.2. Transformation

Transformation into JM109 competent *Escherichia coli* cells (Promega) follows:

1. Gently mix 5 µL of ligation product with 50 µL of JM109 cells and leave on ice for 20 min.
2. Heat shock cells at 42°C for *exactly* (use a timer!) 45 s and return to ice for 5 min.
3. Add 1 mL of LB and shake at 37°C for 1 h.
4. Plate cells onto X-Gal/0.1 *M* Isopropyl β-D-thiogalactopyranoside, Amp100 Agar and leave overnight at 37°C.

The next day, 12 randomly picked bacterial colonies are each used to spike 2 mL Amp100 LB. Grow bacterial cultures at 37°C overnight.

3.8.3. Plasmid Purification

Plasmid is purified from the bacterial cultures using the QIAprep Miniprep kit (QIAGEN).

1. Pellet cultures by centrifugation at 7000*g* for 1 min and resusupend in 250 µL of buffer P1.
2. Add 250 µL of lysis buffer P2 and mix by inversion.
3. Neutralize the reaction within 5 min by the addition of 350 µL of buffer N3. Leaving the alkaline solution for longer will hydrolyze the DNA (see manufacturer's instructions).

4. After centrifugation at 20,000*g* for 10 min, apply the supernatant to the column and leave for 1 min.
5. Centrifuge at 20,000*g* for 1 min
6. Wash once with buffer PB, followed by two washes with buffer PE.
7. Ensure a final centrifugation at 20,000*g* for 3 min before eluting DNA with 100 μL of buffer EB

All plasmids are sequenced in both directions using T7 and SP6 forward and reverse primers. We aim to collect approx 10 clonally related sequences to confidently assess intraclonal variation in FL.

4. Notes

1. When working with RNA, gloves should be worn at all times and touching contaminated surfaces and equipment should be avoided; RNases can be reintroduced by contact with ungloved hands and equipment or with unfiltered air. Use sterile, RNase-free tubes and pipet tips and purchase reagents that are free of RNases. Separate reagents and plasticware used for RNA work from general-use reagents in the laboratory. Place all RNA samples on ice; RNA is susceptible to degradation when left at room temperature.
2. If no amplified products result from the first round of PCR, check cDNA integrity with β-actin primers if not previously performed. If, subsequently, (1) β-actin PCR fails, repeat cDNA synthesis, ensuring that positive and negative controls are run in parallel, and repeat using new cDNA synthesis reagents if necessary. In the event that the β-actin PCR fails again and assuming that cDNA synthesis reagents are viable, proceed to check the quality of the RNA and assess sample collection and storage. (2) If β-actin PCR successful, then the cDNA is viable. Repeat PCR using more cDNA template OR increase the number of PCR cycles OR lower primer annealing temperatures OR try alternative primer combinations OR use the above in combination.
3. If amplified products are weak, repeat PCR using more cDNA template OR increase the number of PCR cycles OR use in combination.
4. If multiple products are amplified from a single primer pair, excise, purify, and sequence each individual band that falls within the expected size range. Alternatively, repeat the PCR using standard (i.e., not "touchdown") cycling conditions and an increased annealing temperature.
5. If the sequencing of PCR product fails, check that the sequencing primer is correct. If not, repeat the sequencing reaction using more template DNA. If this coincides with a low yield of the original PCR product, disregard this product and attempt to increase the yield of product in a repeat PCR (refer to **Subheading 4.2.**) before resequencing.
6. If the sequencing of the PCR product appears clean but does not align to the VBase database, disregard this product. It is not Ig and most probably results from contamination for example from bacterial DNA.
7. If the sequence of the PCR product will (1) align to a V segment but not a J segment or (2) not align to a V or a J segment, examine the electropherogram for the pres-

ence of "double peaks" which indicate the existence of more than one sequence. Pay particular attention to the CDR3 region, from the end of V to constant, which may be polyclonal even if the V segment appears clonal. This PCR product is polyclonal and likely results from the amplification of V genes from normal B-cells, which exist within the tumor cell population.

8. If the cloning of the PCR product yields a low number of related sequences, purify more plasmids from the transformation plate for this PCR product AND/OR clone out the second confirmatory PCR.
9. If cloning of the PCR product yields clonally related sequences but also a second group of sequences (>2) that share a clonally related CDR3 different to that already identified and you are confident that this is not the result of contamination and the tumor is indeed biclonal, purify more plasmids from the transformation plate for this PCR product and determine the dominant clone. We have observed dual light chain rearrangements in approx 8% of FL, whereas we have not found any tumors that proved to be biclonal for V_H.

Acknowledgments

This work was funded by Cancer Research UK and the Wessex Cancer Trust.

References

1. NCI Non-Hodgkin's Classification Project Writing Committee. (1985) Classification of non-Hodgkin's lymphomas: reproducibility of major classification systems: *Cancer* **55,** 457–481.
2. Horning, S. J. (1993) Natural history of and therapy for the indolent non-Hodgkins's lymphoma. *Semin. Oncol.* **20,** 75–88.
3. Ersbøll, J., et al. (1989) Follicular low grade non-Hodgkin's lymphoma: long-term outcome with or without tumor progression: *Eur. J. Haematol.* **42,** 155–163.
4. Simon, R., et al. (1988) The Non-Hodgkin Lymphoma Pathologic Classification Project. Long-term follow-up of 1153 patients with non-Hodgkin lymphomas. *Ann. Intern. Med.* **109,** 939–945.
5. Zukerberg, L. R., et al. (1993) Diffuse low-grade B-cell lymphomas. Four clinically distinct subtypes defined by a combination of morphologic and immunophenotypic features. *Am. J. Clin. Pathol.* **100,** 373–385.
6. Stein, H., et al. (1984) Immunohistological analysis of human lymphoma: correlation of histological and immunological categories. *Adv. Cancer Res.* **42,** 67–147.
7. Harris, N. L., et al. (1984) Immunohistologic characterization of two malignant lymphomas of germinal center type (centroblastic/centrocytic and centrocytic) with monoclonal antibodies. Follicular and diffuse lymphomas of small- cleaved-cell type are related but distinct entities. *Am. J. Pathol.* **117,** 262–272.
8. Stein, H., et al. (1982) The normal and malignant germinal center. *Clin. Haematol.* **11,** 531–559.
9. Harris, N. L., et al. (1994) A revised European-American classification of lymphoid neoplasms: a proposal from the International Lymphoma Study Group. *Blood* **84,** 1361–1392.

10. Johnson, P. W., et al. (1994) Detection of cells bearing the t(14;18) translocation following myeloablative treatment and autologous bone marrow transplantation for follicular lymphoma. *J. Clin. Oncol.* **12,** 798–805.
11. Stamatopoulos, K., et al. (2000) Molecular insights into the immunopathogenesis of follicular lymphoma. *Immunol. Today* **21,** 298–305.
12. Willis, T. G., et al. (2000) The role of immunoglobulin translocations in the pathogenesis of B-cell malignancies. *Blood* 96, 808–822.
13. Lam, K. P., et al. (1997) In vivo ablation of surface immunoglobulin on mature B-cells by inducible gene targeting results in rapid cell death. *Cell* **90,** 1073–1083.
14. Levy, R., et al. (1987) Somatic mutation in human B-cell tumors. *Immunol. Rev.* 43–58.
15. Schroeder, H. J., et al. (1994) The pathogenesis of chronic lymphocytic leukemia: Analysis of the antibody repertoire. *Immunol. Today* **15,** 288–294.
16. Li, Y., et al. (1996) The I binding specificity of human VH4–34 (VH4–21) encoded antibodies is determined by both VH framework region 1 and complementarity determining region 3. *J. Mol. Biol.* **256,** 577–589.
17. Pospsil, R., et al. (1998) CD5 and othr superantigens as 'ticklers' of the B-cell receptor. *Immunol. Today* **19,** 106–108.
18. Silverman, G. J. (1992) Human antibody responses to bacterial antigens: studies of a model conventional antigen and a proposed model B-cell superantigen. *Int. Rev. Immunol.* **9,** 57–78.
19. Bahler, D. W., et al. (1992) Clonal evolution of a follicular lymphoma: evidence for antigen selection. *Proc. Natl. Acad. Sci. USA.* **89,** 6770–6774.
20. Zelenetz, A. D., et al. (1991) Histologic transformation of follicular lymphoma to diffuse lymphoma represents tumor progression by a single malignant B-cell. *J. Exp. Med.* **173,** 197–207.
21. Zhu, D., et al. (1994) Clonal history of a human follicular lymphoma as revealed in the immunoglobulin variable region genes. *Br. J. Haematol.* **86,** 505–512.
22. Malisan, F., et al. (1996) B-Chronic lymphocytic leukemias can undergo isotype switching in vivo and can be induced to differentiate and switch in vitro. *Blood* **87,** 717–724.
23. Efremov, D. G., et al. (1996) IgM-producing chronic lymphocytic leukemia cells undergo immunoglobulin isotype-switching without acquiring somatic mutations. *J. Clin. Invest.* **98,** 290–298.
24. Ottensmeier, C. H., et al. (1998) Analysis of VH genes in follicular and diffuse lymphoma shows ongoing somatic mutation and multiple isotype transcripts in early disease with changes during disease progression. *Blood* **91,** 4292–4299.
25. Stevenson, F., et al. (1998) Insight into the origin and clonal history of B-cell tumors as revealed by analysis of immunoglobulin variable region genes. *Immunol. Rev.* **162,** 247–259.
26. Alizadeh, A. A., et al. (2000) Distinct types of diffuse large B-cell lymphoma identified by gene expression profiling. *Nature.* **403,** 503–511.
27. Hamblin, T. J., et al. (2000) Immunoglobulin V genes and CD38 expression in CLL. *Blood* **95,** 2455–2457.

28. Berek, C. (1992) The development of B-cells and the B-cell repertoire in the microenvironment of the germinal center. *Immunol. Rev.* **5,** 5–19.
29. Limpens, J., et al. (1995) Lymphoma-associated translocation t(14;18) in blood B-cells of normal individuals. *Blood* **85,** 2528–2536.
30. Han, S., et al. (1996) Neoteny in lymphocytes: Rag1 and Rag2 expression in germinal center B-cells. *Science* **274,** 2094–2097.
31. Henderson, A., et al. (1998) Transcriptional regulation during B-cell developmen. *Annu. Rev. Immunol.* **16,** 163–200.
32. Chen, C., et al. (1997) Editing disease-associated autoantibodies. *Immunity* **6,** 97–105.
33. Pelanda, R., et al. (1997) Receptor editing in a transgenic mouse model: site, efficiency, and role in B-cell tolerance and antibody diversification. *Immunity* **7,** 765–775.
34. Radic, M. Z., et al. (1996) Receptor editing, immune diversification, and self-tolerance. *Immunity* **5,** 505–511.
35. Bahler, D., et al. (1991) Ig VH gene expression among human follicular lymphomas. *Blood* **78,** 1561–1568.
36. Stevenson, F. K., et al. (1993) Differential usage of an Ig heavy chain variable region gene by human B-cell tumors. *Blood* **82,** 224–230.
37. Hummel, M., et al. (1994) Mantle cell (previously centrocytic) lymphomas express V(H) genes with no or very little somatic mutations like the physiologic cells of the follicle mantle. *Blood* **84,** 403–407.
38. Stamatopoulos, K., et al. (1997) Follicular lymphoma immunoglobulin kappa light chains are affected by the antigen selection process, but to a lesser degree than their partner heavy chains. *Br. J. Haematol.* **96,** 132–146.
39. Noppe, S. M., et al. (1999) The genetic variability of the VH genes in follicular lymphoma: the impact of the hypermutation mechanism. *Br. J. Haematol.* **107,** 625–640
40. Zhu, D., et al. (2002) Acquisition of potential N-glycosylation sites in the immunoglobulin variable region by somatic mutation is a distinctive feature of follicular lymphoma. *Blood* **99,** 2562–2568.
41. Cleary, M. L., et al. (1986) Clustering of extensive somatic mutations in the variable region of an immunoglobulin heavy chain gene from a human B-cell lymphoma. *Cell* **44,** 97–106.
42. Zelenetz, A. D., et al. (1992) Clonal expansion in follicular lymphoma occurs subsequent to antigenic selection. *J. Exp. Med.* **176,** 1137–1148.
43. Zelenetz, A. D., et al. (1993) A submicroscopic interstitial deletion of chromosome 14 frequently occurs adjacent to the t(14;18) translocation breakpoint in human follicular lymphoma. *Genes Chromosom. Cancer* **6,** 140–150.
44. Wu, H., et al. (1995) A human follicular lymphoma B-cell line hypermutates its functional immunoglobulin genes in vitro. *Eur. J. Immunol.* **25,** 3263–3269.
45. Corbett, S. J., et al. (1997) Sequence of the human immunoglobulin diversity (D) segment locus: a systematic analysis provides no evidence for the use of DIR segments, inverted D segments, "minor" D segments or D-D recombination. J. *Mol. Biol.* **270,** 587–597.

8

Immunoglobulin Gene Mutation Patterns and Heterogeneity of Marginal Zone Lymphoma

Mariella Dono and Manlio Ferrarini

Summary

Marginal zone (MZ) or MZ-like B-cells "home" outside the follicles of peripheral lymphoid tissues. Prototypic examples of these B-cells are those that home the MZ of the spleen, although B-cells with similar phenotypic and functional features can be found in the subepithelial (SE) areas of tonsil, in the Peyer's patches, in the lymph nodes, and in the thymic medulla. MZ-like B-cells also develop in mucosa-associated lymphoid tissue (MALT) and other sites (salivary glands, thyroid) that acquire organized lymphoid tissue after chronic antigenic stimulation, such as Hp infection in gastric maltomas or autoimmune insult in Sjogren's syndrome. Beside the so-called extranodal B-cell MALT lymphoma, the splenic MZ lymphoma with or without circulating villous lymphocytes and monocytoid lymphoma also are thought to originate from MZ B-cells. Normal MZ-like B-cells can be isolated from different tissue sources (tonsil, spleen) by using combination Percoll gradients, magnetic fractionation, and fluorescence-activated cell sorting. Analyses of morphology, phenotype, and functions of these purified MZ B-cells demonstrated that in humans, MZ B-cells are rather heterogeneous, comprising virgin and memory B-cells and of cells specialized in different types of human responses. In this chapter, we review the main procedures used to isolate and test the phenotypic and functional features of the MZ B-cells from human tonsil and spleen in our laboratory and discuss their characteristics by comparing them with the MZ B-cell-derived lymphomas.

Key Words: B-cell subsets; marginal zone; MALT; MZ B-cell lymphomas; VH gene rearrangements; heterogeneity.

1. Introduction

Recent data to from humans have indicated that mature B-cells are heterogeneous and display characteristic phenotype, morphology, and functions depending upon the site of homing in the peripheral lymphoid tissues *(1)*. In secondary lymphoid organs, B-cells are organized in defined structures, the secondary follicles. However, there also are B-cells that home outside the follicle and are generally referred to as extrafollicular B-cells or other names, depending upon the different lymphoid organs (**Fig. 1**). The follicles consist of a germinal cen-

From: *Methods in Molecular Medicine, Vol. 115: Lymphoma: Methods and Protocols*
Edited by: T. Illidge and P. W. M. Johnson © Humana Press Inc., Totowa, NJ

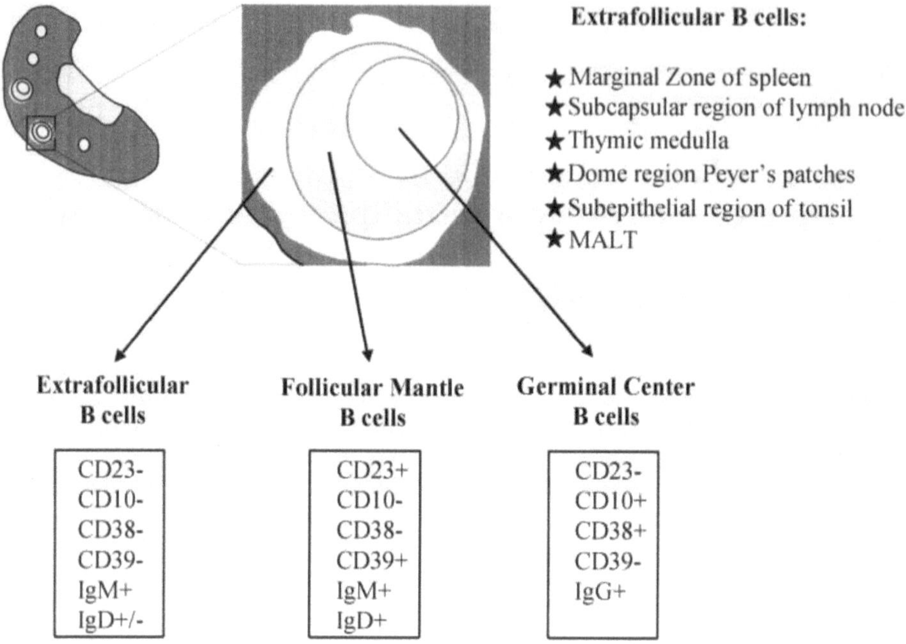

Fig. 1. Schematic representation of a secondary follicle in a lymph node. The different B-cell compartments are indicated together with a summary of the main phenotype of the various B-cell subsets.

ter (GC) and a follicular mantle (FM). B-cells that have been stimulated by T-cell-dependent antigens enter the GC, where they undergo Ig variable (V) gene hypermutation and selection by the stimulating antigen. As a consequence of this process, only B-cells that produce high-affinity antibodies survive and join the memory cell compartment or the long-lived plasma cells pool *(2)*. Somatic hypermutation of Ig V_H genes, therefore, appears to be restricted to those B-cells that have passed through GCs and can be considered the hallmark of GC B-cells and descendants (post-GC B-cells *[3]*). Some of these memory cells home to the extrafollicular areas. FM B-cells primarily comprise virgin B-cells that express unmutated V_H genes. It is conceivable that these cells contribute to the GC B-cell pool after antigenic stimulation, although other B-cell subsets, including extrafollicular B-cells, could migrate into the GC.

The extrafollicular B-cells accumulate in the marginal zone (MZ) of the spleen, in the subepithelial (SE) area of tonsils, in the dome region of the Peyer's patches, in the subcapsular region of lymph nodes, and in the thymic medulla. Also the mucosa associated lymphoid tissue, or MALT, primarily comprises extrafollicular B-cells, and this term is used to indicate the lymphoid tissue that is associated with all the body mucosal linings. Although some of this tissue is normally present at certain sites, such as in Waldeyer's ring, the finding of MALT in certain areas consistently denotes inflammation caused by infection or other events, including autoimmune reactions.

The stomach, for example, normally is devoid of organized lymphoid tissue. This tissue, however, is found in the gastric mucosa that is exposed to chronic infection with *Helicobacter pylori* (Hp) *(4)*. Likewise, salivary glands do not show accumulation of lymphoid tissue unless they are the targets of an autoimmune injury, as occurs in the Sjögren's syndrome *(5)*. The current trend is to refer to all of these extrafollicular B-cells as MZ or MZ-equivalent B-cells.

The initial studies on MZ B-cells, which were conducted in experimental animals, demonstrated that these cells are heterogeneous and are composed of virgin and memory cells. However, these studies also defined a typical feature of MZ B-cells, that is, their capacity to respond to polysaccharides antigens (generally referred to as Ti-2 Ags as opposed to the lipopolysaccharides Ags, which are referred to as Ti-1 Ags *[6,7]*). More recently, the advent of a large panel of mAbs and refined cell separation methods has made it possible to purify and characterize such human MZ B-cells.

1.1. Isolation of MZ B-Cells From Tonsils

In situ studies demonstrated that B-cells in the SE or in the intraepithelial areas of human tonsils displayed a phenotype different from that of B-cells from the GC and FM of the follicles *(8,9)*. For example, SE B-cells express low levels of CD21, CD38, and CD23, which are found on FM (CD23) and GC (CD38, CD21) B-cells. SE B-cells also are composed of some CD39+ or CD69+ cells, indicating the presence of activated cells *(8)*. In addition, anti-IgD antibodies stained a fraction of SE B-cells, whereas FM B-cells were IgD-positive and GC B-cells were IgD-negative *(10)*. A similar phenotype (IgM+ IgD+/– CD10– CD23–) was reported for intraepithelial B-cells, indicating that the two cells were probably of the same subset *(9)*. Owing to their phenotypic differences and state of activation, the three tonsillar B-cell subsets, that is, SE, FM, and GC B-cells, were isolated in suspension using a combination of Percoll gradients, magnetic beads fractionation and FACS sorting (**Fig. 2**) *(8)*. The use of Percoll gradients made it possible to separate B-cells according to the different cellular density that also corresponded to different activation states. Thus, resting cells without activation markers such as CD69 and CD71 could be isolated from the 60% Percoll fractions. Cells with these markers were instead present in the B-cells purified from the 50% Percoll fractions (named activated B-cells) *(11)*. In addition, B-cells of inferior density (large B-cells) could be collected between 30% and 40% Percoll fractions. These were particularly enriched in CD38+ CD10+ GC B-cells (*see* methods section for details) (**8**).

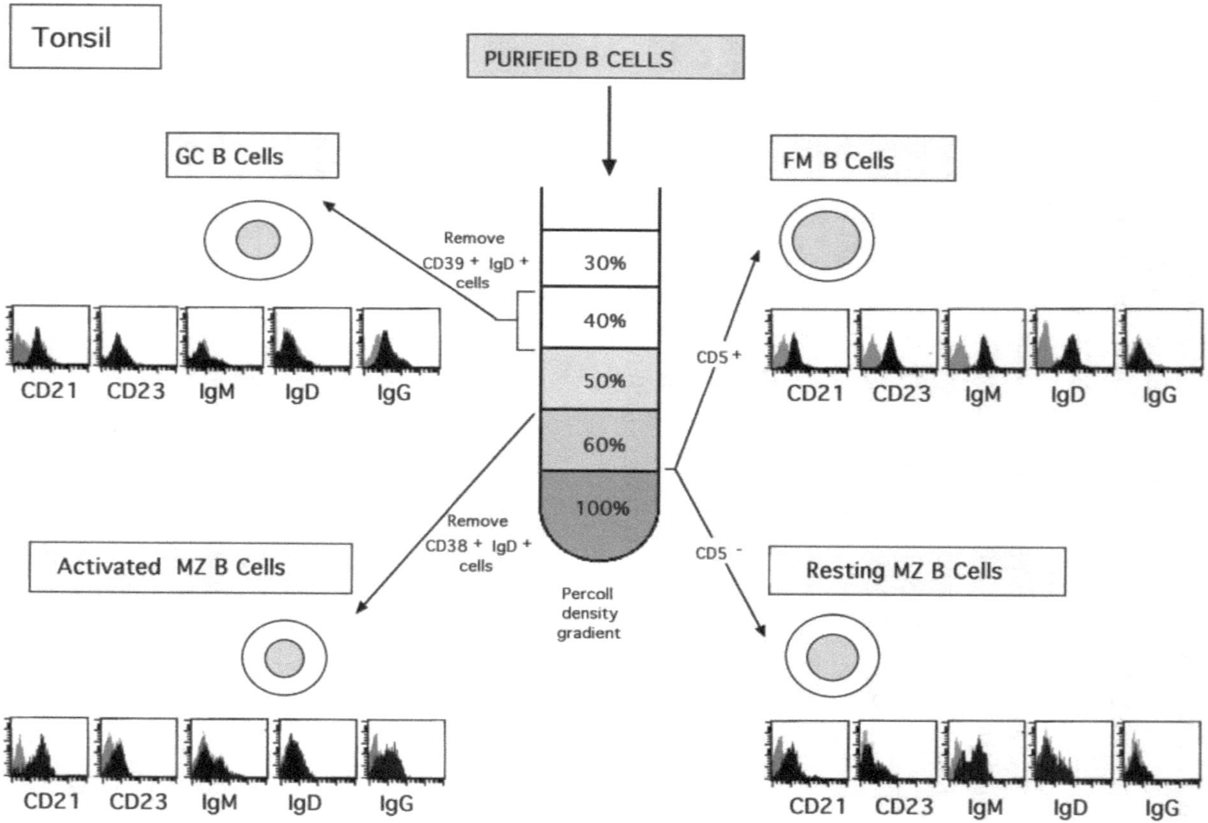

Fig. 2. Summary of the procedures used for the purification of the various B-cell subsets from human tonsils. Each of the B-cell subsets isolated were stained with the indicated mAbs (black areas) or with an unrelated (control) mAb (gray areas) and analyzed by flow cytometry.

Thus, variations in the results of studies on B-cell subset may be in part explained by the different approaches used for their isolation. Indeed, in vivo activated B-cells would conceivably behave in a manner different from resting B-cells in a number of in vitro tests *(12,13)*.

By using the purification strategy described above, a large proportion of SE B-cells were detected in the highest density fractions of Percoll gradients and separated from FM B-cells by cell sorting or magnetic beads (**Fig. 2**) *(8,14)*. This is possible because FM B-cells are CD5+ and CD39+ whereas MZ B-cells were CD5– and CD39–. The MZ B-cells analyzed in suspension did not differ for phenotype and morphology from the same cells studied *in situ (8)*. The overall phenotype was IgM+ IgD+/– CD23– CD10– CD38–. This phenotype is consistent with that of MZ B-cells from the spleen and MZ equivalent B-cells from other tissues. Hence, from now onwards SE B-cells will be referred to as MZ B-cells. A number of MZ B-cells also could be isolated from the 50% Percoll fractions, indicating that they were activated in vivo (**Fig. 2**). These cells were composed of CD5– CD23– CD10– CD38– cells that expressed activation markers such as CD95. These expressed mostly surface IgG and were likely to correspond to the so called "memory "IgG+ B-cells described in other studies on human tonsils *(12,13)*. In contrast to resting MZ B-cells, these activated MZ B-cells have surface co-stimulatory molecules such as CD80 and CD86 *(15)*.

1.2. Subpopulations of MZ B-Cells

The MZ B-cells isolated from the 60% Percoll cell fractions were found to be heterogeneous because they differed for the expression of sIgD. 60–70% of the cells were IgD-negative (IgM-only) and the remaining 30–40% of cells displayed a weak albeit-definitive positive fluorescence (IgD-low)*(14)*. When the two MZ B-cell subsets, that is, IgM-only and IgM+ IgD-low MZ B-cells were sorted and their V_H gene repertoire evaluated, it was found that the IgM-only MZ B-cells expressed primarily unmutated V_H gene segment (96%). These results indicated that they could be virgin B-cells or that they were memory cells that were expanded *in situ* after stimulation by antigen in a T-cell-independent fashion. The findings of multiple molecular variable–diversity–joined (VDJ) clones with the same V_H and the same CDR3 seem to support the latter hypothesis. IgM+ IgD-low MZ B-cells were found to use both unmutated and mutated V_H gene segments (55% and 45%, respectively). This finding also is consistent with the observation that a fraction of IgD-low cells express the CD27 antigen that is a typical memory cell marker. Suspension that was enriched in CD27+ IgD-low MZ B-cells also was enriched in cells that expressed mutated V_H genes compared with the unfractionated (CD27+ve and CD27–ve) IgD-low MZ B-cells. There are different interpretations for the origin of these mutated IgD-low MZ B-cells. These cells could be post-GC B-cells that exited the GC after stimulation/selection. Alternatively, they may have mutated outside germinal center after a T-cell-independent antigenic stimulation. The latter possibility is supported by the finding that patients with X-linked hyper-IgM syndrome who lack a GC have mutated IgM+ IgD+ B-cells *(16)*. By analogy with the IgM-only B-cells, the unmutated MZ B-cells (including the IgD-low and IgD-negative cells) could be virgin B-cells or B-cells stimulated *in situ* by T-cell-independent antigens.

As alluded to previously, a third MZ B-cell population was recovered from the 50% Percoll fractions and comprised cells activated in vivo. Both mutated and unmutated sequences (48% and 52%, respectively) were found in the IgM transcripts of these cells, whereas the majority of the IgG transcripts (81%) were mutated *(14)*. The IgM-expressing cells may represent a stage of activation of the resting IgM-only MZ B-cells described above, whereas the IgG expressing cells may be post GC cells. However, the option has to be considered that these B-cells may have undergone isotype switch and V gene mutation *in situ* upon stimulation with polysaccharides antigens, as it has been described for certain cells of the murine gut mucosa *(17)*.

1.3. Splenic MZ B-Cells

Immunohistochemical studies on human spleens have shown that although FM B-cells stain strongly for CD23 and sIgD, MZ B-cells have a low-to-absent expression of these markers and express CD21 and surface IgM as a major isotype *(18,19)*. Indeed, the combination of anti-IgD and anti-CD23 antibodies has been used to distinguish FM from MZ B-cells in microdissection studies *(20)*. Recently, we demonstrated that isolated human splenic MZ B-cells migrated mainly if not exclusively in the less dense Percoll fractions (50%) (**Fig. 3** *[21]*). This finding is consistent with early *in situ* studies demonstrating the presence of the CD25 marker on splenic MZ B-cells *(22)*, suggesting that these cells are activated in vivo probably, owing to the constant antigenic challenge occurring in the MZ area.

The comparison of the phenotype of splenic and tonsillar MZ B-cells demonstrated remarkable similarity with the exception of the CD21 marker, which was high in the spleen and low in tonsils (*see* **Figs. 2** and **3**). This finding may be explained by the different state of activation or be related to an intrinsic difference of the two cells connected with a particular function of CD21 *(23)*. Notably, the MZ B-cells of mice express high levels of CD21 and this molecule is crucial in certain circumstances in facilitating their stimulation by Ag *(24,25)*.

The majority of the splenic MZ B-cells isolated in suspension express surface IgG like the tonsillar MZ B-cells isolated from the same 50% Percoll density fractions (**Figs. 2** and **3**). However, these splenic MZ B-cells also comprise

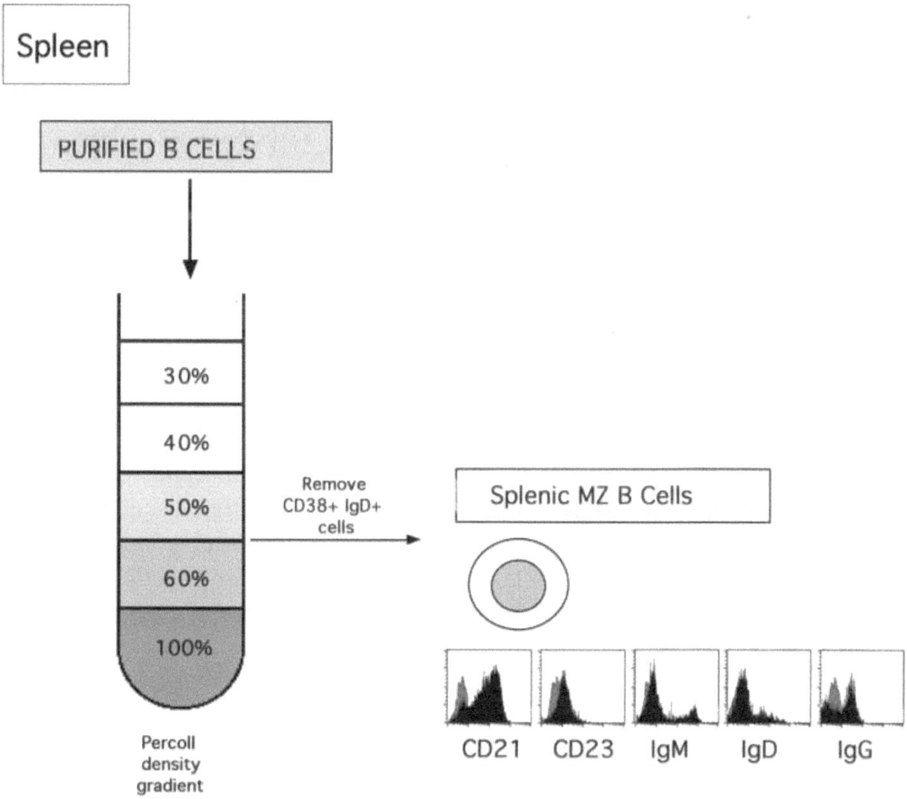

Fig. 3. Protocol of purification of splenic MZ B-cells. The isolated MZ B-cells were stained as indicated in Fig. 2.

IgM+ cells (20–45%, range of three spleens) that have an IgD-negative or IgD-low and CD23-negative phenotype. This finding is apparently in contrast with the *in situ* immunohistochemical studies demonstrating a splenic MZ area populated primarily by IgM+ B-cells. It is possible that technical problems related to the immunostaining of histological sections with anti-IgG antibodies may be responsible at least in part for these discrepancies.

The analysis of V_H gene usage from microdissected MZ B-cells has given different results depending upon the immunostaining used for microdissection. Thus, the studies so far available have indicated that 94% and 62% of microdissected MZ B-cells expressed somatically mutated VH genes ***(20,26)***. However, in the study that reported a higher percentage of mutations, IgD-negative MZ B-cells were taken from splenic sections and are likely to have included both IgM- and IgG-expressing cells, whereas in the other study, MZ

Table 1
Summary of the Main Functional Characteristics of Normal Tonsillar B-cell Subsets

B-cell subset	MZ	FM	GC
Response to			
Polyclonal B-cell activators	–	++	+
TI-1 antigens	–	–	–
TI-2 antigens	+++	–	–
T-cell-dependent antigens	++	+	+
Antigen presentation	++	+/–	nd
Propensity to apoptosis	–	–	++

B-cells were chosen on the basis of their IgM+/IgD– phenotype. This choice likely resulted in the lower percentage of B-cells with mutated sequence. The results of these studies are in line with those on tonsillar B-cells, indicating the existence in the MZ of an IgG+ memory B-cell population together with the IgM-expressing B-cells that may be mutated or unmutated.

1.4. Functional Heterogeneity of MZ B-Cells

The availability of MZ B-cells isolated in suspension has made it possible to investigate some functional features of these cells. Remarkably, MZ B-cells from tonsils were able to respond to TNP-Ficoll, a Ti-2 antigen and of presenting antigens to T-cells efficiently (**Table 1**) *(15)*. A good antigen-presenting activity has been observed for also splenic MZ B-cells from rats and seems consistent with the notion that MZ B-cells are located in areas where exposure to (and picking up of) antigens is facilitated *(27)*. The tonsillar MZ B-cells failed to respond to polyclonal activators, whereas they were induced into proliferation and plasma cell differentiation upon contact with T-cells *(28)*. Thus, as already reported in the experimental animal studies, tonsillar MZ B-cells are capable of both T-independent and T-dependent responses *(6)*. It is possible that these functions associate with different MZ B-cell subsets. Indeed, preliminary data seem to indicate that the ability to produce specific antibodies to Ti-2 antigens segregate primarily with the IgM+ IgD-low B-cells *(22)*.

1.5. Malignancies of Human MZ B-Cells

Lymphomas of the MZ B-cells usually are subdivided into three categories: extranodal, nodal, and splenic. The extranodal entity is represented by the low-grade MALT lymphomas that arise usually in different organs including the stomach, salivary glands, thyroid, lung, and skin *(29)*. Low-grade MALT Lymphoma of the stomach has received special attention because it represents a typical example of a lymphoma associated with antigenic stimulation ***(4,30)***. In this case, a chronic Hp infection, which is present in virtually all patients, causes first the formation of MALT tissue and subsequently the expansion of the lymphoma. In particular, chronic stimulation may promote the expansion of lymphoid cells that have accumulated cytogenetic changes, or alternatively proliferation of B-cells induced by chronic antigenic stimulation may favor the accumulation of cytogenetic changes.

In a few cases of gastric maltomas, it has been possible to investigate the specificity of the Abs produced by the malignant cells ***(31)***. Surprisingly, in no case were those antibodies found to be directed to any known Hp antigens, whereas in certain cases, it was found that they had specificity for autoantigens. Collectively, these data indicate that the newly formed MALT tissue induced by Hp infection also comprises B-cells with specificities for antigens different from the insulting antigen(s). These cells may be recruited at that site and induced to proliferate in the course of the inflammatory reaction that accompanies the Hp infection.

Sequence analyses of the V_H gene regions genes used by MALT lymphoma cells have demonstrated the presence of accumulation of point mutations in the majority of cases, although in some instances, cases with very few or no V gene mutations have been demonstrated ***(32)***. This suggests that both the types of B-cells normally found in the MZ described above are capable of giving rise to lymphomas. In the case of unmutated lymphomas, it is plausible that the cells are transformed while expanding in response to Ti antigens.

Two types of translocations occur in gastric lymphomas, namely t (11; 18), which occur in 48% of the cases, and t (1; 14), which is relatively uncommon ***(29)***. Chromosomal translocation in lymphomas generally are thought to occur in the germinal centers, where the cells are subjected to extensive DNA processing, including mutation of V_H/V_L genes, to switch recombination processes, and also perhaps to V_H/V_L replacement. Errors in these events may result in erroneous genetic recombinations, causing translocations. Therefore, it is plausible that gene translocations took place while the cells were passing through the GCs after antigenic stimulation. This initial stimulation possibly, although not necessarily, occurred at the mucosal level. The cells subsequently moved to GC, where they were transformed and exited from GC to accumulate in the extrafollicular areas. An alternative hypothesis may be that B-cells underwent antigenic stimulation and subsequent selection at the mucosal level, where they also accumulated V gene mutations ***(33)***. If this were the case, the cells would possibly, but not necessarily, acquire the transforming cytogenetic changes outside the GC while responding to Ti-2 Ag in the MZ. In view of the observations that chromosomal translocations in different lymphomas occur primarily while the B-cells pass through the GC, the former hypothesis appears to be more appealing. It is, however, possible that maltomas, in which the cells do not display V gene mutations, undergo a process of malignant transformation that is confined exclusively within the MZ. If this were the case, then it would be interesting to know whether these lymphomas share the same cytogenetic lesions as the ones with V gene mutations.

The identification of tumor cells in gastric MALT lymphoma has implications not only for the diagnosis, eradication, and follow-up of patients, but also for the therapeutic strategy used. However, the molecular diagnosis of Ig rearrangement of this kind of lymphoma may present some difficulties that are primarily related with the quality and quantity of the starting material. Indeed, multiple small biopsies are taken during endoscopy and are usually used for both immunohistochemical diagnosis and Ig gene rearrangement analysis by polymerase chain reaction (PCR; *see* **Subeading 3.**). Tumor cells from low-grade MALT lymphoma generate characteristic lymphoepithelial lesion, although they can often surround and invade pre-existing follicles. Thus, a normal B-cell component of reactive follicles, together with the neoplastic clone, is a common finding in the specimens of gastric MALT lymphoma. Therefore, analysis of Ig V gene rearrangement in the gastric biopsies may often yield an oligoclonal rather than a monoclonal pattern (*see* **Fig. 4**), with consequent difficulties in the identification of the VDJ rearrangements utilized by the lymphomatous cells. The presence of the same VDJ fragments on multiple biopsies taken at different lesion sites would help in identifying the tumor clone. The use of selected tissue sections particularly enriched in cells morphologically indicative of a neoplastic lesion may help in carrying out the analyses.

The monocytoid B-cell lymphoma (MBCL) is characterized by appearance of B-cells with monocytoid morphology. The immunophenotype of MBCL cells detected in tissue sections is IgM+ IgD– CD5– CD10– and the malignant cells use mutated V_H gene ***(34–36)***. They may be derived from the few memory MZ B-cells that are IgM-positive or from the IgM+ IgD+/– cells that have mutated V_H genes because week IgD-positivity may be undetected in the *in situ* studies. However, additional investigation on a larger number of MBCL cases is required to elucidate this issue further. In addition the presence of PCA-1, a plasma cell differentiation antigen, may indicate that the lymphomatous cells retain the potential capacity to differentiate into plasma cells.

Although often included within the MZ Lymphomas, the splenic marginal zone lymphoma (SMZL) is still awaiting definitive classification. Several investigators have suggested that it may be unrelated to the MZ B-cells, although it displays a marginal zone differentiation. The presence of surface IgD (formerly a marker of follicular mantle B-cells) does not appear to help resolving the conundrum, since we have now evidence that also MZ B-cells can express IgD ***(10,14)***. This tumor may be accompanied by a leukemic component the so-

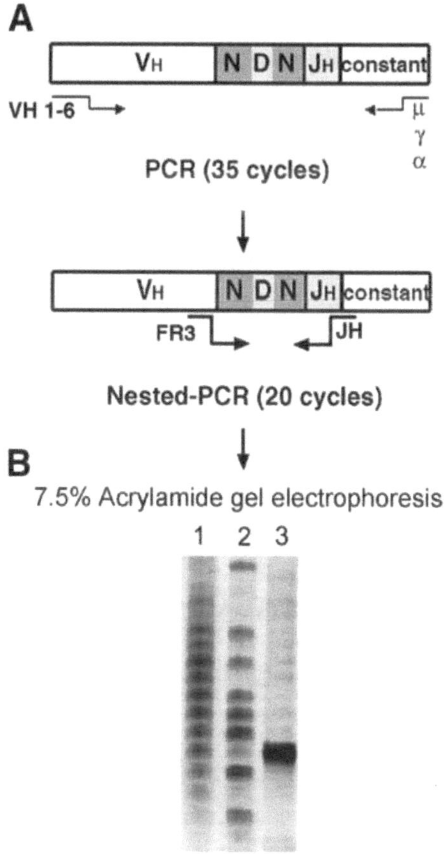

Fig. 4. **(A)** The PCR strategies used to amplify VDJ segments for normal and neoplastic B-cells are represented. **(B)** Typical electrophoretic patterns (lane 1, polyclonal; lane 2, oligoclonal; lane 3, monoclonal) of amplified PCR products obtained as described in **A**.

called "villous lymphocytes" in the peripheral blood (50% of cases). In most cases, the clinical course of splenic MZ lymphoma is indolent, although cases with a more aggressive behavior have been described. The relative heterogeneity of this disease has been pointed out by cytogenetic and molecular studies *(37,38)*. Somatic mutations of BCL-6 and genomic imbalance were commonly found. Genetic losses as well as genetic gains were detected in the majority of the patients (83%). These studies also have outlined that the patients displaying genetic losses (such as 7q31-q32 deletion) had a short survival *(38)*. Early observations on a relatively small number of cases suggested that cells from SMZL could use hypermutated V_H genes *(39,40)*. A subsequent study in which somatic mutation of VH genes and genetic alterations were analyzed in a larger cohort of patients, demonstrated that approximately half of the SMZL expressed unmutated V_H genes and that the 7q31 deletion was more frequent in this group and associated with a shorter overall survival ***(41)***. Furthermore, a preferential usage of V_H1-2 gene segment was noted both in mutated and unmutated cases. Thus, the skewed usage of certain genes may indicate preferential stimulation by certain antigens, autoantigens, or superantigens. The neoplastic transformation may occur during stimulation. Whether the antigenic stimulation/selection and tumor transformation takes place *in situ*, that is, in the MZ area or in a GC, remains unclear, and this issue appears complex. The absence of balanced chromosomal translocations, which are thought to occur in mature B-cells within GC, is consistent with the hypothesis that in splenic MZL neoplastic transformation occurs outside GC in early or late memory B-cells or in MZ B-cells that have never reached the GC.

The aim of this chapter is to summarize the major procedures used in the analyses of "normal" B-cell subsets and of the low-grade MALT-Lymphoma. Because the study of normal B-cells is conducted on fresh material, such as human tonsils, and involves a number of purification steps, the preparation of the B-cell subsets will be detailed in a separate section. This main section will be referred to as "Preparation of Purified Suspension of B-Cell Subpopulations" (**Subheading 3.1.**) and will deal with procedures aimed at isolate pure, viable populations of B-cells that can be used for both functional and molecular studies. In contrast, because MALT-lymphomas material often is obtained from small biopsy specimens, only molecular studies can be performed, which do not require cell purification procedures. The most common techniques used for the analyses of Ig V_H genes will then be described in a separate section referred to as "Molecular analyses of V_H Genes" (**Subheading 3.2.**) In this section, the major techniques used for the study of V_H gene repertoire utilized by both the normal B-cells and the malignant MALT B-cells will be detailed.

2. Materials

2.1. Cell Preparation

1. Ficoll-Hypaque (Seromed, Biochrom AG; Berlin, Germany); store at 4°C.
2. Percoll™ (Amersham Pharmacia Biotech; Uppsala, Sweden); store unopened at room temperature (RT).
3. RPMI (Seromed); store at 4°C.
4. Fetal calf serum (Seromed); deplete of complement by heating 1 h at 56°C, aliquot, and store frozen at –20°C.
5. Glutamine, Penstreptomycin, and Na pyruvate (Seromed); store frozen.
6. Neuraminidase (Dade Behring; Milano, Italy).
7. 10X Hanks Balanced Salt Solution (Gibco BRL; Paisley, Scotland); store unopened at RT.

2.2. B-Cell Subsets Isolation

1. Goat anti mouse Ab (Southern Biotechnology Associates; Birmingham, AL).
2. $CrCL_3$ (Sigma-Aldrich; Steinheim, Germany).
3. Na_2EDTA (Fluka; Buchs, Switzerland).
4. Bovine serum albumin (BSA; Sigma).
5. Goat anti mouse microbeads (Miltenyi Biotec, Bergisch Gladbach, Germany).

2.3. RNA Preparation and cDNA Synthesis

1. RNA-Clean (Tib MolBiol; Genova, Italy).
2. Chloroform (Sigma); store at RT- light sensitive.
3. Propanol Analytical Reagent (Fluka); store at RT.
4. DNTPs (Bohering Mannheim; Germany).
5. MuMLV (Gibco); store at –20°C and keep on ice while in use.

2.4. PCR, Gel Electrophoresis, and End-Labeling

1. Taq DNA polymerase (Perkin-Elmer Biosystem; Milano, Italy).
2. Mastercycler 330 (Eppendorf Scientific, Hamburg, Germany).
3. T4 polynucleotide kinase (Gibco); store at –20°C. Do not leave at RT or at 4°C for prolonged periods!
4. $\gamma\ ^{32}P$-dATP (Amersham); store at –20°C, radiation hazard, use special protections to avoid radioisotope contamination.
5. Boric acid (Fluka).
6. Tris (Fluka).
7. Urea (Fluka).
8. Acetic acid (Fluka); store at RT. Highly corrosive; wear gloves while handling.
9. Acrylamide:bisacrylamide 19:1 (Fluka). Reconstitute in deionized water by stirring overnight and store at 4°C.Light sensitive and toxic; wear glove while handling it.
10. 68% HNO_3 analytical reagent (Prolabo; France).
11. $AgNO_3$ ACS reagent (Sigma). Light sensitive; wear gloves to protect skin.
12. Na_2CO_3 (Sigma).
13. 37% Formaldeide (Sigma), toxic.

2.5. Sequence Analysis

1. TOPO TA vector (Invitrogen; Carlsbad, CA).
2. Sequencing kits (Perkin–Elmer).
3. NUNC TRAP Probe columns (Stratagene; La Jolla, CA).
4. QIAEX II Gel extraction kit (QIAGEN; Germany).

3. Methods

The methods detailed below describe 1) the major steps used to isolate highly purified B-cell subsets from human tonsils and 2) the molecular approach to characterized the V_H gene repertoire of both normal B-cells and MALT B-cells.

3.1. Preparation of Purified Suspension of B-Cell Subpopulations

The isolation and purification of B-cell subsets from tonsils include ordered steps that usually can be performed in 2 d of work. The amount and purity of the isolated B-cells obtained from each experiment varies greatly among tonsils.

3.1.1. Handling of Tonsillar Specimens

Surgically removed tonsils from 5- to 12-yr-old children are stored quickly in a tube containing physiological saline that is kept at 4°C. Before processing, tonsils usually are treated rapidly with 100% ethanol (approx 30 s) to kill bacteria that are possibly adhering to the external surfaces of tonsils and then washed extensively with sterile saline.

3.1.2. Cell Preparation

The tonsils are minced gently with fine needles, and mononuclear cells (MNCs) are isolated on Ficoll–Hypaque (F-H) density gradients by centrifugation at 800*g* for 20 min. This step also is necessary to eliminate the remaining cellular aggregates and the debris. To obtain tonsillar B-cells, T-cells are removed by rosetting the MNCs with neuraminidase-treated sheep red blood cells (SRBC) (*see* **Note 1**). Nonrosetting cells (B-cells) are separated from the rosetting cells (i.e., T and NK cells) on two consecutive F-H gradients. To improve the degree of purification, tonsillar B-cells can be further depleted of contaminant T-cells (CD3+ cells) and monocytes (CD11b+ cells) by magnetic cell separation with monoclonal mAb (*see* **Subheading 3.1.4.**).

3.1.3. Centrifugation on Percoll Gradients

The tonsillar B-cells prepared as above comprise cells at different stages of activation. The B-cells that have a high nucleo/cytoplasm ratio and a high cellular density are usually quiescent, resting cells. Activated B-cells instead display a larger cellular size and a low density. These features vary depending upon the degree of the activation. Thus, these B-cells migrate in multiple density fractions. Separation is conducted on discontinuous Percoll gradients (*see* **Note 2**). Cells with different density will form bands in the different Percoll densities. In general, the high-density resting B-cells are collected on the surface of 100% Percoll; the medium-sized cells are recovered from the 50% Percoll, and the low-density B-cells are recovered in fractions of 30 to 40% Percoll density (*see* **Fig. 2**). Proceed as follows:

1. Mix B-cells (50×10^6) with 2.5 mL of 100% Percoll suspension in a 15-mL conical tube (*see* **Note 3**).
2. Layer sequentially 2.5 mL of five additional Percoll suspensions with 10% increment (60, 50, 40, 30, and 20%) over the 100% fraction.
3. Centrifuge for 20 min in a swing-out rotor at 1500*g* without stop.

3.1.4. B-Cell Subsets Isolation

The isolation of MZ, FM, and GC B-cell subsets from the various Percoll fractions mainly is based on the phenotypic characterization of these human B-cells reported in **Subheading 1**. The most widely used strategy for this isolation is separation with magnetic beads. Details of how perform the isolation steps are in the numbered list that follows. For the isolation of FM B-cells, 60% Percoll fraction is first incubated with anti CD5 mAb and with GAM microbeads. Magnetic-labeled cells retained on a MS column are collected. Resting MZ B-cells are isolated from 60% Percoll fraction by incubating the cells with an anti CD5 mAb and then with GAM microbeads. Labeled cells are then depleted by the passage through a LD column and MZ B-cells recovered as CD5-negative B-cell fraction. For isolation of activated MZ B-cells, the 50% Percoll suspensions are incubated with anti CD5, anti CD38, and anti IgD, followed by GAM microbeads staining. The cells are then passed over a LD column and the resulting flow-through collected. GC B-cells are isolated from the 30+ 40% Percoll fractions by magnetic depletion over a LD column of the CD39+ and IgD+ B-cells stained with the corresponding mAbs and GAM microbeads.

1. Incubate Percoll B-cell fractions (100×10^6/mL) with the corresponding mAb (120–360 ng/10^6 cells depending on the antigen labeled and on the antibody used) for 30 min at 4°C.Wash with a phosphate-buffered saline buffer (pH 7.2) containing 2 m*M* EDTA and 0.5% BSA (*see* **Note 4**).
2. Label cells with Goat anti Mouse Ig microbeads (20 μL/10×10^6) (keep a 1:5 ratio of microbeads to the total labeling volume) for 10–15 min at 4° C and wash with EDTA/BSA buffer.
3. After magnetic labeling, pass the cells through a column placed in a powerful magnet.
4. Recover mAb-negative B-cells by collecting cells not retained on the LD column or mAb+ B-cells that are hold up on the MS column matrix.

As alternative, the classical "immune rosetting" may substitute for magnetic separation. Its advantage is simplicity and relative low cost. Immune rosetting works very nicely and is recommended for the recovery of cells by negative selection. This technique uses ox red blood cells (ORBCs) that have been sensitized with goat anti mouse Ab (GAM; **Note 5**). Cells labeled with a mAb form rosettes when in contact with the GAM-ORBC at cold temperature. The different steps to get isolation of cells are listed below.

1. Incubate Percoll B-cell fractions (100×10^6/mL) with the mAb (120–360 ng/10^6 cells depending on the antigen labeled and on the antibody used) for 30 min at 4°C.
2. Wash cells with 10% FCS medium.
3. Suspend the cells at 10×10^6/mL and add 1 mL of GAM-ORBC.

4. Centrifuge gently at 250*g* for 10 min and keep on ice for 30 min.
5. Discard supernatant and gently resuspend the rosettes by swinging the tube.
6. Isolate rosetting cells (i.e., mAb +ve cells) from nonrosetting cells (i.e., mAb –ve cells) by F-H centrifugation

When combinations of mAbs must be used, flow cytometry and cell sorting technique can be employed. Cells can be labeled with one, two, three (or even more) antibodies coupled with different fluorochromes simultaneously and then sorted on a cell sorter. B-cells are first stained with the appropriate fluorescein isothiocyanate or phycoerythrin or CyChrome-conjugated antibody alone or in combination of at 4°C for at least 30 min, washed with 0.01% Na-Azide/PBS buffer (*see* **Note 6**) in a refrigerate centrifuge and suspend at 10×10^6/mL in 10% FCS medium. Before sorting, stained cells are analyzed to design windows for sorting. Thus undesirable, contaminant cells are discarded, whereas targeted B-cells are gated for sorting.

3.2. Molecular Analyses of V_H Genes

3.2.1. Handling of Gastric Biopsies of MALT Lymphoma Cases

Usually, multiple gastric biopsies are taken during routine endoscopy at different lesion sites. For each of the sites selected by the endoscopist, a couple of samples are taken. This is necessary because one fragment of the couple is used for histopathology and the other fragment is processed for molecular studies. Biopsy specimens are deposed on sterile filter paper wet with saline and processed immediately. In some instances, biopsies can be stored frozen at –80°C in OCT and subsequently used for molecular studies.

3.2.2. RNA Preparation (see **Note 7**) and First-Strand cDNA Synthesis

Multiple fresh or frozen biopsies can be directly used as source of RNA. To purify RNA, RNA-clean (isothiocyanate-phenol solution) or related products are used. After adding the RNA clean solution to biopsies, several passages through needles of different size are recommended to disintegrate the small biopsies. Once gastric specimens are homogenized, 1/10 (v/v) of chloroform is added and the solution vortexed for 1–2 min. This preparation is then kept on ice for 15–30 min and subsequently centrifuged at high speed in a refrigerated rotor for 30 min. With this technique, an aqueous phase containing nucleic acid will separate from the phenolic phase containing proteins, lipids, and debrids. The aqueous phase is recovered, and RNA is precipitated at –20°C overnight by the addition of 1/1 (v/v) of cold isopropanol. After centrifugation at high speed for 30 min, RNA, a white precipitate on the bottom of the tube, is washed by addition of 80% cold ethanol (*see* **Note 8**). Then, RNA is suspended in 20 µL of RNAse-free water.

The B-cell subsets isolated, as described in **Subheading 3.1.**, are instantaneously processed after separation in order to obtain RNA. Because recovery of cells after purification steps may be poor, the amount of cells used can range from 0.5 to 5.0×10^6 cells. RNA is obtained from cells as detailed above.

For first-strand cDNA synthesis, the total RNA yield is reverse transcribed by using oligodT as primer and Murine Myeloblastosis virus reverse transcriptase as follows:

Prepare the following in a sterile tube:

1. Template RNA (*see* **Note 9**).
2. Primer oligo$(dT)_{18}$ 100 pM.

Incubate the mix at 70°C for 5 min and chill on ice. Add the following in the order indicated:

3. 5X reaction buffer (8 µL).
4. 10 m*M* dNTPs, mix 4 µL (1.0 m*M* - final concentration).
5. Ribonuclease inhibitor 20 units.
6. Deionized water (nuclease free) up to 40 µL.

Incubate at 37°C for 5 minutes. Add 20 units of Mu-MLV reverse transcriptase. Incubate the reaction mixture, containing oligo$(dT)_{18}$ at 37°C for 60 min. Stop the reaction by heating at 70°C for 10 min. Chill on ice.

3.2.3. Ig VH PCR

Based on sequence homology, the human V_H gene segments can be grouped into seven different families. Because of high conserved region within the gene members of each V_H family, it is possible to designed upstream family-specific primers and use them together with downstream C_H constant region primers to amplify the expressed genes (*see* **Table 2** and **Fig. 4** for primers details). To perform several parallel reactions, it is recommended the preparation of a master mix containing water, buffer, $MgCl_2$, dNTPs, primers and *Taq* DNA polymerase in a single sterile tube, which can then be aliquoted into individual tubes.

Master mix set up (1 reaction):

dNTPs	200 µ*M*
10X buffer	1:10
$MgCl_2$	1.5 m*M*
V_H primer	25 pmol
C_H primer	25 pmol
Taq gold	2 units
Deionized water	up to 50 µL

Gently vortex sample and briefly centrifuge to collect all drops from walls of tube. Aliquot the mix into the individual PCR tubes and overlay the sample

Table 2
List of V_H-, C_H-, J_H-, and FR3-Specific Primers Used for Ig V_H PCR

V_H leader primers	
V_H 1-7	ATGGACTGGACCTGGAG(GAC)ATCC
V_H 2	ATGGACATACTTTGTTCCACGCTCC
V_H 3	GAGTTTGGGCTGAGCTGG(GAC)TTTT
V_H 4	ATGAAACACCTGTGGTTCTTCCTCC
V_H 5	GGCTGTTCTCCAAGGAGTC
V_H 6	ATGTCTGTCTCCTTCCTCATCTTCC
C_H primers	
μ	CCAAGCTTAAGGAAGTCCTGTGCGAG
γ	GTAGGACAGC(CT)GGGAAGGTGTGCAC
α	CCAAGCTTGAGGCTCAGCGGGAAGACCTT
FR 3 primer	ACACGGC(CT)(AG)TGTATTACTGTGC
J_H primer	CTGA(AG)GAGAC(AG)GTGACC

with mineral oil (half volume of PCR mix) and finally add the cDNA template (1–5 μL). Briefly centrifuge, place samples in a thermocycler, and start PCR. PCR is performed as follows: 1 cycle 95°C for 10 min, 30–35 cycles 94°C of denaturation for 1 min, 59°C of annealing for 50 s, and 72°C of extension for 1 min, followed by 72°C for 10 min. An aliquot of these amplicons is run on ethidium bromide-stained 2% agarose gel at 80 Volts for 45 min and visualized under ultraviolet light.

3.2.4. HCDR3 Length Analyses

After the V_H gene family used by the lymphomatous cells is identified, a nested PCR step can be performed on only one of the samples that contain the relevant VDJ segment amplified in the first step. If this band cannot be identified for the reasons explained in the introduction, a nested PCR can be conducted in all of the samples. The more precise identification of the different lengths of HCDR3 makes possible to identify the band corresponding to the neoplastic cells, although this is not an universal finding. If this is not possible, the tracing of HCDR3 of the malignant cells can be achieved by sequencing the molecular clones as described in **Subheading 3.2.4.** and by determining the frequency of the clones. In our experience, the HCDR3 fragment of the malignant clone is by far the most represented (50% or more of the molecular clones). The first PCR product (1–3 μL), obtained as described in **Subheading 3.2.2.**, is amplified using two nested consensus primers, a sense FR3 and an antisense J_H primer (*see* **Table 2** and **Fig. 4**). PCR reagents are used as above and PCR conditions are the following: 1 cycle 95°C for 10 min; 5 cycles 94°C for 1 min, 55°C for 30 sec, 72°C for 20 s; 15 cycles 94°C for 40 s, 53°C for 30 s, 72°C for 15 s; and a final 72°C extension for 7 min. After this amplification, the products are run on a 7.5% polyacrylamide sequencing gel (*see* **Note 10**) and visualized by a silver staining protocol. With this staining, a double banding pattern (each individual strand) may be evident for each PCR product. For silver staining follow the instructions below:

1. Put the gel that stick on the glass in a basin and start wash with deionized water (10–30 min).
2. Add 10% EtOH for 5 min.
3. Add 1% HNO_3 for 30 min.
4. Wash with deionized water for a few minutes.
5. Add 12 m*M* $AgNO_3$ for 30 min (prepare fresh!).
6. Repeat **step 3**.
7. Develop reaction by adding developing solution (0.28 *M* Na_2CO_3 and 1:100 of 37% formaldehyde, prepare fresh!).
8. When bands start to be visualized, stop reaction by adding 10% acetic acid (2 min).
9. Repeat **step 3** and transfer gel on 3 *M* high-quality paper and let dry on a gel drier for 1–2 h at 80°C.

As alternative, J_H primer can be end-labeled with γ-^{32}P-dATP and T4 polynucleotide kinase and used for the nested PCR at the same conditions described above (*see* **Note 11**).

Set up reaction labeling (20 µL final volume) as follows

1. Deionized water (variable).
2. 2 µL of 10X enzyme buffer.
3. 100 pmol J_H.
4. 1 µL of T4 polynucleotide kinase.
5. 4 µL of γ ^{32}P-dATP (10 mCi/mL).

Add all these reagents in their order and incubate at 37°C for 10–30 min. Stop reaction with 50 µL of 5 *M* NH_4 Ac or in thermostat at 95°C for 10 min. Purify labeled primer in order to discharge unincorporated γ-^{32}P-dATP by using NUNC TRAP Probe Purification columns as described by the manufacturer.

After electrophoresis on the denaturing gel, bands are visualized by exposing dried gel to X-ray film for 1–3 d at –80°C.

3.2.5. cDNA Sequencing

The level and the pattern of somatic mutation of V_H genes can be determined by analyzing the sequences of V_H-expressing molecular clones. To this end, V_H-C_H amplified products obtained as in **Subheading 3.2.3.** are run in a 2% agarose gel and gel-purified by using a kit that allows the melting of the agarose and the isolation of the amplified product of interest by a DNA affinity resin. The purified products are then ligated into a TOPO TA vector (*see* **Note 12**) and transformed into TOP10F competent bacteria. Multiple colonies are picked randomly, purified using Wizard miniprep and sequenced in both directions automatically using the Ready Reaction DyeDeoxy-Terminator or the Big Dye cycle sequencing kit and vector specific primers. The products of the sequencing reaction are then analyzed using the Applied Biosystems Sequenator.

3.2.6. Sequence Analysis

The identification of the V_H, diversity genes (D_H), and junction (J_H) germline gene sequences is performed by using the MacVector software and compared with the V Base Database. This is a comprehensive database of all human Ig germline gene segments. Germline D segments are assigned to the appropriate family by applying the rule of the eight consecutive matches or seven successive matches plus 1 mismatch.

4. Notes

1. Preparation of SRBC (5%)
   - Wash 3X SRBC in saline to eliminate preservative (i.e., ethylenediamine tetraacetic acid, citric acid, etc);
   - Dilute 2.5 mL of SRBC 1/20 in saline; add 0.5 units of Neuraminidase and keep at 37°C for 30 min; and
   - Wash 3X in saline and suspend in 10% FCS culture medium. 1 mL of SRBC is able to rosette 30×10^6 MNCs.
2. Preparation of Percoll gradients. Percoll solution referred to as 100% is obtained by addition nine parts (v/v) of Percoll to one part (v/v) of 10X concentrated cell culture medium, usually Hanks Balanced Salt Solution. All the other Percoll concentrations are obtained by diluting out the 100% Percoll with 1X concentrated culture medium, usually RPMI.
3. We recommend the use of polystyrene plastic tubes because polypropylene tubes are more slippery and may induce mixing of cells with different density during recovery.
4. EDTA serves to prevent cells from clumping. The EDTA/BSA buffer must be degassed to avoid bubble formation in the column matrix during separation. This fact may result in a low purity of purified cells.
5. Preparation of GAM-sensitized ORBC (2.5%)
   - Wash 1 mL of OXRCs 3X in saline;
   - Dilute out 1:1 with saline;
   - Place 200 mL of this suspension in a conical tube;
   - Add 300 mL GAM (1 mg/mL in saline) on the top of suspension;
   - Add 600 mL of 1:10 dilution $CrCl_3$ (1 mg/mL, pH 5.0) drop by drop while vortexing;

- Add 1 mL of saline and kept ORBC at 4°C overnight;
- Wash 3X gently by centrifugation in saline; and
- Suspended in 4 mL of 10% FCS medium. 1 mL of GAM-sensitized ORBC will rosette 15×10^6 cells

6. Na-Azide added to the buffer used for the staining of cells will prevent capping of surface antigen-antibody complexes.
7. RNA is a highly degradable nucleic acid by the RNase ubiquitous enzyme. For this reason all reagents and instrumentation used during manipulation of RNA must be RNase-free. Operator must put on gloves, and glasses must be baked at 200°C. In addition, all solutions to be used must be autoclaved for at least 1 h. It also can be safe to use diethylene pyrocarbonate–water to resupend RNA and to prepare solutions. To this end, add 0.2% of diethylene pyrocarbonate to water, stir/shake vigorously for 1 h, and autoclave before use.
8. When the amount of cells used for the RNA preparation is to low, add 1 µg of glycogen during precipitation with isopropanol. This will help to "see" the RNA after the centrifugation step and to not lose it during EtOH wash.
9. When the amount of RNA recovered is too low, we recommended retrotranscribing all the RNA and to store only the cDNA.
10. Denaturing polyacrylamide gel is prepared by polymerizing acrylamide and bis acrylamide in a 19:1 ratio (40%) and 7 *M* urea added as denaturing agent. It is important to run the gel with 1X TBE at pH 8.3 (Tris base 1 *M*, boric acid 1 *M*, Na_2EDTA 20 m*M*) at 75 Watts. Before loading denatured samples (denaturation is achieved at 95°C for 2 min), prerun the gel for 30–45 min. While prerunning, remove urea that accumulates on the top of the gel by using a syringe or a plastic Pasteur.
11. This "Hot" PCR has a discrete sensibility and thus, the concentration of both FR3 and J_H primers is lowed to 15 pmol/ PCR. After purification, 3 pmol/ 5 µl of hot J_H primer is used together with 12 µL of cold J_H to make the final concentration of 15 pmol/ PCR.
12. Taq polymerase has a nontemplate dependent terminal transferase activity that adds single deoxyadenosine (A) to the 3' ends of the amplified products. The TA vector has deoxythymidine (T) at 3' overhangs. This permits PCR products to be inserted into the vector. However, since these (A)s are easily missed over time, it's recommended to proceed immediately after amplification to cloning of the samples.

References

1. Rajewsky, K. (1996) Clonal selection and learning in the antibody system. *Nature* **381,** 751–758.
2. McHeyzer-Williams, M. G., and Ahmed R. (1999) B-cell memory and long-lived plasma cells. *Curr. Opin. Immunol.* **11,** 172–179.
3. Küppers R., Zhao M., Hansmann M. L., and Rajewsky K. (1993) Tracing B-cell development in human germinal centres by molecular analysis of single cells picked from histological sections. *EMBO J.* **12,** 4955–4967.

4. Nakamura S., Yao T., Aoyagi K. Iida M., Fujishima M., and Tsuneyoshi M. (1997) Helicobacter pylori and primary gastric lymphoma. A histopathologic and immunohistochemical analysis of 237 patients. *Cancer* **79,** 3–11.
5. Bahler DW, Swerdlow SH. (1998) Clonal salivary gland infiltrates associated with myoepithelial sialadenitis (Sjogren's syndrome) begin as non malignant antigen-selected expansions. *Blood* **91,** 1864–72.
6. MacLennan I. C., and Liu Y. J. (1991) Marginal zone B-cells respond both to polysaccharide antigens and protein antigens. *Res. Immunol.* **142,** 346–51
7. Guinamard R., Okigaki M., Schlessinger J., and Ravetch J. V. (2000) Absence of marginal zone B-cells in Pyk-2-deficient mice defines their role in the humoral response. *Nat. Immunol.* **1,** 31–36.
8. Dono M., Burgio V. L., Tacchettic. , Favre A, Augliera A., Zupo S., Taborelli G., Chiorazzi N., Grossi C. E., and Ferrarini M. (1996). Subepithelial B-cells in the human palatine tonsil. I. Morphologic, cytochemical and phenotypic Characterization. *Eur J. Immunol.* **26,** 2035–2042.
9. Morente M., Piris M. A., Orradre J. L., Rivas C., and Villuendas R. (1992) Human Tonsil Intraepithelial B-cells: a marginal zone-related subpopulation. *J. Clin. Pathol.* **45,** 668–672.
10. Dono M., Zupo S., Burgio V. L., Augliera A., Tacchetti C., Favre A., et al. (1997) Phenotypic and functional characterization of human tonsillar subepithelial (SE) B-cells. *Ann. NY Acad. Sci.* **815,** 171–181.
11. Dono M., Zupo S., Masante R., Taborelli G., Chiorazzi N., and Ferrarini M. (1993) Identification of two distinct CD5-B-cell subsets from human tonsils with different responses to CD40 monoclonal antibody. *Eur. J. Immunol* **23,** 873–881.
12. Liu Y. J., Barthelemy C., De Bouteiller O., Arpin C., Durand I., and Banchereau J. (1995) Memory B-cells from human tonsils colonize mucosal epithelium and directly present antigen to T-cells by rapid up-regulation of B7-1 and B7-2. *Immunity* **2,** 239–248.
13. Pascual V., Liu Y-J., Magalski A., de Bouteiller O., Banchereau J., and Capra J. D. (1994) Analysis of somatic mutation in five B-cell subsets of human tonsil. *J. Exp. Med.* **180,** 329–339.
14. Dono M., Zupo S., Leanza N., Melioli G., Fogli M., Melagrana A., Chiorazzi N., and Ferrarini M. (2000) Heterogeneity of tonsillar subepithelial B lymphocytes, the splenic marginal zone equivalents. *J. Immunol.* **164,** 5596–604.
15. Dono M., Zupo S., Augliera A., Burgio V. L., Massara R., Melagrana A., et al. (1996) Subepithelial B-cells in the human palatine tonsil. II. Functional characterization. *Eur. J. Immunol.* **26,** 2043–2049.
16. Weller S., Faili A., Garcia C., Braun M. C., Le Deist F. F., de Saint Basile G. G., et al. (2001) CD40-CD40L independent Ig gene hypermutation suggests a second B-cell diversification pathway in humans. *Proc. Natl. Acad. Sci. USA.* **98,** 1166–1170.
17. Macpherson A. J., Lamarre A., McCoy K., Harriman G. R., Odermatt B., Dougan G., et al. (2001). IgA production without mu or delta chain expression in developing B-cells. *Nat. Immunol.* **2,** 625–631.
18. De Wolf-Peeters C. and Delabie J. (1993) Anatomy and histopathology of lymphoid tissue. *Semin. Oncol.* **20,** 555–569.

19. Van den Oord J. J., de Wolf-Peeters C., De Vos R., and Desmet V. J. (1985) Immature sinus histiocytosis. Light- and electron-microscopic features, immunologic phenotype, and relationship with marginal zone lymphocytes. *Am. J. Pathol.* **118,** 266–277.
20. Tierens A., Delabie J., Michiels L., Vandenberghe P., and De Wolf Peeters C. (1999) Marginal-Zone B-cells in the human lymph node and spleen show somatic hypermutations and display clonal expansion. *Blood* **93,** 226–234.
21. Dono M., Zupo S., Colombo M., Massara R., Gaidano G., Taborelli G., et al. (2004). The human marginal zone B-cell. *Ann. NY Acad. Sci.* **36,** 2105–2111.
22. Hsu S. M. (1985) Phenotypic expression of B lymphocytes. III. Marginal Zone B-cells in the spleen are characterized by the expression of Tac and Alkaline Phosphatase. *J. Immunol.* **135,** 123–130.
23. Timens W., Boes A., and Poppema S. (1989) Human Marginal Zone B-cells are not an activated B-cell subset: strong expression of CD21 as a putative mediator for rapid B-cell activation. *Eur. J. Immunol.* **19,** 2163–2166.
24. Martin F., Kearney J.F. (2000) Positive selection from newly formed to marginal zone B-cells depends on the rate of clonal production, CD19, and btk. *Immunity* **12,** 39–49.
25. Cariappa A., Tang M., Parng C., Nebelitskiy E., Carroll M., Georgopoulos K., et al. (2001) The follicular versus marginal zone B lymphocyte cell fate decision is regulated by Aiolos, Btk, and CD21. *Immunity* **14,** 603–615.
26. Dunn-Walters D. K., Isaacson P. G., and Spencer J. (1995) Analysis of Mutations in Immunoglobulin Heavy Chain Variable region genes of microdissected marginal zone (MGZ) B-cells suggests that the MGZ of human spleen is a reservoir of memory B-cells. *J. Exp. Med.* **182,** 559–566.
27. Oliver A. M., Martin F., and Kearney J. F. (1999) IgM^{high} IgD^{high} lymphocytes enriched in the splenic marginal zone generate effector cells more rapidly than the bulk of follicular B-cells. *J. Immunol.* **162,** 7198–7205.
28. Dono M., Zupo S., Massara R., Ferrini S., Melagrana A., Chiorazzi N., and Ferrarini M. (2001) In vitro stimulation of human tonsillar subepithelial B-cells: requirement for interaction with activated T-cells. *Eur. J. Immunol.* **31,** 752–757.
29. Cavalli F., Isaacson P. G., Gascoyne R. D., and Zucca E. (2001) MALT Lymphomas. *Hematology* 241–258.
30. Parsonnet J., Hansen S., Rodriguez L., Gelb A. B., Warnke R. A., Jellum E., et al. (1994). Helicobacter pylori infection and gastric lymphoma. *N. Engl. J. Med.* **330,** 1267–1271.
31. Hussell T., Isaacson, P. G., Crabtree, J. E., Dogan, A., and Spencer, J. (1993) Immunoglobulin specificity of low grade B-cell gastrointestinal lymphoma of mucosa-associated lymphoid tissue (MALT) type. *Am. J. Pathol.* **142,** 285–292.
32. Tierens A., Delabie J., Pittaluga S., Driessen A., and DeWolf-Peeters C. (1998) Mutation analysis of the rearranged immunoglobulin heavy chain genes of marginal zone cell lymphomas indicates an origin from different marginal zone B lymphocyte subsets. *Blood* **91,** 2381–2386.

33. Wang D., Wells S. M., Stall A. M., and Kabat E. A. (1994) Reaction of germinal centers in the T-cell-independent response to the bacterial polysaccharide alpha(1->6)dextran. *Proc. Natl. Acad. Sci. USA* **91,** 2502–2510.
34. Miranda R.N., Cousar J.B., Hammer R.D., Collins R.D., and Vnencak-Jones C.L. (1999) Somatic mutation analysis of IgH variable regions reveals that tumor cells of most parafollicular (monocytoid) B-cell lymphoma, splenic marginal zone B-cell lymphoma, and some hairy cell leukemia are composed of memory B lymphocytes. *Hum Pathol.* **30,** 306–312.
35. Ngan B. Y., Warnke R. A., Wilson M., Takagi K., Cleary M. L., and Dorfman R. F. (1991) Monocytoid B-cell lymphoma: a study of 36 cases. *Hum. Pathol.* **22,** 409–421.
36. Kuppers R., Hajadi M., Plank L., Rajewsky K., and Hansmann M. L. (1996) Molecular Ig gene analysis reveals that monocytoid B-cell lymphoma is a malignancy of mature B-cells carrying somatically mutated V region genes and suggests that rearrangement of the kappa-deleting element (resulting in deletion of the Ig kappa enhancers) abolishes somatic hypermutation in the human. *Eur. J. Immunol.* **26,** 1794–1800.
37. Mateo M. S., Mollejo M., Villuendas R., Algara P., Sanchez Beato M., Martinez P., et al. (2001) Molecular heterogeneity of splenic marginal zone lymphomas: analysis of mutations in the 5'non-coding region of the bcl-6 gene. *Leukemia* **15,** 628–634.
38. Sole F., Salido M., Espinet B., Garcia J.L., Martinez Climent J. A., et al. (2001) Splenic marginal zone B-cell lymphomas: two cytogenetic subtypes, one with gain of 3q and the other with loss of 7q. *Haematologica.* **86,** 71–77.
39. Zhu D., Oscier D. G., and Stevenson F. K. (1995) Splenic lymphoma with lymphocytes involves B-cells with extensively mutated Ig heavy chain variable region genes *Blood* **85,** 1603–1607.
40. Dunn-Walters D. K., Boursier L., Spencer J., and Isaacson P. G. (1998) Analysis of immunoglobulin genes in splenic marginal zone lymphoma suggests ongoing mutation *Human Pathol.* **29,** 585–593.
41. Algara P., Mateo M. S., Sanchez-Beato M., et al. (2002) Analysis of the IgV(H) somatic mutations in splenic marginal zone lymphoma defines a group of unmutated cases with frequent 7q deletion and adverse clinical course. *Blood* **99,** 1299–1304.

9

T-Cell Receptor Molecular Diagnosis of T-Cell Lymphoma

Elizabeth Hodges, Anthony P. Williams, Susan Harris, and John L. Smith

Summary

Malignant and reactive lymphoproliferations in most cases can be distinguished by histology and immunohistology alone; however, in T-cell lymphoproliferations and lymphoproliferations of unknown origin, histology often is inconclusive, and there is no reliable protein marker of malignancy. At the genomic level T-cell neoplasms clonally rearrange T-cell receptor (TCR) genes that can serve as clonal markers. In comparison with Southern blot analysis, polymerase chain reaction (PCR) techniques increasingly are being used to detect these rearrangements because PCRs are rapid, easy to perform, and can be used to amplify poor-quality deoxyribonucleic acid (DNA) from paraffin-embedded formalin-fixed biopsies. Nevertheless there are a number of problems associated with the detection of gene rearrangements using PCR. The foremost of these is improper primer annealing that will lead to false-negative or false-positive PCR results that may arise from poor primer design, especially for TCRB genes with an extensive variable (V), diversity (D), and joined (J) gene repertoire. There also can be difficulty in discriminating between clonal and polyclonal PCR products unless specific methods such as heteroduplex analysis or gene scanning are used. In this chapter, we describe methods, derived from a recent European collaborative BIOMED-2 program, for the detection of TCRG, B, and D rearrangements. TCRB VJ and DJ gene rearrangements are detected using 23 VB primers, 13 JB primers, and 2 DB primers in 3 multiplex tubes. TCRG VJ gene rearrangements are detected with four VG and two JG primers in two multiplex tubes, and TCRD VJ, VD, DJ, and DD rearrangements are detected with six VD primers, four JD primers, and two DD primers in one multiplex tube. Gaussian distributions of polyclonal PCR products are seen at specific size ranges for both TCRB and TCRG. Interpretation of TCRD rearrangements is more complex because of the wide range in PCR product size and often low numbers of TCRGD cells in target tissue. For all loci, some indication of gene usage can be ascertained by labeling the primers with different fluorochromes and gene scan analysis of PCR products. Furthermore the complementarity of the TCR loci affords an unprecedented high clonal detection rate. In addition, we also describe a set of control gene primers designed to amplify amplicons of 100, 200, 300, 400, and 600 bp for the assessment of the integrity and amplifiability of DNA. This set of primers is particularly useful for the assessment of DNA extracted from paraffin-embedded biopsies.

Key Words: T-cell lymphomas; TCR gene rearrangements; BIOMED-2; PCR; gene scanning; heteroduplex analysis.

From: *Methods in Molecular Medicine, Vol. 115: Lymphoma: Methods and Protocols*
Edited by: T. Illidge and P. W. M. Johnson © Humana Press Inc., Totowa, NJ

1. Introduction

Lymphoid malignancies are a heterogeneous group of disease that result from the neoplastic transformation of T, B, or natural killer (NK) cells at different stages of ontogeny and development. The classification of such malignancies has recently been standardized through the efforts of the World Health Organization *(1)*.

The clinical diagnosis of such lymphoid malignancies is supported by a range of laboratory investigations. Traditionally, these investigations involved morphological analysis of the lymphocytes in conjunction with monoclonal antibody staining of cell surface and intracellular/nuclear antigens. B-cell clonality clearly is demonstrated by immunoglobulin (Ig) light chain restriction; however, there is no analogous surface protein for T-cell clonality. The advent of new molecular techniques, such as Southern blot and polymerase chain reaction (PCR) analysis, together with the identification and sequencing of the T-cell receptor alpha, beta, gamma, and delta genes, has facilitated the development of T-cell clonality techniques *(2–9)*. Such techniques also are applied to Ig gene analysis and chromosomal translocations *(2,4)*. During the 1990s, the focus on T- and B-cell clonality for the diagnosis of lymphoid malignancy gathered momentum and was supported by advances in basic science. The greater availability of reagents for the detection of B-cell neoplasms through the detection of monoclonal surface immunoglobulin and the paucity of such reagents for T-cell studies led to other approaches being explored for the characterization of T-cell clonality. Although TCRVβ antibody studies can be used as an initial screening method for the detection of expanded families and/or skewing of the T-cell repertoire in various disease states, molecular analysis still is required to assess the clonality of the expanded T-cell population *(10)*. During the last 5–7 yr, molecular studies have addressed this diagnostic imbalance through the use of sequence specific PCR multiplex technology that is directed towards TCR beta, alpha, gamma, and delta gene families *(4–8)*. More recently, new TCR primer sets and protocols have been assessed as part of the BIOMED-2 concerted action *(11,12)* and will be addressed in this chapter. However, it is first worth reviewing the gene structure and properties of TCR rearrangements that lend themselves to the identification of T-cell clonality through multiplex PCR technology.

T-cell and B-cell receptors are similar in their structure comprising of disulfide-linked heterodimers that are constructed from variable (V) and constant (C) genes regions. The TCR is typically a heterodimer of alpha (α) and beta (β) chains (approx 95% of T-cells), with a minor fraction bearing the gamma (γ)/delta (δ) heterodimer *(13)*. The α- and δ-chain genes are located on chromosome 14q11, and the β-chain genes are located on chromosome 7q34. The γ chain genes are on chromosome 7p15 *(9)*. There is a preordained order for

TCR gene rearrangements with the δ gene rearranging first followed sequentially by the γ, β and, finally, α genes. Each germline configuration contains multiple exons for the variable region and constant regions of the TCR. The variable regions consist of V, diversity (D), and joining (J) gene segments and are usually located 5' of the C gene segment. The complexity and the number of V, D, J, and C gene segments available for recombination is different for each TCR loci (**Table 1**) *(9)*. The process of gene segment rearrangement is again sequential, with initial juxtaposition of a D segment to a J segment, with deletion of the intervening non-coding deoxyribonucleic acid (DNA). In the same way, a V region is next apposed to a DJ segment, with cleavage of the intervening DNA to form a VDJ gene segment *(14)*. Prior to the joining of the VDJ coding segment with the C gene segment, the whole region is transcribed to a mitochondrial ribonucleic acid (mRNA) template. Finally, splicing of the VDJ region to the C region occurs, and the completed TCR receptor chain is transcribed into the TCR polypeptide chain for assembly on the cell surface (**Fig. 1**). For the TCRG and TCRA genes, direct VJ joining occurs, attributed to the absence of D segments at these loci. Therefore, diversity of the T-cell repertoire is not only a consequence of different V, D, and J recombinations but also as a result of nucleotide insertion and deletion at junctional sites thereby increasing diversity for recognition of a vast array of antigens.

The molecular approaches of Southern blot and PCR amplification use this ordered approach to gene recombination for the assessment of the clonality of the T-cell population. Clonal populations with unique gene rearrangements and CDR3 sequences can be identified through identical VDJ/VJ rearrangements, which contrasts with the multiple different gene recombinations seen in normal T-cells. Southern blot analysis largely has been replaced by PCR because PCR is quicker to perform and poor-quality DNA can be used. The type of PCR approach will depend on whether DNA- or RNA-based methods are applicable. Paraffin-embedded material often is the only material available in routine diagnostic pathology laboratories; therefore, protocols are restricted to DNA-based methods and the amplification of small (<250 bp) PCR fragments. Both DNA and RNA methods are suitable for fresh material. After amplification with specific TCR primers, amplified products are detected by a variety of methods, which include heteroduplex analysis and/or by gene scanning *(6–8)*. Both detection methods exploit the heterogeneity of the size of the PCR fragments, but heteroduplex analysis also exploits the conformation of the PCR products and, therefore, clonal T-cell populations are clearly distinguishable from polyclonal reactive T-cell populations.

These molecular approaches, which have also been applied to B-cell neoplasms, have numerous advantages over traditional approaches used in the diagnosis and classification of T-cell lymphoma. We will highlight these advantages

Table 1
Diversity of TCR Repertoire

TCR	α	β	γ	δ
V segments	54(41)	65(30)	15(4)	8
D segments	0	2	0	3
J segments	61	13(2)	5(3)	4
VDJ recombinations	3294	1690	75	96
N regions	1	2	1	2–4
V domains	10^6	10^9	10^4	10^{13}
V domain pairs	10^{15}		10^{17}	

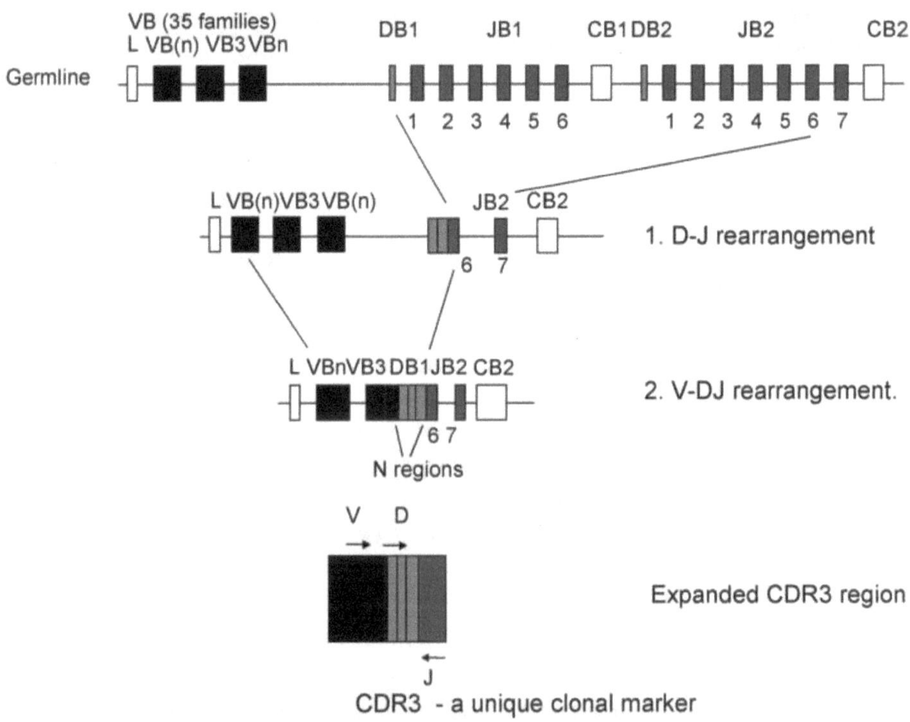

Fig. 1. TCRB gene rearrangement. Schematic diagram showing the two-step recombination process of TCRB gene rearrangement. First, one of the two D genes (D1) joins to one J gene (J2.6), followed by the joining of one V gene (V3) to the DJ coding block. The hatched boxes indicate N regions. The conserved sequences of the, V, D, and J genes (or flanking regions) serve as primer binding sites whilst the complementarity determining region (CDR) 3 serve as a unique clonal marker for each cell.

in this chapter and discuss how this information may be integrated with the clinical, morphological, genetic, and immunophenotyping data for the accurate diagnosis and follow-up of T-cell lymphoma. The TCR primer sets and the molecular techniques described in this chapter were designed as part of the BIOMED-2 concerted action (BMH4-CT98-3936), which was involved in the design and standardization of PCR primers and protocols for the detection of TCR as well as Ig gene rearrangements and chromosomal translocations in suspect lymphoproliferations *(11,12)*. As part of the BIOMED-2 program, the newly designed primer sets have been comprehensively tested against a series of T- and B-cell lymphoproliferations that had been characterized previously by immunohistology, immunophenotype, and Southern blot analysis, and the high detection rates found have been unprecedented.

2. Materials

2.1. Preparation of DNA From Peripheral Blood Mononuclear Cells (PBMCs)

1. QIAamp mini blood kit (QIAGEN, Crawley, West Sussex, United Kingdom).
2. Absolute ethanol (Hayman Ltd, Witham, Essex, United Kingdom).

2.2. Preparation of DNA From Paraffin Sections

1. QIAamp mini blood kit (QIAGEN).
2. Absolute ethanol (Hayman Ltd).
3. Proteinase K @10 mg/mL (QIAGEN).
4. Xylene.

2.3. Multiplex PCR Amplification of TCRB, TCRG, TCRD, and Control Genes

A DNA engine thermal cycler is used in the laboratory to perform all our PCRs. All primer mixes are aliquoted and stored at –20°C. All buffers, dNTPs, magnesium chloride, and Taq polymerase are all stored at –20°C.

1. Water: sterile deionized water (molecular grade).
2. Oligonucleotide primers (Available from In Vivo Scribe, specific primer sequences available from Professor JJM van Dongen *[12]*) all are stored at a concentration of 100 pmol/µL for dilution to 10 pmol/0.1 µL for all PCRs.
3. 10X Buffer II: complete with magnesium at 1.5 m*M* (Applied Biosystems International (ABI), Warrington, Cheshire, UK).
4. dNTPs: 1.25 m*M* of each deoxyribonucleoside triphosphate [dNTP] is stored at –20°C. (Amersham-Pharmacia-Biotech, Little Chalfont, Buckinghamshire, UK).
5. Taq polymerase; AmpliTaq Gold (5 U/µL; ABI).
6. DNA template: 100 ng per 50-µL reaction.

2.4. Heteroduplex Analysis

Heteroduplex analysis is used to discriminate between heterogeneous and homogeneous PCR products. Clonal PCR products will anneal to form homoduplexes after heat denaturation and rapid cooling whereas polyclonal PCR products will form heteroduplexes. The homoduplexes can be separated from the heteroduplexes on a nondenaturing polyacrylamide gel as they migrate more rapidly through the gel whereas the heteroduplexes from a background smear of slower-migrating species. In addition to the materials listed below, a vertical electrophoresis tank, glass plates, power pack transilluminator, and photoimager are necessary for heteroduplex analysis.

1. Accugel mix (29:1; National Diagnostics, Hessle, Yorkshire, UK).
2. Ammonium persulphate (AMP; Sigma, Poole, Dorset, UK).
3. TEMED (Sigma).
4. Sucrose (Sigma).
5. Bromophenol blue (Sigma).
6. Ethidium bromide (Sigma).
7. pBR322 HAE III DNA ladder (Sigma).
8. 10X TBE (National Diagnostics).

2.5. Genescanning

Genescanning is a capillary electrophoresis system that allows for automated, high-throughput fragment analysis. The principal of the detection system is that primers are 5' labeled with fluorescence dyes that fluoresce when excited with an argon laser. The emitted fluorescence is then collected on a CCD camera and may be compared with control fragments of known length (Rox molecular weight marker). The detection cell supports the identification of five fluorescent dyes. We use the dyes 6-FAM (blue), HEX (green), and NED (yellow).

1. ABI PRISM 3100 Genetic Analyser for Gene Scanning (ABI).
2. Fluorescent-labeled primer (available from In Vivo Scribe).
3. GeneScan software (ABI).
4. HiDi formamide Rox 400 HD molecular weight marker (ABI).

3. Methods

3.1. Preparation of DNA From PBMCs

Genomic DNA (gDNA) is prepared from whole blood and other bodily fluids using the commercially available QIAGEN mini blood kit, according to the manufacturer's protocol (*see* **Notes 1–3**). This approach is fast, reliable, and ensures that gDNA is free from protein, nucleases, and other contaminants/inhibitors. DNA quantitation is undertaken by spectrophotometric analysis using a UV 1101 Spectrophotometer. Five microliters of the gDNA sample is added to 495 µL of distilled water and mixed thoroughly (*see* **Note 4**). The reading at 260 nm allows the concentration of gDNA in the sample to be calculated whereas the ratio of the reading at 260 nm and 280 nm provides an estimate of the purity of the gDNA.

3.2. Preparation of DNA From Paraffin Sections

We routinely cut our own sections from paraffin-embedded samples.

1. Wash the microtome knife holder thoroughly with xylene and then return to the microtome block. Insert a new knife blade into knife holder (*see* **Note 5**). The thickness setting is set to 15 µm and cut 6 × 15-µm sections.
2. Each section is transferred with a sterile needle or forceps to a microcentrifuge tube labeled with the patient's name, biopsy number, and date.
3. In a fume hood, add 1 mL of xylene to each microcentrifuge tube and mix gently until the paraffin wax has dissolved (*see* **Note 6**). The sample is then centrifuged at 6000*g* for 5 min.
4. The xylene is then removed and the pellet resuspended in 1 mL of absolute ethanol and centrifuged again at top speed.
5. The pellet is then washed with 0.5 mL of absolute ethanol and centrifuged again prior to drying the pellet at 56°C for 30 min.
6. The gDNA is then prepared from the pellet using the commercially available QIAGEN QIAamp DNA mini blood kit, according to the manufacturer's protocol (*see* **Note 3**).

3.3. Multiplex PCR Amplification of TCRB, TCRG, TCRD, and Control Genes

3.3.1. PCR Amplification of TCRG Chain Genes

1. Two multiplex PCR tubes are used to analyze different VJ recombinations of the TCRG chain genes. Both tube A and tube B are set up similarly with the same J primers but different V primers (**Fig. 2**). The J1.3/2.3 primer is labeled with FAM, and the J1.1/2.1 is labeled with HEX (*see* **Note 7**). The tubes (*see* **Note 8**) are set up (in a total reaction volume of 50 µL) as follows:

	TCRG mix
Sterile water (*see* **Note 9**)	33.4 µL
10X buffer II	5 µL
dNTP mix (1.25 m*M*)	8 µL (0.2 m*M*)
$MgCl_2$ (25 m*M*)	3 µL (1.5 m*M*)
TCRG primers[a]	0.4 µL (10 pmol of each primer)
AmpliTaq Gold	0.2 µL (1U)
100 ng of DNA	

[a]TCRG tube A: VF1, V10, J1.3/2.3, J1.1/2.1; for [a]TCRG tube B: V9, V11, J1.3/2.3, J1.1/2.1.

For storage of PCR reagents, see Notes 10 and 11, for general PCR set up, and for validity of data, *see* **Notes 12–20**.

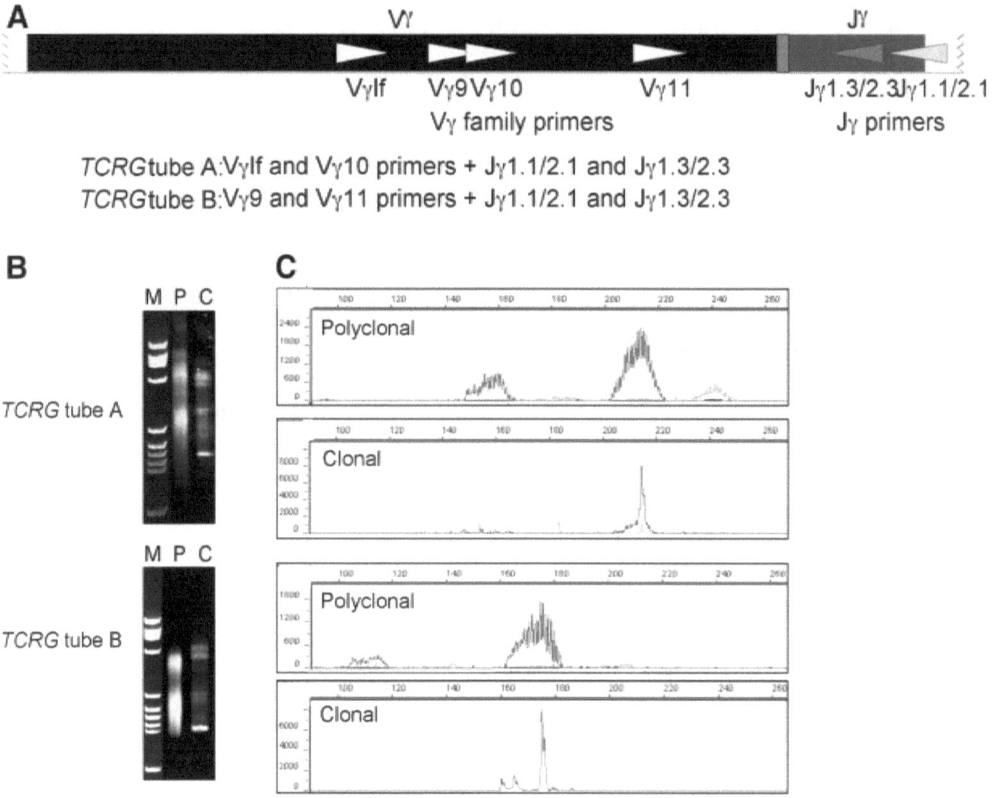

Fig. 2. PCR analysis of *TCRG* gene rearrangements. **(A)** Schematic diagram indicating the appropriate position and designation of V and J region primers for TCRG PCR analysis. The hatched boxes represent N regions. **(B)** Heteroduplex analysis of PCR products from both tube A and B PCRs. M, molecular weight marker; P, polyclonal peripheral blood DNA; C, clonal T-cell lymphoma DNA. Such analysis exploits the differences in the sizes of the PCR products as well as the variation in sequences. Heteroduplexes of imperfectly matched junctional sequences are seen as ill defined smears retarded in the gel whereas homoduplexes of identical junctional sequences are identified as narrow bands within the appropriate size range. **(C)** Genescan analysis of the same samples as shown in **(B)**. PCR fragment size is plotted against fluorescent intensity. TCRG analysis of polyclonal samples for both tube A and B demonstrate four Gaussian distributions representing different gene recombinations in varying magnitudes. For tube A, PCR analysis identifies a clonal population (narrow peak) representing Vf1–J1.3/2.3 gene recombination. A different clonal sample for tube B analysis demonstrates a V9–J1.3/2.3 gene recombination. *See* **Color Plate 6**, following page 270.

2. The standardized cycling conditions are: 94°C for 10 min, then 35 cycles of 94°C for 1 min/60°C for 1 min/72°C for 1 min. The samples are then heated to 72°C for 10 min for a final extension, prior to holding at 8°C.

3.3.2. PCR Amplification of TCRB Chain Genes

1. Three multiplex PCR tubes are required to analyze partial and complete TCRB chain gene rearrangements (**Fig. 3**). All JB primers are labeled with FAM or for distinction between different J gene usage JB1 primers can be labeled with FAM and JB2 primers with HEX (*see* **Note 7**). The PCRs are set up (in a total reaction volume of 50 µL) as follows (*see* **Note 8**):

	TCRB-A mix	TCRB-B mix
Sterile water (*see* **Note 9**)	27.4 µL	27.9 µL
10X buffer II	5 µL	5 µL
dNTP mix (1.25 m*M*)	8 µL (0.2 m*M*)	8 µL (0.2 m*M*)
$MgCl_2$ (25 m*M*)	6 µL (3.0 m*M*)	6 µL (3.0 m*M*)
TCRB primers	3.2 µL (10 pmol of each primer[a])	2.7 µL (10 pmol of each primer[b])
AmpliTaq Gold	0.4 µL (2U)	0.4 µL (2 U)
100 ng DNA		

	TCRB-C mix
Sterile water (*see* **Note 9**)	33.2 µL
10X buffer II	5 µL
dNTP mix (1.25 m*M*)	8 µL (0.2 m*M*)
$MgCl_2$ (25 m*M*)	3 µL (1.5 m*M*)
TCRB primers	1.5 µL (10 pmol of each primer[c])
AmpliTaq Gold	0.2 µL (1U)
100 ng DNA	

[a]TCRB A mix (32 primers): 23 VB primers, 6 JB1 primers (JB1.1-1.6), and 3 JB2 primers (JB2.2, 2.6, 2.7).
[b]TCRB B mix (27 primers): 23 VB primers and 4JB2 primers (JB2.1, 2.3, 2.4, 2.5).
[c]TCRB C mix (15 primers): DB1, DB2 primers and 6 JB1 primers (JB1.1–1.6) and 7 JB2 primers (JB2.1–2.7).
For storage of PCR reagents, *see* **Notes 10** and **11**, and for general PCR set up and validity of data, *see* **Notes 12–20.**

2. The PCR cycling conditions are as noted previously.

3.3.3. PCR Amplification of TCRD Chain Genes

1. Only one multiplex PCR tube is necessary to analyze full and partial TCRD gene rearrangements (including VDJ, DJ, DD, and VD). There are six V primers (VD1, VD2, VD3, VD4, VD5, VD6), three J primers (JD1, JD2, JD3), and two D prim-

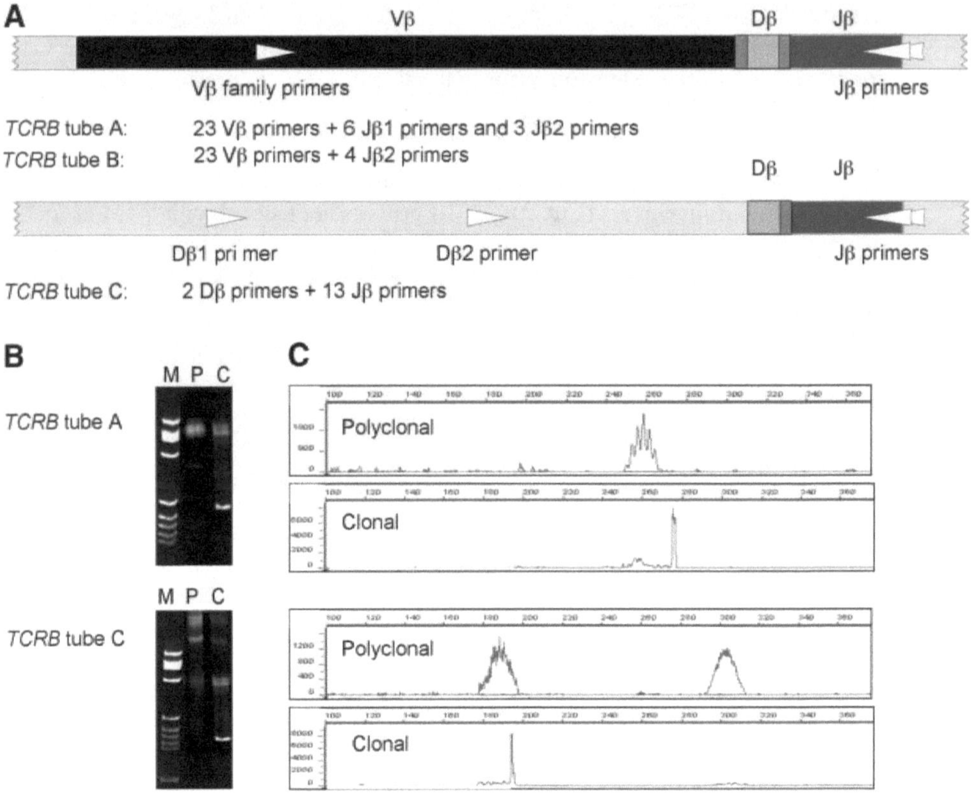

Fig. 3. PCR analysis of *TCRB* gene rearrangements. **(A)** Schematic diagram indicating the appropriate position and designation of V, D, and J region primers for the analysis of complete and partial TCRB gene rearrangements. The hatched boxes represent N regions. **(B)** Heteroduplex analysis of PCR products from tube A and C PCR reactions. M, molecular weight marker; P, polyclonal peripheral blood DNA; C, clonal T-cell lymphoma DNA. **(C)** Genescan analysis of the same samples as shown in **B**. TCRB analysis of polyclonal peripheral blood DNA identifies one Gaussian distribution in tube A and two in tube C. A complete TCRB VDJ rearrangement is identified in the clonal sample for tube A analysis whereas a clonal peak identifying a D2-J recombination is identified for tube C analysis. *See* **Color Plate 7**, following page 270.

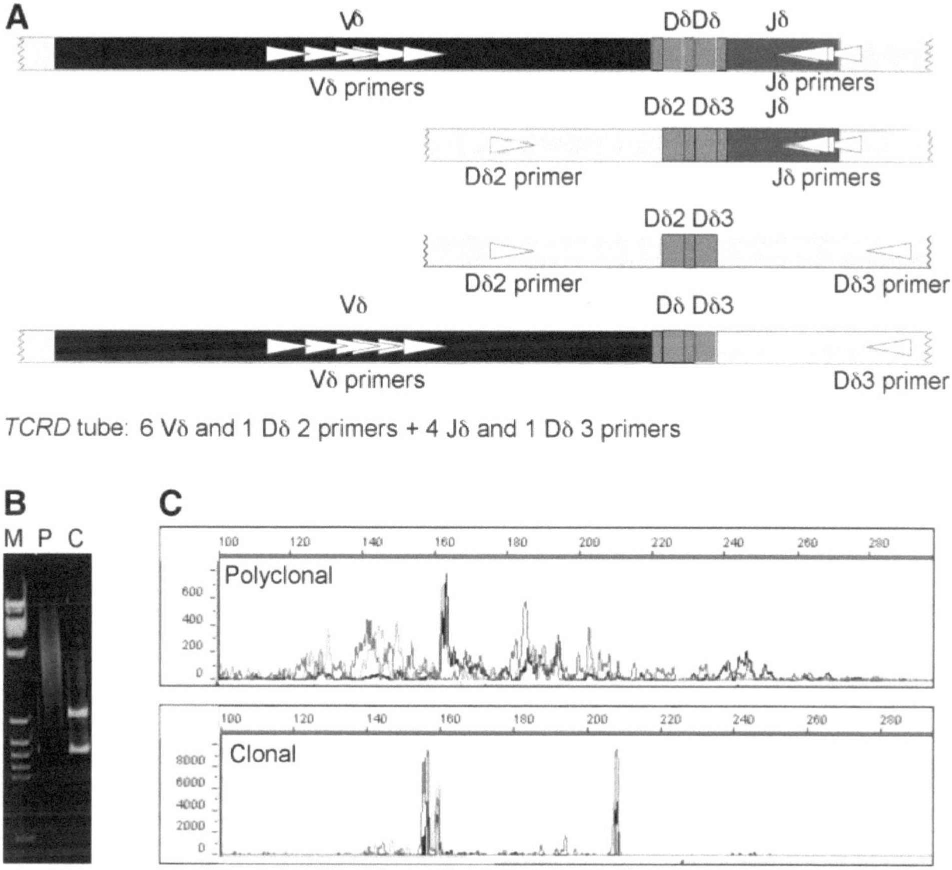

Fig. 4. PCR analysis of *TCRD* gene rearrangements. (**A**) Schematic diagram indicating the appropriate position and designation of V, D, and J region primers for complete (VDJ) and partial (DJ, DD, VD) TCRD PCR analysis. The hatched boxes represent N regions. (**B**) Heteroduplex analysis of PCR products from the single multiplex tube used for TCRD analysis. M, molecular weight marker; P, polyclonal peripheral blood DNA; C, clonal T-cell lymphoma DNA. (**C**) Genescan analysis of the same samples as shown in **B**. The fluorescent profile of a polyclonal sample is distinct from a normal Gaussian distribution (seen in **Figs. 2C** and **3C**) as a consequence of the large range in TCRD PCR product sizes. However, clonal products are easily identified as shown for the representative clonal DNA from a T-cell lymphoma showing a partial DJ and full VDJ clonal rearrangement. *See* **Color Plate 8**, following page 270.

ers (one 5' D2 and one 3' D3; **Fig. 4**; *see* **Note 7**). To identify different partial and full TCRD recombinations, JD1 is labeled with HEX, JD2-JD4 with FAM, and 3'D3 with NED. The PCR set up (in a total reaction volume of 50ul) as follows (*see* **Note 8**):

	TCRD mix
Sterile water (*see* **Note 9**)	31.5 µL
10X buffer II	5 µL
dNTP mix (1.25 m*M*)	8 µL (0.2 m*M*)
$MgCl_2$ (25 m*M*)	4 µL (2.0 m*M*)
TCRD primer mix	1.35 µL (10 pmol of each primer)
AmpliTaq Gold	0.2 µL (1U)
100 ng DNA	

For storage of PCR reagents, *see* **Notes 10** and **11**, and for general PCR set up and validity of data, *see* **Notes 12–20**.

2. The standardized cycling conditions as noted previously are used.

3.3.4. PCR Amplification of Control Genes

To assess DNA quality and amplifiability, PCR is performed on the specimen DNA with primer pairs designed to amplify amplicons of 100, 200, 300, and 400bp (and 600 bp if required).

1. One multiplex PCR is required to analyze the control genes. Primer mix A contains 0.25 µL of forward and reverse primers for the following genes: TBXAS1 (exon 9), RAG1 (exon 2), PLZF (exon 1), and AF4 (exon 11) to give amplicons of 100, 200, 300, and 400 bp, respectively. This PCR is suitable for assessment of DNA extracted from paraffin-embedded samples. Primers that amplify a fragment of 600 bp can be added if required for high-quality DNA (mix B). The PCR reaction is set up as follows (*see* **Note 8**):

	Control tube mix A
Sterile water (*see* **Note 9**)	29.8 µL
10X Buffer II	5 µL
dNTP mix (1.25 m*M*)	8 µL (0.2 m*M*)
$MgCl_2$ (25 m*M*)	4 µL (2.0 m*M*)
Primer mix A	2.0 µL (2.5pmol of each primer)
AmpliTaq Gold	0.2 µL (1U)
100 ng DNA	

If required, 0.5 mL (2.5 pmol) of forward and reverse primers for AF4 (exon 3) can be added to amplify amplicons of 600 bp to the above reaction mix and is then designated mix B.

For storage of PCR reagents, *see* **Notes 10** and **11**, and for general PCR set up, *see* **Notes 12–19**.

2. The standardized cycling conditions are used as noted previously.

3.4. Heteroduplex Analysis

3.4.1. Gel Preparation

1. Ensure that the glass plates are scrupulously clean before starting by cleaning with absolute alcohol and then rinsing in deionized water.
2. For a 6% gel, add 8.58 mL of deionized water, 12.5 mL of TBE, 3.72 mL of Accugel mix (29:1) and, finally, 150 µL of 20% AMP and 22.5 µL of TEMED (*see* **Note 21**).
3. Using a 20-mL syringe, transfer the gel mix between the two plates, insert the comb, and leave to stand for 30 min.

3.4.2. Sample Preparation and Gel Electrophoresis

1. Remove the comb from the gel and rinse the wells with 1X TBE.
2. Mix 1 µL of the DNA ladder with 2 µL of the 6X loading dye and 10 µL of 0.5X TBE.
3. Heat the PCR product at 95°C for 5 min and then remove and place immediately on ice to induce duplex formation (*see* **Notes 22** and **23**).
4. Incubate the tubes on ice at 4°C for 1 h, before adding 4 µL of the 6X loading dye (also at 4°C) to 20 µL of the PCR sample.
5. Place 0.5X TBE into top and bottom chambers and run for 2 h at 240 volts.
6. Disconnect from power pack and remove gel by separating the plates with a plastic el separator.
7. Place the gel in a staining plastic tray of 0.5ug/mL of ethidium bromide in 0.5X TBE for 5 min.
8. Read the gel using a UV image transilluminator and recorder.

3.5. Genescanning

1. Add 1 µL of each PCR sample to 10 µL of HIDi formamide (containing 0.5 µL of the Rox 400HD molecular weight marker) (*see* **Note 22**).
2. Each gene scan run is performed in groups of 16 on a 96-well plate and any empty wells need to be filled with 10 µL of HiDi.
3. Once loaded, the plate is sealed and heated to 95°C fro 5 min before immediately cooling to 4°C.
4. The plate is then centrifuged to remove air bubbles and the seal removed.
5. The plate is then placed into the 3100 gene scanner for analysis according to the manufacturer's instructions.

3.6. Analysis of TCR PCR Products

3.6.1. Heteroduplex Analysis

Clonal products with identical junctional regions (homoduplexes) are visualized as sharp narrow bands within the appropriate size range whereas polyclonal products are seen as ill defined smears (heteroduplexes) retarded at higher molecular weight due to conformational differences of duplexes of less perfectly matched junctional regions.

3.6.2. Genescanning Analysis

Clonal products are seen as narrow peaks because of identically sized products, whereas polyclonal products give a gaussian distribution of the differently sized products within the appropriate size ranges.

3.6.3. Analysis of TCR Loci

For TCRB and TCRG loci, both heteroduplex and gene scanning analysis are suitable and complement each other (*see* **Subheadings 3.7.1.** and **3.7.2.**). For TCRD, heteroduplex analysis is preferred; however, genescanning analysis may be used if the user is aware of potential problems (*see* **Subheadings 3.7.3.**).

3.6.4. Complementary and Detection Rates of TCR PCR

It has been shown that TCRG+TCRB (>TCRD) should be used to analyze any suspect T-cell lymphoproliferations, and in a series of 18 histologically, immunphenotypically, and Southern blotted defined T-cell malignancies, a detection rate of 100% of detectable clonal TCR gene rearrangements has been demonstrated *(**12**)*.

3.7. Interpretation of TCR Data

Data should always be interpreted in the context of complete clinical, histological and phenotypical data. Furthermore, known positive, and polyclonal, and negative controls should always be set up for each multiplex TCR PCR tube.

3.7.1. Interpretation of TCRG Data

The optimal assessment of TCRG gene rearrangements requires both heteroduplex and genescanning analysis. Heteroduplex alone may be associated with false-negative results because of sensitivity issues whereas genescanning alone will increase the risk of false-positive results as a consequence of variable CDR3 sequences of uniform length migrating as an apparent clonal population. Because of the differently labeled JG primers and the different size range for each VG recombinations, different VJ recombinations are easily visible (**Fig. 2, Table 2**): in tube A FAM (blue), profiles indicate J1.3/2.3 recombinations (V10 gene usage at 140–170 bp and VF1 gene usage at 200–230 bp) and HEX (green) profiles indicate J1.1/2.1 recombinations (V10 gene usage at 180–200 bp and VF1 at 230–250 bp). In tube B FAM profiles indicate J1.3/2.3 recombinations (V11 gene usage at 100–120 bp and V9 gene usage at 160–190 bp) and HEX profiles indicate J1.1/2.1 recombinations (V11 gene usage at 130–150 bp and V9 at 200–220 bp). VF1/V9/V10 – J1.3/2.3 and VF1-J1.1/2.1 polyclonal repertoires are detectable to variable extents whereas polyclonal V9/V10–J1.1/2.1 and V11–J1.3/2.3 are less frequent and clearly identifiable Gaussian distributions may be rare.

Table 2
Details of TCR PCR Product Sizes and Sensitivity Levels

TCR	Gene recombination (PCR product size in bp)[b]				Gene sensitivity[a]
TCRG	**J1.1/2.1**	**J1.3/2.3**			
V10	180–200	140–170			1–10%
VF1	230–250	200–230			
V11	130–150	100–120			
V9	200–220	160–190			
TCRB	**J**				
V	250–290				1–10%
D1	290–321				
D2	170–191				
TCRD	**J1/J2**	**J3**	**J4**	**D3–3'**	
V1	170–210	180–220	160–200	220	0.5–10%
V2	200–240	200–240	190–230	240	
V3	230–270	240–280	220–260	280	
V4	180–220	190–230	170–210	230	
V5	220–260	230–270	210–250	270	
V6	200–240	210–250	190–230	250	
D2–5'	130(J1), 140(J2)	150	130	190	

[a]Sensitivity experiments performed with dilutions of clonal DNA in peripheral blood mononuclear cell DNA mononuclear cell DNA. Sensitivity levels are dependent on the size of the clonal product relative to the polyclonal Gaussian distribution and the complexity of the polyclonal repertoire.

[b]Non-specific products: TCRB; 150 bp (tube A and B), 273 bp (tube A), 221 bp (tube B), 128 bp, 337 bp (tube C), TCRD; 90 bp.

3.7.2. Interpretation of TCRB Data

Analysis of complete TCRB VJ gene rearrangements in a polyclonal T-cell population give rise to a single Gaussian profile (250–290 bp) in tubes A and B whereas analysis of partial TCRB DJ gene rearrangements give rise to two Gaussian profiles because of the recombinations of D2J at 170–190 p and D1J at 290–320 bp. Thus partial clonal rearrangements can be identified as D2 or D1 recombinations (**Table 2**). Likewise, if the JB2 primers are labeled with HEX (data not shown), identification of J1 or J2 family gene recombinations is possible. Because of the vast number of VB primers, on occasions when the clonal population is less than 10%, the clonal products may not be apparent above the Gaussian distribution. In such cases where TCRVB expression is known from monoclonal cell surface antibody studies, PCR analysis using individual VB primers with the JB mixes may provide confirmation of such a population since experiments of singleplex reactions have shown sensitivity levels of 0.1–1%. In addition, TCRG PCR complements TCRB analysis and should identify such populations.

3.7.3. Interpretation of TCRD Data

Heteroduplex analysis is the preferred detection method however genescanning can be used, but because of the large size range of TCRD products there is no classical Gaussian distribution for polyclonal samples and pseudoclonality may be seen in samples as a consequence of limited usage of TCRD (**Fig. 4, Table 2**). Again by labeling different TCRD primers with different fluorochromes, specific gene recombinations can be identified (i.e., JD1 is labeled with HEX, JD2-JD4 with FAM and 3'D3 with NED).

3.8. Interpretation of Control Gene Data

These analyses give some indication of the integrity of the DNA; however, it gives no indication of the numbers of target T and B-cells.

3.9. Analysis of DNA Extracted From Paraffin-Embedded Samples

PCR amplification of DNA extracted from paraffin blocks may be improved by diluting the DNA and using 50 ng per PCR amplification because this dilutes any inhibitors present. However, experiments have shown that if the DNA is very degraded, dilution of the DNA has no influence on the amplifiability. Furthermore, duplicate PCRs should be performed for reproducibility and to avoid any misinterpretation of pseudoclonality of any of the loci.

3.10. Applications

TCR clonality assays are useful for establishing the presence of clonal T-cell populations in suspect lymphoid malignancies. In particular clonality analyses complement routine immunohistology/immunophenotyping for the diagnosis of lymphoid malignant lymphoproliferations where other definitive markers may be lacking and are essential for establishing clonality in T-cell lymphoproliferations. Clonality analyses are also of value in assessing the nature of lymphoproliferative disease where it occurs in immunosuppressed transplant recipients and are useful for the characterization of lymphocyte populations following bone marrow grafts, where poor reconstitution may be reflected in restricted T- and B-cell repertoires. Furthermore, T-cell clonality has an important role in the assessment of suspect T-cell lymphoproliferative lesions in common variable immunodeficiency.

TCRG gene rearrangements can be used as markers of clonality, not only in TCRγδ+ve malignancies (where the rearrangements are functional) but also in TCRαβ+ve malignancies where nonfunctional TCRG gene rearrangements are observed as a consequence of the ordered hierarchy of TCR loci gene rearrangements. The TCRB locus is the locus of choice for establishing clonality of TCRαβ-expressing tumors, which comprise more than 90% of lymphoid malignancies. The TCRA locus has proved too complex for suitable DNA clonal analyses. However, the newly designed BIOMED-2 primer sets have shown an extremely high TCRB + TCRG detection rated in cases previously characterized by histology, immunophenotype, and Southern blot analysis. Analysis of TCRD genes is mainly restricted to TCRγδ+ve malignancies, which are fairly rare, because TCRD genes are deleted in the majority of TCRαβ+ve T-cell malignancies. The comprehensive nature of the BIOMED-2 primer sets allows a robust analysis of TCR loci where complimentarity of the loci is key to the interpretation of the data.

4. Notes

1. Plugged pipet tips must be used when pipetting blood products and clean tips used between all liquid transfers.
2. The preferred anticoagulant for blood or bone marrow is ethylenediamine tetraacetic acid.
3. Short-term DNA storage should be at 4°C; long-term storage at –20°C.
4. Spectrophotometric curvettes should be well rinsed in distilled water before and after use.
5. To avoid cross-contamination of tissues for PCR analysis from other tissues routinely cut on histopathology microtomes, the old knife blade should be removed, the knife holder thoroughly cleaned with xylene, and then a new blade carefully inserted.
6. For the extraction of DNA from paraffin-embedded material, vigorous vortexing should be avoided because DNA from formalin-fixed tissues is fragile and will easily shear.
7. Primers must be quality controlled using known positive controls with specific rearrangements and polyclonal peripheral blood controls.
8. Plastics can be UV irradiated for 10 min before use.
9. Ultrapure water should be used for all PCRs.
10. Bulk primer mixes can be made, aliquoted, and stored at –20°C.
11. Buffer, dNTP, magnesium chloride, and Taq must be stored at –20°C.
12. Gloves must be worn for all procedures and discarded before leaving the PCR areas.
13. Plugged pipet tips must be used for all stages of the PCR method.
14. All working areas should be cleaned with alcohol before and after use.
15. All procedures must be conducted using aseptic technique.
16. All components of the master mixes except DNA, primers and Taq can be UV irradiated in an Amplirad for 10 min prior to making up reaction mixes.
17. Care must be taken to avoid contamination at any stage of the PCR procedure by defining pre- and post-PCR areas. These areas require dedicated pipet sets, pipet tips, and racks that should never be transferred from one area to another.

18. The pre-PCR area should have dedicated equipment for handling primers and preparing master mixes, all of which should be DNA free. No DNA or amplified products must be brought into this area.
19. The PCR set-up area is for preparing DNA and adding samples. To avoid contamination, for no reason should PCR products be handled in this area.
20. Known positive and polyclonal controls as well as a water alone control must always be set up for each multiplex TCR PCR tube for validity of data.
21. When preparing the polyacrylamide gel mix, care must be taken to avoid the introduction of air bubbles into the gel mix. Components of the gel mix are mixed gently and the AMP and TEMED must be added last.
22. A post-PCR area should be set aside for gel preparation and the handling of all post-PCR products, including gene scanning.
23. Samples must remain on ice at 4°C for 1 h to induce duplex formation, and samples must not be allowed to warm up to room temperature.

Acknowledgments

This work was supported by a BIOMED-2 Concerted Action (BMH4-CT98-3936). We thank all colleagues involved in this program, especially Professor J. J. M. van Dongen, Dr. A. Langerak, Professor E. R. Macintyre, Dr. F. L. Lavender, Dr. M. Brüggeman, Dr. H. E. White, and Dr. H. van Krieken. This work was also supported by the Leukaemia Research Fund (LRF).

References

1. Tumours of haematopoietic and lymphoid tissues, in *WHO Classification of Tumours*, (Jaffe, E. S., Harris, N. L., Stein, H., Vardiman, J. W., eds). IARC Press, Lyon, France, 2001.
2. van Dongen, J. J. M., and Wolvers-Tettero, I. L. M. (1991) Analysis of immunoglobulin and T-cell receptor genes. Part II: possibilities and limitations in the diagnosis and management of lymphoproliferative diseases and related disorders. *Clin. Chim. Acta* **198,** 93–174.
3. Griesser, H. (1995) Gene rearrangements and chromosomal translocations in T-cell lymphoma- diagnostic applications and their limits. *Virchows Arch.* **426,** 323–338.
4. Slack, D. N., McCarthy, K. P., Wiedemanm, L. M., et al. (1993) Evaluation of sensitivity , specificity, and reproducibility of an optimised method for detecting clonal rearrangements of immunolglobulin and T-cell receptor genes in formalin fixed, paraffin embedded sections. *Diag. Mol. Pathol.* **2,** 223–232.
5. McCarthy, K. P., Sloane, J. P., Kabarowski, J. H. S., et al. (1992) A simplified method of detection of clonal rearragements of the T-cell receptor γ chain gene. *Diagn. Mol. Pathol.* **1,** 173–179.
6. Langerak, A. W., Szczepanski, T., van der Burg, M., et al. (1997) Heteroduplex PCR analysis of rearranged T-cell receptor genes for clonality assessment in suspect T-cell proliferations. *Leukemia* **11,** 2192–2199.

7. Kneba, M., Boilz, I., Linke, B., et al. (1995) Analysis of rearranged T-cell receptor beta-chains by polymerase chain reaction (PCR) DNA sequencing and automated high resolution PCR fragment analysis. *Blood* **86,** 3930–3937.
8. Delabesse, E., Burtin, M. L., Millien, C., et al. (2000) Rapid, multifluorescent TCRG Vgamma and Jgamma typing application to T-cell acute lymphoblastic leukaemia and to the detection of minor clonal populations. *Leukaemia* **14,** 1143–1152.
9. Lefranc, M-P. (2000) Locus maps and genomic repertoire of the human T-cell repertpoire. *The Immunoloogist.* **8,** 72–78.
10. Langerak, A. W., van den Beemd, R., Wolvers-Tettero, I. L., et al. (2001) Molecular and flow cytometric analysis of the Vbeta repertoire for clonality assessment in mature TCRalphabeta T-cell proliferations. *Blood* **98,** 165–73.
11. van Dongen, J. J. M., Langerak, A. W., San Miguel, J. F., et al. (2001) PCR-based clonality studies for early diagnosis of lymphoproliferative disorders: Report of the BIOMED-2 concerted action. *Blood* **98,** p505a (Abstract 543).
12. van Dongen, J. J. M., Langerak, A. W., Brüggeman, M., et al. (2003) Design and standardization of PCR primers and protocols for detection of clonal immunoglobulin and T-cell receptor gene rearrangements in suspect lymphoproliferations. Report of the BIOMED-2 concerted Action BMH4-CT98–3936. *Leukaemia* **17,** 2257–2317.
13. Clevers, H., Alarcon, B., Wileman, T. et al. (1988) The T-cell receptor/CD3 complex: a dynamic protein ensemble. *Annu. Rev. Immunol.* **6,** 629–662.
14. Alt, F. W., Oltz, E. M., Young, F., et al. (1992) VDJ recombination. *Immunol. Today* **13,** 306–314.

10

Cloning of Immunoglobulin Chromosomal Translocations by Long-Distance Inverse Polymerase Chain Reaction

E. Loraine Karran, Takashi Sonoki, and Martin J. S. Dyer

Summary

Many subtypes of B-cell malignancy are characterized by chromosomal translocations that target the immunoglobulin loci. Molecular cloning of such translocations continues to allow the identification of genes whose deregulated expression plays a pivotal role in the pathogenesis of B-cell malignancy. The clustering of breakpoints within the immunoglobulin loci has allowed the development of rapid and robust polymerase chain reaction methods for cloning. We discuss in this chapter the use of long-distance inverse polymerase chain reaction methods to clone immunoglobulin chromosomal translocation breakpoints from clinical material. These methods have been successfully applied to several other types of chromosomal translocation including those involving other genes such as *BCL6*, *ETV6*, and *MYC*.

Key Words: Chromosomal translocations; immunoglobulin gene loci; polymerase chain reaction; oncogenes.

1. Introduction

Malignancy is a genetic disease. Sequential, somatic changes to several "key" genes, including dominant transforming oncogenes and tumor suppressor genes, result in synergistic effects on pathways controlling cell growth, death, and differentiation and are necessary for the emergence of the final neoplastic phenotype.

Within the hematological malignancies, identification of the key molecular alterations has been successfully achieved for the acute leukemias. In these diseases, all the common translocations have been cloned, and cytogenetic/molecular cytogenetic recognition of chromosomal translocations now forms the basis of stratified therapy. Furthermore, the presence of the t(9;22)(q34;q11) in chronic myeloid leukemia also has allowed the rational

From: *Methods in Molecular Medicine, Vol. 115: Lymphoma: Methods and Protocols*
Edited by: T. Illidge and P. W. M. Johnson © Humana Press Inc., Totowa, NJ

development of new forms of therapy. The challenge is now to repeat this paradigm for the other forms of hematological malignancy. However, many genes of primary importance remain to be identified. For the B-cell non-Hodgkin's lymphoma (B-NHL), cytogenetic analysis has been hampered by a number of considerations. In contrast to the acute leukemias, which are usually characterized by a single chromosomal translocation, B-NHLs exhibit a large number of complex genetic alterations, reflecting their long natural history. Cytogenetic investigations are not performed routinely in B-NHL. Also, many recurrent abnormalities in B-NHL are either deletions or amplifications. Even with the completion of the human genome sequence, identification of the key genes associated with deletions and amplifications remains difficult, since the regions of DNA involved may be large (*1* but *see* **refs.** ***2,3***).

In B-NHL, molecular analysis of chromosomal translocations continues to allow the rapid identification of novel, dominantly-acting oncogenes. In this chapter, we discuss the use of long-distance inverse polymerase chain reaction (LDI-PCR) methods to clone chromosomal translocations targeted to the immunoglobulin loci.

1.1. Immunoglobulin Translocations in B-NHL

In mature B-cell diseases, and in particular in the various subtypes of B-NHL, an important and probably "primary" event is the translocation of oncogenes to the immunoglobulin (Ig) loci (reviewed in **refs.** ***4*** and ***5***). These are located on chromosome 14q32.33 in the case of the heavy chain (*IGH*) locus (this is at the very telomere of the long arm of chromosome 14), chromosome 2p12 for the kappa light chain, and 22q12 for the lambda light chain locus. All are involved in recurrent translocations with a wide variety of partner genes. *IGH* translocations are recognized cytogenetically as an additional band on the long arm of chromosome 14 (designated 14q+). However, several translocations are cytogenetically "cryptic" and need fluorescence *in situ* hybridization (FISH) or spectral karyotyping to be identified. The 14q32.3 translocations are usually reciprocal and bring genes on other chromosome fragments into close apposition of *IGH* locus.

Many *IG* translocations are found at high frequency in specific types of B-NHL, suggesting disease-specific mechanisms that operate in specific subsets of mature B-cells. Examples include the presence of the t(14;18)(q32.3;q21.3) in approx 85% of follicular B-NHL, t(11;14)(q13.3;q32.3) probably in all cases of mantle cell B-NHL, and t(8;14)(q24.1;q32.3) in all cases of Burkitt lymphoma. Multiple translocations either to both *IGH* loci or to the *IGH* and the *IGL* loci within the same clone are common and may account for the loss of expression of surface *IG* expression. The genes involved are mostly concerned with the control of proliferation and programmed cell death and/or apoptosis and include *BCL2* (chromosome 18q21.3) and *MYC* (chromosome 8q24.1). The consequences of *IG* translocations are 1) deregulated expression of an incoming oncogene caused by the proximity of potent B-cell transcriptional enhancers within the *IG* loci and in some instances and 2) mutation caused by the actions of the somatic hypermutation mechanism present in mature B-cells, which normally allow for the affinity maturation of the immunoglobulin response.

Interestingly, at least some *IG* translocations may be found at low levels in many normal individuals. The possible clinical significance of this finding remains to be assessed. Whether all Ig translocations occur in normal individuals at low level is not known.

1.2. LDI-PCR for the Detection of IG Translocation Breakpoints

Therefore, the detection of *IG* translocations may be of possible diagnostic, prognostic, and therapeutic value, with deregulated expression making these genes suitable targets for various therapeutic approaches. However, routine detection is hindered not only by the lack of cytogenetics but also by the large number of possible partner genes and the variability of the breakpoints within the incoming oncogene. Once recurrent breakpoints have been cloned, FISH assays can detect *IG* translocations in clinical samples, either on fresh tissues or in paraffin-embedded sections. However, for several applications, the DNA sequence of the breakpoint may be required; moreover, many recurrent translocations remain to be cloned.

We have devised LDI-PCR methods to clone *IG* translocations ***(6–8)***. These methods exploit the observation that most *IG* breaks are clustered within specific *IG* sequences, usually either the joining (J) or switch (S) region gene segments. LDI-PCR has been used to detect virtually all translocations to the *IGHJ* segments and more recently to *IGHS* translocations. It may therefore be possible to classify the B-NHL on the presence of specific *IG* translocations in the absence of conventional cytogenetics. Similar LDI-PCR methods also have been used to clone recurrent translocations involving the *ETV6* locus in acute leukemia and *BCL6* in B-NHL ***(9,10)***.

1.3. Structure of IgH Locus and Its Recombinations

To understand the basis for the *IGH* LDI-PCR method, it is necessary to understand something of the structure of the *IGH* locus and its normal recombination events. The *IGH* locus comprises 51 functional variable (V_H) segments, 27 diverse (D_H) segments, 6 joining (J_H) segments, and 9 constant (C_H) segments (**Fig. 1**). Each C_H segment (except Cδ) is preceded by repetitive DNA sequences or switch (S) segments, which play a role in isotype class switch recombination. To generate *IG* diversity, two major somatic gene recombination events occur during normal B-cell differentiation. The first step is VDJ

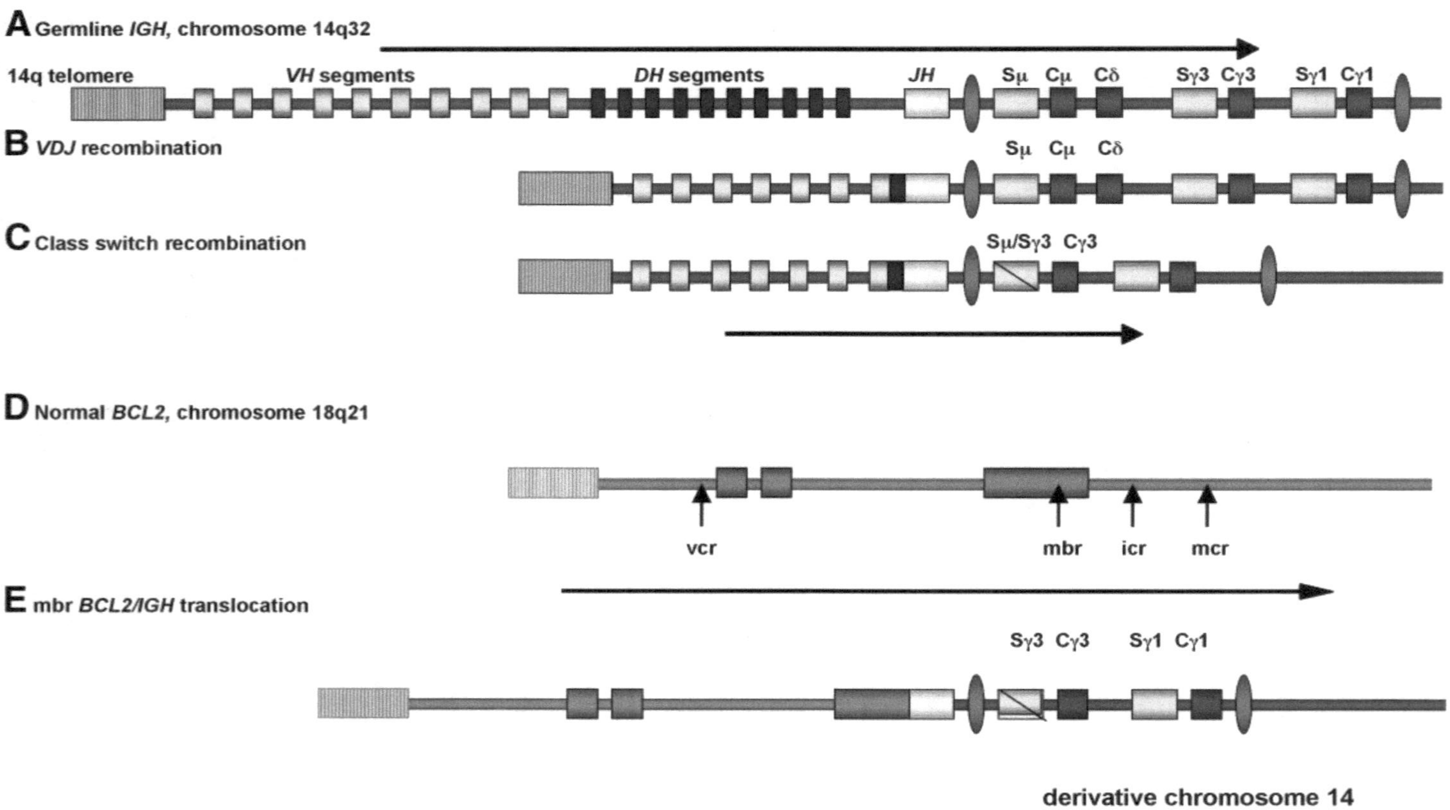
A Germline IGH, chromosome 14q32
14q telomere
VH segments
DH segments
JH
Sμ
Cμ
Cδ
Sγ3
Cγ3
Sγ1
Cγ1
B VDJ recombination
Sμ
Cμ
Cδ
C Class switch recombination
Sμ/Sγ3
Cγ3
D Normal BCL2, chromosome 18q21
vcr
mbr
icr
mcr
E mbr BCL2/IGH translocation
Sγ3
Cγ3
Sγ1
Cγ1
derivative chromosome 14

rearrangement to generate the variable domain of the immunoglobulin heavy chain molecule. The V, D, and J segments undergo recombination at specific DNA sequences that are called recombination signal sequences. The second type of recombination is class-switch recombination. In this process, Sμ recombines with the S segment in front of a downstream C_H segment resulting in isotype switching. VDJ recombination occurs within the bone marrow in B-cell precursors, whereas class switching occurs within the germinal centre of the lymph node after the onset of V_H somatic hypermutation (for additional references on somatic recombination, please *see* **refs. *5*** and ***11***).

Most translocation breakpoints of the *IGH* locus are clustered. The tumors arising from pre- or early germinal center B-cells usually bear breakpoints within the *IGHJ* segments, whereas in contrast, tumors arising from postgerminal center B-cells often have breakpoints within *IGHS* segments. Thus, molecular cloning of chromosome *IGH* translocations has proceeded on the assumption that in most instances the translocation will involve either the *IGHJ* or the *IGHS* regions. However, this is not always the case, and Ig translocations may involve rearranged and un-rearranged V_H/V_L genes, D_H segments and fall within the J_H-C_μ intron. In B-cell precursor acute lymphoblastic leukemia, the breaks would appear to occur frequently within the Cδ-Cγ3 intron. Moreover, some

---

Fig. 1. (*opposite page*) Schema showing the structure of the rearrangements within the immunoglobulin heavy chain (*IGH*). **(A)** The unrearranged *IGH* locus is composed of dispersed variable (V_H), diversity (D_H), and joining (J_H) region segments that have to recombine to produce a functional V_H gene. **(B)** VDJ recombination occurs within the bone marrow in B-cell precursors. Cells that fail to undergo this process successfully die from apoptosis within the marrow. **(C)** Class switch recombination occurs following recombination between switch regions that occur immediately upstream of most constant region genes and allows the generation of antibodies with different effector functions. This occurs within the germinal centre of the lymph node after encounter with antigen and after the onset of somatic hypermutation—the two processes appear to be mechanistically similar. **(D)** Schema of the *BCL2* gene on chromosome 18q21.3. *BCL2* is composed of three exons separated by an intron of approx 250 kb. The transcriptional orientation of the gene is the same as that for the IgH locus as shown by the horizontal arrow. Breaks adjacent to *BCL2* are not random, but clustered within specific regions both 5' and 3' of the gene as indicated (vertical arrows). **(E)** Schema of a typical *IGHJ* translocation. The most common *BCL2* break occurs within the *BCL2* mbr, which lies within the 3' UTR of the gene; this region becomes juxtaposed to an *IGHJ* segment (usually J_H6) in the t(14;18)(q32.3;q21.3) resulting in a fusion messenger ribonucleic acid product comprising full-length *BCL2* and derived *IG* sequences. Interestingly, nearly all *BCL2/IGHJ* translocations are found in *IGH* alleles that would appear to have already undergone class-switching. *See* **Color Plate 9**, following page 270.

14q32 translocations may not involve the *IGH* locus but some as yet-unidentified centromeric locus; this is particularly so in chronic lymphocytic leukemia, where *IGH* translocations are very rare ***(11)***. It is therefore advisable to perform FISH assays to confirm the direct involvement of the *IGH* locus before embarking on any attempt at cloning new translocation breakpoints involving chromosome 14q32.

2. Materials

1. High Molecular Weight DNA: At least 50 µg of high molecular weight DNA should be prepared. Approximately 1 µg is required for each LDI-PCR. However, it should be noted that much smaller amounts of DNA (as little as 50 ng) may be used. The quality of the DNA is an important factor when amplifying long distance targets, but conventional high molecular weight DNA extraction methods are adequate (see Maniatis). Genomic DNA in TE (10 m*M* Tris, pH 7.5; 1 m*M* ethylenediamine tetraacetic acid, pH 8.0) is stable at 4°C for at least 2 yr. DNA from paraffin-embedded samples has not yet proved suitable for LDI-PCR (*see* **Note 1**). It is advisable to perform Southern blotting in parallel with the LDI-PCR experiments because this will allow the identification of artifactual amplification products. It is necessary to show comigration of rearranged *IGH* and novel amplified sequences by Southern blot to confirm that the fragment amplified genuinely represents the chromosomal translocation breakpoint. Alternatively, FISH assays can be used to confirm that the breakpoint has been cloned (*see* **Note 2**).
2. Restriction Endonucleases: *Bgl*II, *Hind*III, *Pst*I, and *Xba*I are suitable enzymes for LDI-PCR amplification from *IGHJ* because they have sites in the intronic enhancer. Digests of the genomic DNA are conducted by following the enzyme manufacturer's instructions and by using the buffers provided. The digested DNA can be stored for up to 1 yr at –20°C.
3. T4 Ligase: The concentration of the digested DNA (*see* **Subheading 3**) used in the self-ligation step is crucial as excess may inhibit circle formation. The ligated DNA pool will be stable for up to 1 yr at –20°C. DNA ligases and buffers are used from commercially available kits.
4. Silica-Based DNA Purification: Before LDI-PCR, the self-ligated circular DNA must be purified to remove excess salt from the self-ligation mixture. Silica-based DNA purification kits are commercially available for this purpose. After purification, the circular DNA is eluted in distilled/sterilized water and may be stored in –20°C for up to 1 yr.
5. Thermostable DNA Polymerase and Primers: Many thermostable DNA polymerases for long template amplification are suitable for LDI-PCR. The first-round PCR does not yield a band on agarose gel electrophoresis, and nested PCR is necessary to obtain sufficient product. The first round PCR product can be stored at –20°C for at least 1 yr. The primers for LDI-PCR from *IGHJ* are listed in **Table 1.**

A 100 µ*M* stock solution of the primers is made in water for storage at –20°C (up to 2 yr) and diluted to the working solution of 10 µ*M*. The nested PCR prod-

Table 1
DNA Oligonucleotide Primers for LDI-PCR From IGHJ

	Primer	Nucleotide sequence	Application
JH	J6E	CCCACAGGCAGTAGCACAAAACAA	External J6 primer
	J6I	GCAGAAAACAAAGGCCCTAGAGTG	Internal J6 primer
	JBE	GAAGCAGGTCACCGCGAGAGT	External primer for *Bgl*II
	JBI	CTTCTGGTTGTGAAGAGGGGTTTTG	Internal primer for *Bgl* II
	JHE	TGGGATGCGTGGCTTCTGCT	External primer for *Hind*III
	JHI	GCCCTTGTTAATGGACTTGGAGGA	Internal primer for *Hind* III
	JXE	CACTGGCATCGCCCTTTGTCTAA	External primer for *Xba*I or *Pst*I
	JXI	CCCATGCCTTCCAAAGCGATT	Internal primer for *Xba*I or *Pst*I

ucts are analyzed by agarose gel electrophoresis and the size of the bands compared with those obtained by the Southern blot to identify the band corresponding to the rearranged *IGH* restriction fragment. Typically, the LDI-PCR method should yield enough product for direct sequencing of the excised band.

Inverse PCR is a method involving the amplification of restriction endonuclease-digested DNA self-ligated at low concentrations to form monomeric circles; it is a simple strategy for amplifying DNA sequences flanked on one side by a region of known sequence. By combining this with techniques for long-distance PCR and using oligonucleotide primer pairs complementary to sequences within the *IGH* enhancer and *IGHJ6* regions, it has been possible to detect virtually all translocations to the *IGHJ* segments. The procedure is outlined in **Fig. 2**. *BCL9* and *BCL10* were cloned from t(1;14)(q21;q32) and t(1;14)(p22;q32), respectively, using this technique ***(12,13)***. We have subsequently cloned a large number of other breakpoints from cases with *IGH* translocations (unpublished observations). Others have used the technique to clone the *LHX4* gene from t(1;14)(q25;q32) from B-cell precursor acute lymphoblastic leukemia ***(14)***.

Subsequently, we developed LDI-PCR methods for *IGHS* regions. These regions have been applied for molecular cloning of translocation breakpoints in the Sμ and Sγ regions as described (and manuscript in preparation). We describe here only the method for amplification from *IGHJ*; this is a simple and robust method, which in our experience has not produced many artifactual amplification products. In contrast, amplification from *IGHS* is more difficult and more prone to artifacts. Additional information for protocols for amplification from *IGHS* may be obtained on request.

An interesting feature of the method is that both IgH alleles are amplified in the one PCR, even when the two alleles are of different size.

3. Methods

Detailed methods for preparation of high molecular weight DNA, Southern blot analysis, and DNA sequencing may be obtained elsewhere. We recommend preparing a premix to avoid contamination during experimental procedures. Here, we describe a premix for three samples.

3.1. Digestion of High Molecular Weight DNA With Restriction Endonucleases

Use 20 units of endonuclease for 1 μg of DNA. Excess enzymatic activity may cause "star" (nonspecific cleavage of DNA) activity and, therefore, high concentrations of enzymes should be avoided. Prepare the following reaction premix in a 1.5-mL microcentrifuge tube on ice.

	Reaction mix	Reaction premix (X3.2)
10X buffer	2 μL	6.4 μL
Endonuclease (20 unit/μL)	1 μL (20 units)	3.2 μL
DNA (0.5 μg/μL)	2 μL	(-)
Distilled sterile H_2O	15 μL	48 μL
Total	20 μL	18 μLX3.2

(Several enzymes may require small amount of bovine serum albumin for maximum activity. Follow the manufacturer's instructions for the enzyme.) Mix the reaction premix with gentle inversion and spin down the contents by brief centrifugation at 4°C. Then, aliquot 18 μL in a 1.5-mL tube and add 2 μL (1 μg) of the DNA into the reaction premix. After gentle mixing, spin the tube briefly. Incubate the reaction mix at the appropriate temperature for 18–24 h.

Fig. 2. (*opposite page*) Overview of LDI-PCR procedures. High molecular weight DNA is digested with appropriate endonucleases. The digested DNA is reacted with T4-ligase at low DNA concentration to promote self-ligation and thus generate circular DNA. After purification of the ligation mix using silica-based column, long-distance PCR using thermostable DNA polymerase, which allows amplification up to 7 kb is performed; the maximal size fragment that can be obtained with this procedure has not been determined. Analysis on agarose gel usually shows the presence of two rearranged fragments.

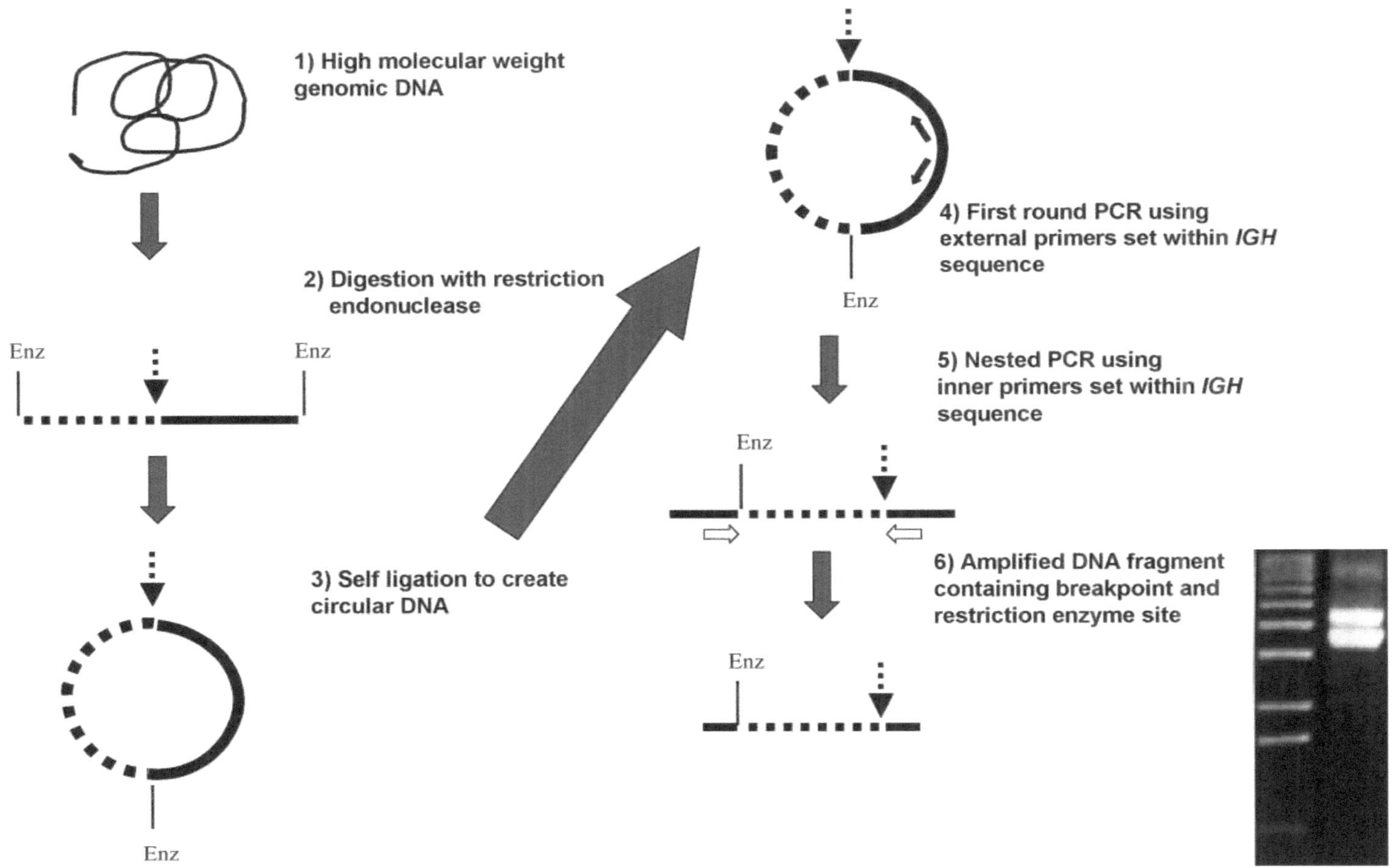
1) High molecular weight genomic DNA
2) Digestion with restriction endonuclease
Enz
Enz
3) Self ligation to create circular DNA
Enz
4) First round PCR using external primers set within *IGH* sequence
Enz
5) Nested PCR using inner primers set within *IGH* sequence
Enz
6) Amplified DNA fragment containing breakpoint and restriction enzyme site
Enz

It is important at this stage to check that the DNA has been digested to completion by agarose electrophoresis of a small aliquot on a minigel. When the DNA is digested with completion, it shows as a smear with typical satellite bands of approx 1 kb when using some enzymes such as *Hind*III. Heat inactivation of the enzymes at a suitable temperature for 20 min is recommended because DNA may be lost during phenol/chloroform inactivation. The final DNA concentration of the reaction mix should be about 50 ng/μL.

3.2. Self-Ligation

Several T4-ligase kits are commercially available and all are suitable for the self-ligation step. We have used a T4-DNA ligation kit from New England Biolabs. Prepare the following reaction premix in a 1.5-mL microcentrifuge tube on ice.

	Ligation mix	Reaction premix (X3.2)
10X buffer	12.5 μL	40 μL
Digested DNA	2 μL(100 ng)	(-)
T4 ligase (3 U/μL)	.5 μL	1.6 μL
Distilled sterile water	110 μL	352 μL
Total	125 μL	123 μL X3.2

Mix the reaction premix by inversion of the tube and collect by brief centrifugation. Aliquot 123 μL of the premix into a 1.5-mL microtube and add 2 μL (100 ng) of the digested DNA. Mix the reaction components by gentle inversion of the tube and briefly centrifuge. Incubate the reaction mix at 15°C for 16–24 h. The final DNA concentration should be 0.8 ng/μL.

3.3. Purification of the Ligation Mix Using a Silica-Based Column Method

Before using the self-ligated circular DNA as a template for LDI-PCR, purification of the ligated DNA must be conducted to remove excess salts. Various silica-based column kits are available; for instance, we have used a PCR purification kit (QIAGEN) for this purpose. The detailed procedure is according to the manufacturer's instructions. The purified DNA is eluted with 50 μL of sterile distilled water and can be stored at –20°C.

3.4. LDI-PCR

The reaction components of the LDI-PCR should be made according to the thermostable DNA polymerase manufacturer's instructions. In particular, the manufacturers have optimized the Mg concentration and annealing/extension time corresponding to the size of DNA target. The annealing and extension temperature should be fixed at 68°C to amplify specific and long DNA targets. A procedure for LDI-PCR of purified self-ligated circular DNA using primers to amplify from the *IGHJ* region is as follows.

	PCR reaction mix	Premix (X3.2)
3.3X GeneAmp XL Buffer II	15 µL	48 µL
10 m*M* dNTPs	1 µL	3.2 µL
10 µ*M* forward primer	1 µL	3.2 µL
10 µ*M* reverse primer	1 µL	3.2 µL
purified circular DNA	5 µL (10 ng)	(-)
25 m*M* $Mg(OAc)_2$	5 µL	(-)
rTth thermostable DNA polymerase	1 µL (1U)	3.2 µL
Distilled sterile water	21 µL	67.2 µL
Total	50 µL	40 µL X3.2

Prepare the reaction premix in 1.5-mL microcentrifuge tube on ice. To achieve a hot-start PCR method, avoid addition of $Mg(OAc)_2$ at this stage. Mix by gentle inversion and collect the components by brief centrifugation. Transfer 40 µL of the premix into a thin walled PCR tube then add 5 µL (10 ng) of the purified circular DNA. Heat the reaction mix at 85°C for 3 min and then add 5 µL of 10X $Mg(OAc)_2$. The PCR program is 94°C for 5 min, followed by 30 cycles of 94°C for 1 min and 68°C for 6 min, followed by a terminal extension at 68°C for 7 min. One microliter of the PCR reaction is then reamplified for 30 cycles using identical conditions with nested primers. Amplification was performed on a programmable heating block (Biometra TRIO Thermoblock; Biometra, Göttingen, Germany).

3.5. DNA Sequencing

Take 5 µLof the 50 µL PCR product and analyze it on a 0.8% agarose gel in 1X TAE buffer. When a PCR product of interest is obtained, run the total nested PCR product on an agarose gel and isolate the DNA from a gel slice using an appropriate silica-based DNA purification kit, such as the Gel Purification system from QIAGEN. The DNA sequence can be determined using nested primers.

The PCR product is usually sufficient to analyze by direct sequencing, but when the PCR product of interest is low level or of a large size, cloning into a plasmid is recommended. The TA cloning kit from Invitrogen is ideal for these purposes.

Direct sequencing using nested primers sometimes fails to reach the *IGHJ* translocation breakpoint. In such cases, further primers will be required for determination of the breakpoint.

3.6. Analysis of Results

If LDI-PCR and Southern blotting are performed on patient samples, it is likely that germline bands and products will be seen as well as productive and rearranged alleles. The sizes of these germline bands for all the suggested enzyme digests are shown below.

Digest Probe	Germline *IGH* fragment	Germline LDI-PCR product
*Hind*III	9.9 kb	[a]
*Pst*I	4.4 kb	2.2 kb
*Bgl*II	3.7 kb	2.7 kb
*Xba*I	5.7 kb	3.5 kb

[a]*Hind*III digestion may not produce a germline band in many LDI-PCR reactions due to the large size (8.0 kb) of the product.

After sequencing, standard NCBI BLAST programs (http://www.ncbi.nlm.nih.gov/BLAST/) are used to identify the *IGHJ* regions and any additional unknown sequence in the LDI-PCR product. A full description of the methods necessary to analyze the sequences obtained is beyond the scope of this chapter. However, the advent of the draft of the human genome sequence has greatly simplified this phase of a cloning project; if the sequence contains the translocation breakpoint, this should become rapidly apparent by blasting the derived sequence against the genome (http://www.ncbi.nlm.nih.gov/genome/seq/page.cgi?F=HsBlast.html&&ORG=Hs). This usually allows the involved gene to be readily identified because the breaks may fall either immediately 5' or 3' of the target gene. Two potential problems should be noted. Firstly, many translocation breakpoints fall in regions of the genome that are "unstable" for whatever reason and may not have been sequenced. In this case, additional cloning and large-scale sequencing may be required (e.g., **ref. 7**). Second, translocation breakpoints may fall several hundred kilobases either centromeric or telomeric of the target gene, which may again confound analysis.

4. Notes

1. LDI-PCR is a surprisingly robust method for cloning rearrangements and translocations. The key to the method is obtaining circular DNA, and for this, quality high molecular weight DNA has to be available. In our hands, it has not proved possible to use paraffin-embedded material. If there are any concerns over this issue, then it is worthwhile running out some undigested DNA on a gel to check for degradation. We have used normally processed clinical samples for cloning without any problems and routine methods for DNA extraction can be used. Once circular DNA has been obtained then it should be relatively straightforward to obtain PCR products and the method can be used almost routinely on large numbers of samples ***(10)***.

2. For cloning translocations, it is best to have cytogenetic and FISH analyses performed beforehand to confirm that the breakpoint genuinely involves the *IGH* locus. Translocations involving *IGHJ* can be cloned "blind" without corroboration from southern blot data, but it is necessary to confirm the breaks in *IGHS* by southern since these methods tend to generate more artefacts. If problems with this technique persist, then we would be more than willing to assist in any way possible!

Acknowledgments

The LDI-PCR technique was developed by Dr Tony Willis whilst a PhD student at the Institute of Cancer Research, Sutton UK. We gratefully acknowledge the generous financial support from the Bud Flanagan Leukaemia Fund, the Kay Kendall Leukaemia Fund, the Cancer Research Campaign and the Leukaemia Research Fund. Additional references and offprints of selected articles may be obtained on request to M.J.S.D.

References

1. Devilee, P., Cleton-Jansen, A., Cornelisse, C. J. (2001) Ever since Knudson. *Trends Genet.* **17,** 569–573.
2. Balmain, A. (2001) Cancer genetics: from Boveri and Mendel to microarrays. *Nat. Rev. Cancer* **1,** 77–82.
3. Davies, H., Bignell G.R., Cox C., Stephens, P., Edkins, S., Clegg, S., et al. (2002) Mutations of the *BRAF* gene in human cancer. *Nature* **417,** 949–954.
4. Willis, T. G.. and Dyer, M. J. S. (2000) The role of immunoglobulin translocations in the pathogenesis of B-cell malignancies. *Blood* **96,** 808–822.
5. Kuppers, R., and Dalla-Favera, R. (2001) Mechanisms of chromosomal translocations in B-cell lymphomas. *Oncogene* **20,** 5580–5594.
6. Willis, T. G., Jadayel, D. M., Coignet, L. J., Abdul-Rauf, M., Treleaven, J. G., Catovsky, D., and Dyer, M. J. S. (1997) Rapid molecular cloning of rearrangements of the J locus using long-distance inverse polymerase chain reaction. *Blood* **90,** 2456–2464.
7. Sonoki, T., Harder, L., Horsman, D. E., Karran, L., Taniguchi, I., Willis, T. G., et al. (2001) Cyclin D3 is a target gene of t(6;14)(p21.1;q32.3) of mature B-cell malignancies. *Blood* **98,** 2837–2844.
8. Satterwhite, E., Sonoki, T., Willis, T. G., Harder, L., Nowak, R., Arriola, E. L., et ak. (2001) The *BCL11* gene family: involvement of *BCL11A* in lymphoid malignancies. *Blood* **98,** 3413–3420.
9. Wiemels, J. L., and Greaves, M. (1999) Structure and possible mechanisms of *TEL-AML1* gene fusions in childhood acute lymphoblastic leukemia. *Cancer Res.* **59,** 4075–4082.
10. Akasaka, H., Akasaka, T., Kurata, M., Ueda, C., Shimizu, A., Uchiyama, T., et al. (2000) Molecular anatomy of *BCL6* translocations revealed by long-distance polymerase chain reaction-based assays. Cancer Res. **60,** 2335–2341.

11. Dyer, M. J. S., and Oscier, D. G. (2002) The configuration of the immunoglobulin genes in B-cell chronic lymphocytic leukemia. *Leukemia* **16,** 973–984.
12. Willis, T. G., Zalcberg, I. R., Coignet, L. J.A., Wlodarska, I., Stul, M., Jadayel, D. M., et al. (1998) Molecular cloning of translocation t(1;14)(q21;q32) defines a novel gene (*BCL9*) at chromosome 1q21. Blood **91,** 1873–1881.
13. Willis, T. G., Jadayel, D. M., Du, M. Q., Peng, H., Perry, A. R., Abdul-Rauf, M., et al.(1999) *Bcl10* is involved in t(1;14)(p22;q32) of MALT B-cell lymphoma and mutated in multiple tumor types. *Cell* **96,** 35–45.
14. Kawamata, N., Sakajiri, S., Sugimoto, K. J., Isobe, Y., Kobayashi, H., and Oshimi, K. (2002) A novel chromosomal translocation t(1;14)(q25;q32) in pre-B acute lymphoblasticleukemia involves the LIM homeodomain protein gene, *Lhx4*. *Oncogene* **21,** 4983–4991.

11

Sequential Fluorescence *In Situ* Hybridization Analysis for Trisomy 12 in B-Cell Chronic Lymphocytic Leukemia

Viktoria Hjalmar

Summary

Tumor-specific chromosomal abnormalities are attracting a large interest owing to the diagnostic, prognostic, and therapeutic importance. The development of molecular techniques, e.g., fluorescence *in situ* hybridization (FISH), have improved the detection of specific chromosomal abnormalities in chronic lymphocytic leukemic (CLL). By using FISH, the problem with tumor cells with low mitotic rate is avoided since this method readily detects clonal aberrations also in nondividing, interphase cells. Three different types of probes are used: (1) centromeric probes for numerical chromosome abnormalities, (2) whole chromosome paints, and (3) locus-specific probes. The DNA probes are labeled with fluorochromes and the signals yielded are strong enough to enable analysis of interphase cells. These DNA probes may be directed towards any defined chromosomal region and this chapter will in detail describe the FISH method as a detector of trisomy 12 in CLL.

Key Words: Fluorescence *in situ* hybridization (FISH); protocol; CLL; trisomy 12.

1. Introduction

1.1. Background

Tumor-specific chromosomal abnormalities have attracted a large interest since the 1960s, when the Philadelphia chromosome, that is, the translocation between chromosomes 9 and 22 t(9;22), was found in chronic myelogenous leukemia. The interest is now even larger as a result of the new therapeutic opportunity of the ABL tyrosine kinase inhibitor STI571, directed against the tyrosine kinase resulting from the t(9;22). Early studies of metaphase analyses of either unstimulated bone marrow cells or phytohemagglutinin A-stimulated blood cells from patients with chronic lymphocytic leukemia (CLL) resulted in either no mitosis or normal karyotypes. In the 1970s it was concluded that chromosomal abnormalities were not found in CLL *(1)*. It has later been shown

From: *Methods in Molecular Medicine, Vol. 115: Lymphoma: Methods and Protocols*
Edited by: T. Illidge and P. W. M. Johnson © Humana Press Inc., Totowa, NJ

that most of these normal metaphases obtained were nonleukemic B-cells and T-cells *(2–4)*. The reason for these early negative results is that in tumor-cells from indolent/low-grade lymphomas, for example, CLL, standard cytogenetic methods are hampered by the fact that the tumor B-cells have a low mitotic rate and are difficult to stimulate in vitro *(2,3)*. In the 1980s, improved stimulation methods with polyclonal B-cell activators were introduced, inducing division of the malignant B-cells *(2,4–7)*. These improved methods resulted in detectable chromosomal clones in approximately half of the CLL cases.

1.2. Fluorescence In Situ *Hybridization*

The development of molecular techniques, for example, fluorescence *in situ* hybridization (FISH), has further improved the detection of specific chromosomal abnormalities in CLL. By using FISH, the problem of tumor cells with low mitotic rate is avoided because this method also readily detects clonal aberrations in nondividing, interphase cells. A variety of nucleic acid sequences are used as probes to cellular deoxyribonucleic acid (DNA) targets, leading to visualization of specific chromosomal regions. Three different types of probes are used: (1) centromeric probes for numerical chromosome abnormalities; (2) whole chromosome paints; and (3) locus-specific probes *(8)*. The DNA probes are labeled with fluorochromes and the signals yielded are strong enough to enable analysis of interphase cells. These DNA probes may be directed towards any defined chromosomal region and this chapter will in detail describe the FISH method as a detector of trisomy 12 in CLL.

In successful metaphase analysis, it is possible to detect any clonal aberration, whereas the FISH method provides results only of the aberrations studied, depending on probes used, for example, trisomy 12. Many studies have now demonstrated a discrepancy between conventional G-banding metaphase analyses and FISH regarding the prevalence of trisomy 12 in CLL, with a higher prevalence using FISH *(9–14)*. The explanation to these findings is that trisomy 12 detected by FISH also have been found in cases with a normal metaphase analysis *(9–14)*.

1.3. Sequential FISH Analysis

Repeat metaphase cytogenetics and FISH analyses have shown that clonal evolution occurs in CLL. Sequential FISH analyses with a median time of 32 mo between analyses were undertaken in 60 patients diagnosed with CLL without trisomy 12. The results indicated that the aberration most likely did not appear during the course of the disease *(15)*. Expansion of the trisomy 12 clone was observed in all patients with trisomy 12 and progressive lymphocytosis *(15)*. Patients with a clinical response to therapy exhibited a decrease of the clone *(15)*. Interestingly, in six patients with CLL in complete remission after chemotherapy, the trisomy 12-positive clone was still detectable when using FISH ***(10)***. Another FISH study showed no acquisition of trisomy 12 during the 13–73 mo that the 15 patients with CLL cases were followed ***(16)***. In the same study, a persistent mosaicism of the trisomy 12 clone was found in four cases, with the percentages of trisomic tumor cells remaining constant during a period of 15 to 81 mo ***(16)***. In three other FISH studies, trisomy 12 was found in a total of seven patients with CLL who all progressed to a morphologically more aggressive disease with prolymphocytes or Richter's syndrome ***(13,17,18)***. Because the clonal evolution was associated with morphological transformation, it was suggested that trisomy 12 was correlated with disease progression ***(18)***. In this study by Garcia-Marco et al., all 13 patients with trisomy 12 had an increase of clonal cells during follow-up ***(18)***. In contrast, Auer et al. found no significant change in the percentage of trisomic cells observed during a 4-yr period, even in CLL patients with disease progression ***(19)***.

A consensus is thus emerging for the role of FISH in studying chromosomal aberrations in CLL. The method is described in this chapter should be simple, sensitive, and reproducible when used for the detection of trisomy 12 and other chromosomal abnormalities in CLL. By analyzing unstimulated lymphocytes, the abnormalities detected are probably inherent to the malignant clone and are of biological and clinical significance. Sequential analyses allow us to follow the malignant clone during the course of the disease and finally minimal residual disease is readily detected. The clinical importance of trisomy 12 in CLL has been extensively investigated and atypical CLL, defined as either atypical morphology or atypical immunophenotype, has been found to be strongly associated with trisomy 12 ***(14,20–30)***. Despite the association between trisomy 12 and atypical CLL morphology, it has been shown by combined conventional staining Mary-Grünwald-Giemsa and FISH (MGG/FISH) studies of individual cells that the aberration is not restricted to lymphocytes with atypical morphology ***(31)***. Patients with advanced disease have been shown to have a higher incidence of trisomy 12 than newly diagnosed asymptomatic patients ***(10,25,26)***. Patients with trisomy 12 have a shorter treatment-free survival ***(10,22,29)*** but whether trisomy 12 detected by FISH is associated with poor survival in CLL is still debated ***(10,22,26,29,32)***. This chapter will focus on the FISH protocols used to detect trisomy 12 in patients with CLL.

2. Materials

All buffers, reagents, and solutions used are shown in **Table 1**. Their storage conditions, stability, and, if known, toxicity is noted. It is advisable to always use protective gloves during the experiment to reduce possible biological and chemical hazards.

Table 1
FISH Protocol for Chromosome 12 Materials Needed

	Buffers/solutions/ reagents	Manufacturer	Storage conditions	Working conditions	Stability	Toxicity
Gradient separation of MNC	Histopaque-1077	Sigma-Aldrich, St. Louis, MO	refrigerated	room temperature		
	PBS		refrigerated	room temperature		
Fiaxation	Methanol:acetic acid 3:1		room temperature	freshly made		
Dehydration	Ethanol 70%		room temperature			
	Ethanol 95%		room temperature			
	Ethanol 99%		room temperature			
Postfixation	Neutral-buffered formaldehyde 1%		room temperature			
	Formaldehyde 4%		room temperature			
	Tris buffered saline		refrigerated			
Hybridisation	Probe chromosome 12	Oncor, Gaithersburg, MD	frozen in –20°C			
	Hybrisol VI	Oncor	room temperature			
Stringency wash	1X SSC		refrigerated			
	Tris buffered saline		refrigerated			
	Tween-20, 0.05%		refrigerated			
Antigen retrieval/ detection	FITC	Boerhinger Mannheim	refrigerated		light-sensitive	
	FITC-anti-sheep Ig	Dakopatts	refrigerated			
Counter stain	Dapi		refrigerated protect from light		light-sensitive	carcinogenic

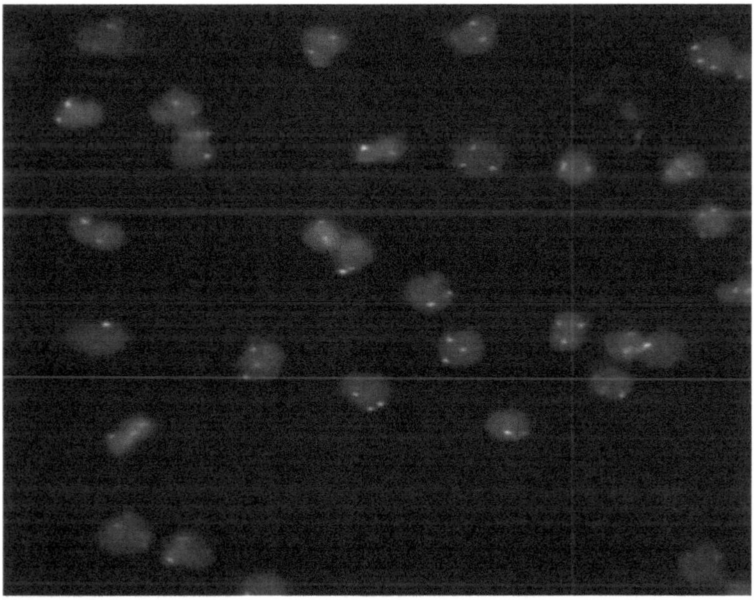

Fig. 1. FISH for trisomy 12 in peripheral blood from a patient with CLL. *See* **Color Plate 11**, following page 270.

3. Methods

To purify the tumor cells, gradient separation of MNCs from peripheral blood, bone marrow, lymph node, or tumor bulk specimens is performed before storage or immediate after FISH analysis. After thawing, the MNCs are hybridized with 175 bp of large alpha-satellite probe specifying the centromeric region of chromosome 12 (Oncor) Antigen detection is performed by using, for example, anti-digoxigenin-fluorescein Fab (FITC) antibodies, and thereafter the slides should be ready for analysis with a fluorescence microscope (**Fig. 1**). The FISH method for detection of trisomy 12 in CLL is described in detail below ***(15,22,31,33)***.

1. Sample peripheral blood with standard heparinized syringes.
2. Gradient separated peripheral blood MNCs are obtained using Histopaque-1077 (Sigma-Aldrich).
3. Re-suspend the MNC fraction in PBS (*see* **Note 1**) to a concentration of approx 5 $\times 10^9$ MNCs/L.
4. Drop one or two drops of this cell suspension on slides (approx 2×10^5 MNCs/slide) and allow to air dry.
5. Freeze the films wrapped in aluminium foil paper and store at –20°C until use.
6. Thaw the slides in room temperature (*see* **Note 2**).
7. Mark the area of the MNC drop with a diamond pen (*see* **Note 3**).

8. Fixate the cells in a cuvette with freshly made methanol:acetic acid, 3:1, for 15 min at room temperature (*see* **Note 4**).
9. Dehydrate in 70% ethanol for 1 min, 95% ethanol for 1 min, and finally 99% ethanol for 1 min.
10. Dry in front of a fan for approx 5 min.
11. Post-fixate in 1% NBF (neutral buffered formaldehyde) for 10 min (*see* **Note 5**).
12. Wash twice in TBS for 1 min each time (*see* **Note 6**).
13. Dehydrate in 70% ethanol for 1 min, 95% ethanol for 1 min, and finally 99% ethanol for 1 min.
14. Dry in front of a fan for 15 min or longer.
15. Take the digoxigenin labeled probe for chromosome 12 (Oncor) from the freezer and warm in 37°C warm chamber for 5 min.
16. Take 1.5 µL of the probe and mix it with 15 µL of hybridization medium (Hybrisol VI) in an Eppendorf plastic Vacutainer (*see* **Note 7**).
17. Put all (16.5 µL) on the slide within the diamond pen marked area.
18. Cover the slide with an 18 × 18-mm cover slip (*see* **Note 8**).
19. Put ordinary "rubber" glue around the cover slip.
20. Denaturate for 5 min in 82–84°C on a hot plate.
21. Hybridize 16–24 h in a moist chamber of 37°C.
22. Warm the water-bath till 72°C.
23. Put a cuvet with 1X SSC in the water bath (*see* **Note 9**).
24. Take the slides from the moist chamber and remove glue and cover slip.
25. Wash in 1X SSC of 72°C for 2 min (*see* **Note 10**).
26. Wash in TBS with 0.05% Tween-20 for 3 min (*see* **Note 11**).
27. Add 40 µL of FITC per slide (*see* **Note 12**).
28. Cover with a 24 × 32-mm cover slip and incubate in a moist chamber of 37°C for 30 min.
29. Wash 3times in TBS with Tween-20 for 1 min each time.
30. Add 40 µL of FITC-anti-sheep Ig (*see* **Note 13**).
31. Cover with a 24 × 32-mm cover slip.
32. Incubate in a moist chamber of 37°C for 5 min (*see* **Note 14**).
33. Wash with TBS three times with Tween-20 for 1 min each time.
34. Counter stain with 16 µL of Dapi (1 µg/mL) per slide.
35. Cover with a 24 × 32-mm cover slip.
36. After antigen detection, the slides should be protected from light to maintain the potency of the fluorescence (*see* **Note 15**).
37. Analyze the slides in a dark room with a fluorescence microscope (e.g., Zeiss EPI-Fluorescence Axioskop 20).
38. In each case we score 500 well spread cells. Cells with three distinct fluorescent signals are counted as trisomic (**Fig. 1**).
39. In our material of peripheral blood, a sample was considered positive for trisomy 12 if more than 1.3% (mean of normal controls + 3SD) of the cells showed three fluorescent signals. This cutoff limit was chosen after analyzing 10 peripheral blood samples from healthy individuals. The proportion of MNCs with three sig-

nals in normal controls was 0.2% ± 0.3 (mean ± SD), range 0–1.0%. Zero signals were found in 0%, one signal in 7.0% ± 2.3, range 1.2–8.8%, and 2 signals in 92.7% ± 2.2, range 91.2–98.3% in the normal controls.

Most authors analyze at least 200 well-spread cells. We analyze, if possible, 500 cells, to increase the reproducibility. Also, different cutoff levels by FISH, from 1.4% to 5%, for trisomy 12 are reported in the literature ***(10–14,16,20,22)***. The critical point here is to use a cutoff limit that corresponds to your own normal range laboratory results gained from healthy blood donors. If you use archived material, which successfully have been used 10 yr after sampling ***(12)***, the controls must have been stored the same way since the normal values will vary compared with fresh material due to degeneration of nuclei.

4. Notes

The hybridization protocol has to be slightly modified, from time to time, to obtain optimal hybridization signals. This is probably due to changes of the material analyzed and the environmental conditions. If the signals are too weak they might be enhanced by adding pronase and /or pepsin to increase the cell membrane permeability. If a direct labeled probe for chromosome 12 is used (Vysis), **steps 16–26** can be omitted.

1. To make 1000 mL of PBS, pH 7.35, add 8 g of NaCl, 1.4 g of di-saline-hydroxy-phosphate $2H_2O$, 0.2 g of KCl, 0.2 g of potassium-di-hydroxy-phosphate, and 0.2 g of azid to 1000 mL of sterile water.
2. It is important that the slides are free from damp (condensation); therefore, it might be preferable to thaw the slides in front of a fan.
3. This is optional but reduces the volume of probe needed. It is preferable to mark the backside of the slide.
4. We make 40 mL (30 mL of methanol and 10 mL of acetic acid) at a time.
5. We make 40 mL (30 mL TBS and 10 mL of 4% formaldehyde) at a time.
6. 12. 1000 mL of 0.05 *M* TBS, pH 7.6, is made of 60.56 g of Tris (hydroxy-metyl-amino-metan) diluted in 500 mL of sterile water. Add HCl until a pH of 7.6 is reached, and after that, add sterile water until a total volume of 1000 mL is achieved. One part of this solution is added to nine parts of NaCl 9 g/L.
7. This volume is per slide.
8. Extra care must be taken to avoid air-bubbles when covering.
9. To make 250 mL 2X SSC, take 25 mL of 20X SSC and dilute with 225 mL of sterile water. 40 mL 1X SSC is made of 20 mL 2X SSC and 20 mL of sterile water. The 1X SSC used in the protocol should be 75°C because the temperature drops till approx 72°C when the slides are put in.
10. If the background is too prominent, wash for up to 5 min each time to reduce it.
11. Mix 0.5 g of Tween-20 with 1000 mL of TBS. The use of Tween is optional, but it is the method we prefer to increase to cell membrane permeability.

12. If you, for example, are analysing eight slides (8 × 40 µL = 320 µL), take 80 µL of FITC and dilute with 240 µL of TBS with Tween-20. This yields a concentration of 1:4 FITC:TBS with Tween-20. Antigen detection might also be performed with anti-digoxigenin-rodamine Fab fragment using the same protocol, to yield a red fluorescein signal instead of a green.
13. For example, if eight slides are to be analyzed (8 × 40 µL = 320 µL), take 16 µL of FITC-anti-sheep Ig and dilute with 304 µL of TBS with Tween-20. This yields a concentration of 1:20 FITC-anti-sheep Ig:TBS with Tween-20.
14. The slides may, as an alternative, be incubated in room temperature for 30 min.
15. If the slides are to be stored for a longer period, we put "rubber" glue around the cover slip and store in a freezer of –20°C.

Acknowledgments

The author sincerely thanks Professor Robert Hast, Department of Hematology, Karolinska Institutet at Karolinska Hospital, and Associate Professor Eva Kimby, Department of Hematology, Karolinska Institutet at Huddinge University Hospital, for fruitful collaboration and Mrs. Ingrid Arvidsson, Department of Hematology, Karolinska Institutet at Karolinska Hospital, Stockholm, Sweden, for excellent knowledge of the FISH technique.

References

1. Crossen, P. E. (1975) Giemsa banding patterns in chronic lymphocytic leukaemia. *Humangenetik.* **27,** 151–156.
2. Autio, K., Turunen, O., Pentillä, O., Erämaa, E., de la Chapelle, A., and Schröder, J. (1979) Human chronic lymphocytic leukemia: karyotypes in different lymphocyte population. *Cancer Genet. Cytogenet.* **1,** 147–155.
3. Knuutila, S., Elonen, E., Teerenhovi, L., Rossi, L., Leskinen, R., Bloomfield, C. D., and de la Chapelle, A. (1986) Trisomy 12 in B-cells of patients with B-cell chronic lymphocytic leukemia. *N. Engl. J. Med.* **314,** 865–869.
4. Autio, K., Elonen, E., Teerenhovi L., and Knuutila, S. (1987) Cytogenetic and immunologic characterization of mitotic cells in chronic lymphocytic leukaemia. *Eur J Haematol.* **39,** 289–298.
5. Gahrton, G., Robèrt, K. H., Friberg, K., Zech, L., and Bird, A. G. (1980) Nonrandom chromosomal aberrations in chronic lymphocytic leukemia revealed by polyclonal B-cell-mitogen stimulation. *Blood.* **56,** 640–647.
6. Nowell, P., Shankey, T. V., Finan, J., Guerry, D., and Besa, E. (1981) Proliferation, differentiation and cytogenetics of chronic leukemic B lymphocytes cultured with mitomycin-treated normal cells. *Blood.* **57,** 444–451.
7. Robèrt, K. H., Gahrton, G., Friberg, K., Zech, L., and Nilsson, B. (1982) Extra chromosome 12 and prognosis in chronic lymphocytic leukaemia. *Scand. J. Haematol.* **28,** 163–168.
8. Kearney, L. (1999) The impact of the new FISH technologies on the cytogenetics of haematological malignancies. *Br. J. Haematol.* **104,** 648–658.

9. Döhner, H., Pohl, S., Bulgay-Mörschel, M., Stilgenbauer, S., Bentz, M., Lichter, P. (1993) Trisomy 12 in chronic lymphoid leukemias—a metaphase and interphase cytogenetic analysis. *Leukemia* **7,** 516–520.
10. Escudier, S. M., Pereira-Leahy, J. M., Drach, J. W., Weier, H. U., Goodacre, A. M., Cork, M. A., et al. (1993) Fluorescent in situ hybridization and cytogenetic studies of trisomy 12 in chronic lymphocytic leukemia. *Blood.* **81,** 2702–2707.
11. Perez Losada, A., Wessman, M., Tiainen, M., Hopman, A. H., Willard, H. F., Sole, F., et al. (1991) Trisomy 12 in chronic lymphocytic leukemia: an interphase cytogenetic study. *Blood.* **78,** 775–779.
12. Anastasi, J., Le Beau, M. M., Vardiman, J. W., Fernald, A. A., Larson, R. A., and Rowley, J. D. (1992) Detection of trisomy 12 in chronic lymphocytic leukemia by fluorescence in situ hybridization to interphase cells: a simple and sensitive method. *Blood* **79,** 1796–1801.
13. Cuneo, A., Wlodarska, I., Sayed Aly, M., Piva, N., Carli, M. G., Fagioli, F., et al. (1992) Non-radioactive in situ hybridization for the detection and monitoring of trisomy 12 in B-cell chronic lymphocytic leukaemia. *Br. J. Haematol.* **81,** 192–196.
14. Que, T. H., Garcia Marco, J., Ellis, J., Matutes, E., Babapulle, V. B., Boyle, S., et al. (1993) Trisomy 12 in chronic lymphocytic leukemia detected by fluorescence in situ hybridization: analysis by stage, immunophenotype and morphology. *Blood* **82,** 571–575.
15. Hjalmar, V., Hast, R., and Kimby, E. (2001) Sequential fluorescence in situ hybridization analyses for trisomy 12 in chronic leukemic B-cell disorders. *Haematologica.* **86,** 174–180.
16. Raghoebier, S., Kibbelaar, R. E., Kleiverda, J. K., Kluin-Nelemans, J. C., van Krieken, J. H., Kok, F., et al. (1992) Mosaicism of trisomy 12 in chronic lymphocytic leukemia detected by non-radioactivity in situ hybridization. *Leukemia* **6,** 1220–1226.
17. Brynes, R. K., McCourty, A., Sun, N. C., and Koo, C. H. (1995) Trisomy 12 in Richter's transformation in chronic lymphocytic leukemia. *Am J Clin Pathol.* **104,** 199–203.
18. Garcia-Marco, J. A., Price, C. M., and Catovsky, D. (1997) Interphase cytogenetics in chronic lymphocytic leukemia. *Cancer Genet Cytogenet.* **94,** 52–58.
19. Auer, R. L., Bienz, N., Neilson, J., Cai, M., Waters, J. J., Milligan, D. W., and Fegan, C. D. (1999) The sequential analysis of trisomy 12 in B-cell chronic lymphocytic leukaemia. *Br. J. Haematol.* **104,** 742–744.
20. Criel, A., Wlodarska, I., Meeus, P., Stul, M., Louwagie, A., Van Hoof, A., et al. (1994) Trisomy 12 is uncommon in typical chronic lymphocytic leukaemias. *Br. J. Haematol.* **87,** 523–528.
21. Criel, A., Verhoef, G., Vlietinck, R., Mecucci, C., Billiet, J., Michaux, L., et al. (1997) Further characterization of morphologically defined typical and atypical CLL: a clinical, immunophenotypic, cytogenetic and prognostic study on 390 cases. *Br. J. Haematol.* **97,** 383–391.
22. Hjalmar, V., Kimby, E., Matutes, E., Sundström, C., Jakobsson, B., Arvidsson, I., et al. (1998) Trisomy 12 and lymphoplasmacytoid lymphocytes in chronic leukemic B-cell disorders. *Haematologica.* **83,** 602–609.

23. Hjalmar, V. (2001) *Chronic leukemic B-cell disorders and trisomy 12: A study of surface markers, protein expression and clinical course.* Thesis, Stockholm.
24. Hjalmar, V., Hast, R., and Kimby, E. (2002) Cell surface expression of CD25, CD54 and CD95 on B- and T-cells in chronic lymphocytic leukaemia in relation to trisomy 12, atypical morphology and clinical course. *Eur. J. Haematol.* **67,** 1–14.
25. Knauf, W. U., Knuutila, S., Zeigmeister, B., and Thiel, E. (1995) Trisomy 12 in B-cell chronic lymphocytic leukemia: Correlation with advanced disease, atypical morphology, high levels of sCD25, and with refractoriness to treatment. *Leuk. Lymphoma.* **19,** 289–294.
26. Matutes, E., Oscier, D., Garcia-Marco, J., Ellis, J., Copplestone, A., Gillingham, R., et al. (1996) Trisomy 12 defines a group of CLL with atypical morphology: correlation between cytogenetic, clinical and laboratory features in 544 patients. *Br. J. Haematol.* **92,** 382–388.
27. Oscier, D. G., Matutes, E., Copplestone, A., Pickering, R. M., Chapman, R., Gillingham, R., et al. (1997) Atypical lymphocyte morphology: an adverse prognostic factor for disease progression in stage A CLL independent of trisomy 12. *Br. J. Haematol.* **98,** 934–939.
28. Su'ut, L., O'Connor, S. J., Richards, S. J., Jones, R. A., Roberts, B. E., Davies, F. E., et al. (1998) Trisomy 12 is seen within a specific subtype of B-cell chronic lymphoproliferative disease affecting the peripheral blood/bone marrow and co-segregates with elevated expression of CD11a. *Br. J. Haematol.* **101,** 165–170.
29. Tefferi, A., Bartholmai, B. J., Witzig, T. E., Jenkins, R. B., Li, C. Y., Hanson, C. A., et al. (1997) Clinical correlations of immunophenotypic variations and the presence of trisomy 12 in B-cell chronic lymphocytic leukemia. *Cancer Genet. Cytogenet.* **95,** 173–177.
30. Woessner, S., Sole, F., Perez-Losada, A., Florensa, L., and Vila, R. M. (1996) Trisomy 12 is a rare cytogenetic finding in typical chronic lymphocytic leukemia. *Leuk. Res.* **20,** 369–374.
31. Hjalmar, V., Kimby, E., Matutes, E., Sundström, C., Wallvik, J., and Hast, R. (2000) Atypical lymphocytes in B-cell chronic lymphocytic leukemia and trisomy 12 studied by conventional staining combined with fluorescence in situ hybridization. *Leukemia Lymphoma.* **37,** 571–576.
32. Döhner, H., Stilgenbauer, S., Benner, A., Leupolt, E., Kröber, A., Bullinger, L., et al. (2000) Genomic aberrations and survival in chronic lymphocytic leukemia. *N. Engl. J. Med.* **343,** 1910–1916.
33. Jacobsson, B., Bernell, P., Arvidsson, I., and Hast, R. (1996) Classical morphology, esterase cytochemistry and interphase cytogenetics of peripheral blood and bone marrow smears. *J. Histochem. Cytochem.* **44,** 1303–1309.

12

Splenic Marginal Zone Lymphoma

7q Abnormalities

Rachel E. Ibbotson, Anton E. Parker, and David G. Oscier

Summary

7q abnormalities are the most common cytogenetic or genetic aberrations found in splenic marginal zone lymphoma. The molecular methods whereby these regions of genetic loss can be characterized are discussed in this chapter. Emphasis is given to careful experimental design, for example sample purification and optimization, that is, ensuring that only target sequences are amplified. There also is discussion of result interpretation, pitfalls that may be encountered, and alternative visualization techniques that might be used.

Key Words: Splenic marginal zone lymphoma (SMZL), splenic lymphoma with villous lymphocytes (SLVL), 7q, microsatellites, loss of heterozygosity (LOH).

1. Introduction

Splenic marginal zone lymphoma (SMZL) is a chronic B-cell disorder diagnosed on the basis of splenic histology, which shows that the splenic white pulp is infiltrated by an inner zone of small lymphocytes and an outer zone of larger cells with abundant pale cytoplasm. The tumor cells are positive for surface immunoglobulin (Ig)M and IgD and express CD20, CD22, and CD79a but not CD5, CD10, CD23, or cyclin D1. Patients usually present with splenomegaly without peripheral lymphadenopathy. Bone marrow and blood involvement is common. Circulating tumor lymphocytes frequently have a characteristic villous appearance and in such cases in which splenectomy is not indicated clinically, are diagnosed as splenic lymphoma with villous lymphocytes (SLVLs) *(1,2)*.

Analysis of V_H genes from a small number of cases with SMZL or SLVL has shown that most have undergone somatic mutation with or without intraclonal heterogeneity. However, a subset of cases with unmutated V_H genes

From: *Methods in Molecular Medicine, Vol. 115: Lymphoma: Methods and Protocols*
Edited by: T. Illidge and P. W. M. Johnson © Humana Press Inc., Totowa, NJ

has recently been described *(3)*. This would be consistent with the derivation of SMZL from the heterogeneous population of normal splenic marginal zone B-cells, which includes both naïve and memory B-cells.

No consistent cytogenetic or genetic abnormality that defines SMZL has so far been described. Occasional patients with reciprocal chromosome translocations involving the immunoglobulin loci have been documented. The partner chromosomes include 7q21 resulting in juxtaposition of the CDK6 gene to the kappa light chain locus, and 6p12, with juxtaposition of cyclin D3 to the immunoglobulin heavy chain locus *(4)*.

Approximately 50% of patients with SMZL or SLVL have a deletion of chromosome 7q. Although different regions of loss of 7q have been reported the majority of cases have a deletion of 7q31.3 – 32 *(5)*. The molecular consequence of this deletion is unknown.

Microsatellite analysis is a valuable tool for detecting loss of heterozygosity (LOH) in regions with candidate tumor suppressor genes *(6)*, In this chapter we will discuss the microsatellite analysis methods we have used to look for LOH and hence determine the commonly deleted region (CDR) of chromosome 7q in our series of SMZL/SLVL patients. Cytogenetic techniques will not be discussed, but the results of karyotyping and fluorescent *in situ* hybridization (FISH) often provide an excellent method of identifying chromosomal regions of interest before beginning the search for a CDR by molecular techniques. Southern blotting will also not be discussed, however labeled restriction fragment-length polymorphism (RFLP) analysis is a very useful tool in the confirmation of microsatellite LOH results and hybridization analysis also may be used to investigate homozygous loss in a newly defined CDR *(7,8)*.

Microsatellites are tandem repeats of simple di-, tri-, tetra-, penta-, or hexanucleotide sequence (2–6 bases), which occur abundantly and at random throughout most eukaryotic genomes. They are typically short (often less that 100 bp long) and embedded within unique sequence, thus being ideal for designing flanking primers for in vitro amplification by the polymerase chain reaction (PCR). The high degree of polymorphism (attributable to variation in the number of repeat units) displayed by microsatellites is especially advantageous because the majority of samples will be heterozygous (otherwise said to be informative) at the locus of interest. In addition, very small amounts of tissue are required for microsatellite analysis, as typically only 100 ng of template DNA is used compared with 10 μg for a Southern blot, meaning that archival material also can be exploited *(9)*.

For LOH studies, it is imperative that there is access to matched normal and tumor tissue so that direct comparison between the two can be made. In our own studies, we have analyzed peripheral blood lymphocytes using granulocytes as matched controls. Also, it should be emphasized that these matched

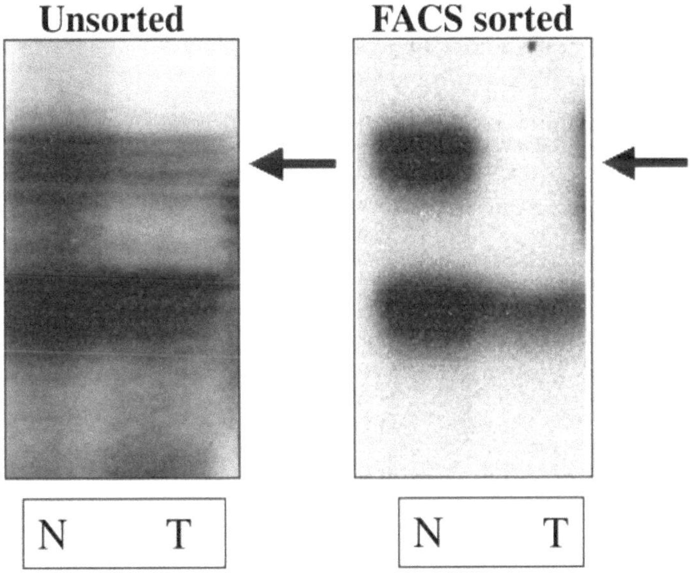

Fig. 1. Autoradiogram of polyacrylamide gel electropheresis (PAGE) of ^{32}P labeled PCR products. Microsatellite analysis on normal (N) and tumor (T) derived DNA from unsorted and FACS sorted cell populations. The arrow indicates the additional band arising from DNA from normal cells contaminating the tumor cell population. LOH is clearly demonstrated when DNA from FACS sorted cells is analyzed.

samples must be purified to greater than 85%, that is, the tumor sample should not be contaminated with normal material and vice versa; otherwise, problems will be encountered during the result interpretation (**Fig. 1**).

Sample pairs are scored as follows: heterozygous, not deleted (two different alleles present in both normal and tumor tissue); heterozygous, deleted (two alleles present in normal tissue, but only one present in tumor tissue); homozygous, not informative (two alleles of the same size present in both normal and tumor tissue).

2. Materials

2.1. Sample Purification

2.1.1. Sample Processing

The starting material is heparinised peripheral blood, which is centrifuged through a Histopaque (Sigma Diagnostics, UK) gradient to separate the lymphocytes and granulocytes.

1. 20 mL heparinised blood.
2. 50 mL conical based tubes (Bibby, UK).
3. Histopaque-1077 (Sigma Diagnostics, UK).
4. Plastic Pasteur pipets.
5. Phosphate buffered saline (PBS).
6. Deionised water.
7. Centrifuge to spin 50 mL tubes at 400*g*.

2.1.2. Fluorescent Assisted Cell Sorting (FACS)

1. Flow cytometer with sort facility plus associated equipment and consumables.
2. Mouse anti-human monoclonal antibodies specific for the tumor clone of interest (*see* **Note 1**).

2.1.3. Magnetic Microbead Purification

1. MACS CD19 microbeads (Miltenyi Biotec, Germany) plus associated equipment and consumables.

2.2. DNA Extraction

2.2.1. Extraction Method for Sorted Cell Fractions

1. 50 m*M* sodium hydroxide.
2. Hot block at 100°C.
3. 1 *M* Tris-HCl pH 7.5.
4. 1.5 mL micro-centrifuge tubes

2.2.2. Extraction Method for Granulocytes

1. Same as **Subheading 2.2.1.** above.

2.3. Amplification of Microsatellites, Resolution, and Detection

The details given in this section assume that the fluorescently labeled primer method will be followed. *See* **Note 2** for details for the radioactive and fluorescent dCTP incorporation methods.

1. Genomic DNA from tumor and normal tissue.
2. dNTP mix (Pharmacia).
3. 10X PCR buffer (supplied with enzyme).
4. $MgCl_2$ solution (supped with enzyme).
5. Thermoprime *Taq* DNA polymerase (Applied Biotechnologies, UK).
6. Microsatellite primers (*see* **Note 3**; Oswel, UK).
7. 0.2-mL Microcentrifuge tubes (Perkin Elmer).
8. 0.5-mL Genetic Analyser sample tubes (Applied Biosystems).
9. Septa for 0.5-mL Sample tubes (Applied Biosystems).
10. PCR machine (Perkin Elmer).
11. ABI PRISM 310® Genetic Analyser (Applied Biosystems; *see* **Note 4**).

12. De-ionised formamide (Applied Biosystems).
13. TAMRA-500 size standard (Applied Biosystems).
14. GeneScan® Analysis Software V3.1 (Applied Biosystems; *see* **Note 4**).

3. Methods

3.1 Sample Purification

3.1.1. Sample Processing

1. Carefully overlay 20 mL blood onto 20 mL histopaque and spin in an un-braked centrifuge for 30 min at 400*g*.
2. Remove the lymphocytes which form a layer at the interphase between the histopaque and the plasma using a plastic Pasteur pipet and transfer to a clean tube.
3. Remove the granulocytes which form a layer on top of the red blood cell pellet underneath the histopaque at the base of the tube using a plastic Pasteur pipet and transfer to a clean tube.
4. Wash the lymphocytes with 30 mL PBS and the granulocytes with 30 mL water (to lyse the red blood cells).
5. Pellet cells, decant supernatant, and repeat this washing step.
6. Re-suspend the cells in residual fluid after decanting the second time.
7. Make a 1/100 dilution in PBS of the lymphocytes and count the number of cells either by using a haematology analyser such as an Advia 120 (Bayer, UK) or in Neubauer counting chamber. The lymphocytes are now ready for purification by either of the two suggested methods.
8. Transfer a small volume (20 μL) of the granulocyte suspension to a 1.5 mL micro-centrifuge tube in preparation for genomic DNA extraction. The remaining granulocyte pellet should be stored at –20°C.

3.1.2. FACS

Refer to the manufacturer's instructions on how to sort specific populations on the chosen machine. The sorted cells are analyzed by flow cytometry to verify the purity of the separation (**Fig. 2**).

3.1.3. Magnetic Micro-Bead Purification

Miltenyi CD19 micro-beads are supplied with a detailed protocol sheet, which is simple and straightforward. We access the purity of our samples by labelling 1×10^6 cells, both before and after the column purification, with CD5 FITC and CD20 RPE mouse antihuman monoclonal antibodies (Dako, Denmark) and analysing by flow cytometry (*see* **Note 5**).

We recommend the micro-bead purification method because it is less labor-intensive and the yield is higher; however, the limitation is that it is difficult to sort on more than one parameter at a time.

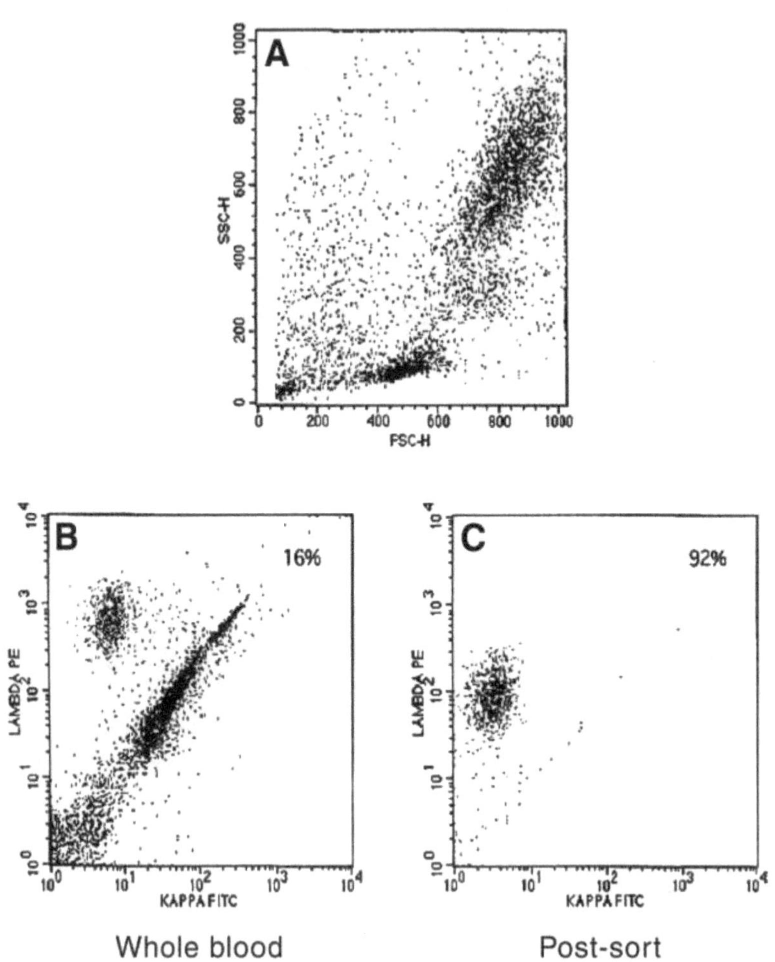

Fig. 2. FACS plots of peripheral blood from SLVL patient, **(A)** forward scatter versus side scatter of whole blood **(B)** whole blood labeled with κ and λ light chain mouse monoclonal antibodies (Dako, Denmark) before FACS sorting; **(C)** the same cells as in **(B)** but after FACS sorting for the clonal λ population.

3.2. DNA Extraction

3.2.1. Sorted Cell Fractions

1. Transfer sorted cells into a 1.5 mL micro-centrifuge tube and pellet at 400*g* for 3 min.
2. Decant supernatant; add 100 µL of 50 m*M* NaOH and vortex to mix for 15 s.
3. Incubate for 5 min at 100°C in a hot block.

4. Add 20 μl of 1 *M* Tris, pH 7.5, vortex, and spin to collect any debris at the bottom of the tube.
5. Decant the supernatant (DNA solution) into a fresh tube and store at –20°C.

3.2.2. Granulocyte Cell Pellet

1. Follow the same procedure as in **Subheading 3.2.1.** above.
2. The genomic DNA from the granulocytes is likely to be more concentrated than that extracted from the sorted cell fraction and will need to be diluted to a comparable concentration (*see* **Note 6**).

3.3. Microsatellite Selection

Once the genomic region of interest has been identified, appropriate microsatellites for investigation must be selected, either from previously identified microsatellites listed in the databases or from novel microsatellites. It is possible to database search for the presence of novel microsatellites by using computer programs. However, public databases with comprehensive lists of known microsatellite loci are also available (e.g., National Centre for Biotechnology Information [NCBI] at http://www.ncbi.nlm.nih.gov/), which provide data on hetrozygosity rates and suggested primer sequences in addition to the locations and flanking sequences.

3.4. Microsatellite Analysis

Microsatellite polymorphism is quantified by PCR and electrophoresis. There are several resolution procedures that can be used for visualizing the PCR products. Incorporation of radioactive ^{32}P followed by polyacrylamide gel electrophoresis (PAGE) has long been a standard technique, and details are discussed in previous books in this series. Advances in fluorescent chemistry and automated sequencing by using PAGE or, more recently, capillary electrophoresis, have fueled the widespread adoption of fluorescent microsatellite assays. The incorporation of fluorescence into the PCR products can be achieved by the use of fluorescent dye-labeled primers or fluorescent dNTPs ([F] dNTPs).

3.4.1. LOH at Microsatellite Markers on Chromosome 7 in Peripheral Blood Lymphocytes and Granulocytes

1. PCR amplifications are set up as follows using one unit of Thermoprime *Taq* DNA polymerase, 50–100 ng of template DNA; 50 μ*M* of each of dCTP, dATP, dTTP, and dGTP, 1.75–2.5 m*M* Mg^{2+}, 20 pm 5' fluorescent-labeled forward primer; and 20 pm unlabeled reverse primer (*see* **Note 7**) in a total volume of 25 μL.
2. Standard PCR parameters are 25 cycles of denaturation at 94°C for 30 s; annealing at 58°C for 30 s; and extension at 72°C for 30 s, with a final extension of 10 min at 72°C followed by a hold at 4°C until ready to analyze (*see* **Note 7**).

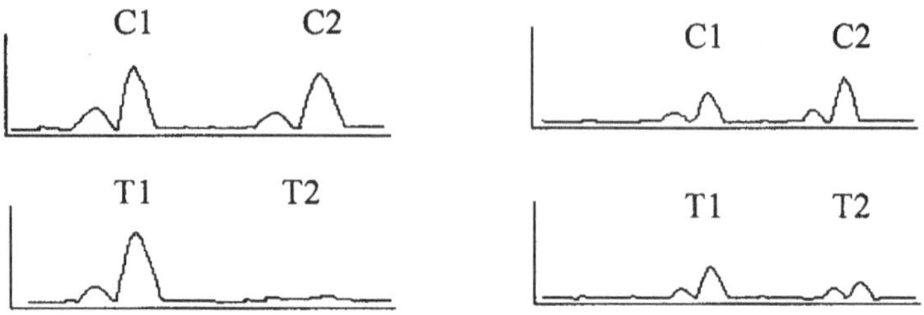

Fig. 3. Schematic representation of Genescan Eletrophrogram traces showing LOH. **(A)** LOH at D7S2486. C1 = 12846, C2 = 13125, T1 = 14547, T2 = 183, CR= 0.98, TR= 79.5, CR/TR = 0.01. **(B)** LOH at D7S643. C1 = 7274, C2 = 8667, T1 = 7834, T2 = 2219, CR= 0.84, TR= 3.53, CR/TR = 0.24.

3. Mix 1 μL PCR product with 12 μL of deionized formamide and 1 μL of TAMRA-500 size standard in a 0.5 mL sample tube covered with a septa. Denature at 92°C for 2 min and keep on ice until ready to load on the ABI-310 genetic analyser®
4. Run samples for 24 min at 60°C using GeneScan®.
5. It is recommended that all PCRs be performed in duplicate to verify results.

As stated previously, microsatellite markers that show distinct peaks from two alleles in the electropherogram of the constitutional DNA were considered to be informative (*see* comment in **Note 8**). For all informative samples, peak areas were calculated for C1 and C2, which represent the short and long alleles in the constitutional (C) DNA and for T1 and T2 representing the short and long alleles in the tumor (T) DNA (**Fig. 3**). Peak area ratios for the constitutional sample (CR) and tumor sample (TR) were calculated, where CR = C1/C2 and TR = T1/T2. If the value of CR fell outside of the range 0.8–1.2, then the sample was considered unsuitable for assessment for LOH. The ratio of CR/TR was then calculated: if CR/TR was <0.25 or >4, then this indicated that the total peak area of one allele in the tumor sample was reduced by greater than 75% relative to the peak area of the remaining allele and was thus scored as LOH. Homozygous loss should not be determined by this method because DNA from residual normal cells in the tumor DNA fraction will interfere with interpretation of the results.

4. Notes

1. We typically label lymphocytes with a triple-color combination of κ FITC/λ RPE /CD19 RPE-Cy5 (Dako, Denmark) and sequentially gate first on the basis of forward/side scatter, second on the CD19 positive population, and third on the surface immunoglobulin. We recommend referring to the instructions supplied by the manufacturer of the flow cytometer.

2. For fluorescent nucleotide incorporation, the only additional requirement will be the R110 Fluorescent [F]dCTP (ABI).. For radioactive nucleotide incorporation, the additional requirements are [^{32}P]dCTP (10 µCi/µL) (ICN), 10X TBE: 0.9 *M* Tris borate, 20 m*M* EDTA; sequencing apparatus; sequencing gel dryer; Hydrotech vacuum pump (all Bio-Rad); X-ray film; and autoradiograph cassettes. Special consideration should be given to working with radioactive chemicals and the local radiation protection advisor must be contacted for advice.
3. Whether uniplex or multiplex reactions are to be performed, care should be taken in designing sets of primer pairs with similar properties, that is, 50% GC rich, not self complimentary or complementary to each other, between 17 and 24 bp and with a product size <350 bp. When using fluorescent labeled primers, a fluorochrome should be attached to the 5' end of only one of the paired primers. The use of different fluorochromes for primers with similar sized products is essential in multiplex experiments.
4. More information on the ABI PRISM 310® and GeneScan® software can be found at http://www.appliedbiosystems.com/products/.
5. We have found that labeling with CD5 and CD20 gives a good indication of how many B-cells (CD20+) and T-cells (CD5+) are in your purified sample. Do not use CD19 for labeling the post column sample, as staining will be significantly reduced, as the specificity is the same as that of the microbead.
6. It is difficult to quantify the concentration of genomic DNA extracted from the sorted cells as it is so dilute; however, to produce comparable results the concentration of DNA extracted from the granulocytes should be approximately equal. To overcome this, the granulocyte DNA should be serially diluted and used in trial PCRs to evaluate the optimal dilution necessary to produce equivalent results.
7. As with all PCR based techniques, it is of primary importance to ensure optimum template DNA quality and to spend time optimizing the reaction conditions for each microsatellite loci, that is, annealing temperature and Mg^{2+}, template and primer concentrations. The presence of a correctly sized, distinct band on an agarose gel is a clear indication that a PCR product is being produced but sequencing of the product is advised to check it is the expected sequence.
8. The generation of stutter peaks, byproducts of the PCR amplification differing in length from the original allele by one or more repeat units, is a well known problem with the amplification of short tandem repeat loci. It is often especially apparent in PCR from degraded DNA where the generation of these by-products can be intensified, resulting in shadow bands that can exceed the peak height or band intensity of the real allele. Generation of shadow bands during the amplification process can be reduced by changing parameters of the denaturation and elongation steps or adjustment of the A/T: G/C ratio of the dNTP mix according to the sequence amplified.

Acknowledgments

The Bournemouth Leukaemia Fund and the Leukaemia Research Fund supported the work in the authors' laboratory, and we thank Mary Tiller for her excellent technical assistance.

References

1. Jaffe, E. S., Harris, N. L., Stein, H., and Vardiman, J. W. (2001)Pathology and genetics of tumors of haematopoietic and lymphoid tissues, in WHO Classification of Tumors. WHO, Geneva.
2. Chacon, J. L., Mollegjo, M., Munox, E., Algara, P., Mateo, M., Lopez, L., et al. (2002) Splenic marginal zone lymphoma: clinical characteristics and prognostic factors in a series of 60 patients. *Blood* **100,** 1648.
3. Algara, P., Mateo, M. S., Sanchez-Beato, M., Mollejo, M., Navas, I. C., Romero, L., et al. (2002) Analysis of the IgV_H somatic mutations in splenic marginal zone lymphoma defines a group of unmutated cases with frequent 7q deletion and adverse clinical course. *Blood* **99,** 1299.
4. Corcoran, M. M., Mould, S. J., Orchard, J. A., Ibbotson, R. E., Chapman, R. M., Boright, A. P., et al. (1999) Dysregulation of cyclin dependent kinase 6 expression in splenic marginal zone lymphoma through chromosome 7q translocations. *Oncogene* **18,** 6271–6277.
5. Mateo, M., Mollejo, M., Villuendas, R., Algara, P., Sanchez-Beato, M., Martinez P., et al. (1999) 7q31-32 allelic loss is a frequent finding in splenic marginal zone lymphoma. *Am. J. Pathol.* **154,** 1583–1589.
6. Jones M. H.,Nakamura Y. (1992) Detection of loss of heterozygosity at the human TP53 locus using a dinucleotide repeat polymorphism. *Genes Chromosomes Cancer* **5,** 89–90.
7. Tripputi P., Cassani B., Alfano R., Graziani D., Cigognini D., Doi P., et al. (1993) Detection of human chromosomes in somatic cell hybrids by PCR analysis. *Cytogenet Cell Genet.* **62,** 1–4.
8. Corcoran M. M., Rasool O., Liu Y., Iyengar A., Grander D., Ibbotson R. E., et al. (1998) Detailed molecular delineation of 13q14.3 loss in B-cell chronic lymphocytic leukaemia. *Blood* **91,** 1382–1390.
9. Pabst T., Schwaller J., Tobler A., Fey M. F. (1996) Detection of microsatellite markers in leukaemia using DNA from archival bone marrow smears. *Br. J. Haematol.* **95,** 135–137.

13

BCL-6

Rearrangement and Mutation in Lymphoma

Simon D. Wagner and Jaspal S. Kaeda

Summary

BCL-6 is a zinc finger transcription factor that is highly expressed in normal germinal center B-cells. Its function is to prevent differentiation and apoptosis and allow growth. BCL-6 also is expressed in various lymphoproliferative conditions, for example, diffuse large cell lymphoma, Burkitt's lymphoma, and follicular lymphoma as well as lymphocyte predominant Hodgkin's disease. Expression also has been demonstrated in some T-cell lymphomas. In diffuse large cell lymphoma, BCL-6 is involved in translocations with a number of different translocation partners but most commonly the immunoglobulin heavy chain locus. The first intron of BCL-6 is heavily mutated, and detailed analysis reveals two "hotspots." The mutated region appears to be within a transcriptional control region, and there is the potential for alterations to contribute to overexpression of BCL-6. Methods for deoxyribonucleic acid extraction from lymphoma samples and amplification by polymerase chain reaction of the hypermutated intronic region are described.

Key Words: Lymphoma; transcription factor; germinal center; translocation; somatic hypermutation.

1. Introduction

1.1. Function in Normal B-Cell Development

The consistent chromosomal translocations found in lymphoproliferative diseases are the focus of intense study because they provide an avenue to understanding the mechanism by which these conditions develop. For example, constitutive activation of c-MYC to the immunoglobulin heavy chain enhancer by the translocation t(8;14) of Burkitt's lymphoma maintains the cell in cycle, and the resulting proliferation is likely to promote lymphomagenesis. BCL-6 was cloned from a similar translocation between the immunoglobulin heavy chain enhancer and chromosome 3q27 *(1)*.

From: *Methods in Molecular Medicine, Vol. 115: Lymphoma: Methods and Protocols*
Edited by: T. Illidge and P. W. M. Johnson © Humana Press Inc., Totowa, NJ

The important elements of BCL-6 structure are a deoxyribonucleic acid (DNA) binding domain comprising six zinc fingers and at the other end of the molecule a pox virus zinc finger (POZ) effector domain. The latter recruits corepressors and histone deacetylase to accomplish transcriptional repression *(2)*. Between the POZ domain and the DNA binding domain is a central regulatory region containing three PEST domains, which are involved with targeting the protein for degradation *(3)*.

During the course of normal development, B-cells are produced in the bone marrow, selected into the peripheral blood, and then migrate to the lymph nodes *(4)*. In a normal immune response, B-cells follow diverging paths: if activated by a T-independent antigen, they proliferate for a few days in the extrafollicular areas and subsequently differentiate to plasma cells. If, on the other hand, B-cells are activated by T-dependent antigens, they undergo sustained proliferation for 3 to 4 wk within a germinal center and differentiate to produce long-lived plasma cells and memory cells. BCL-6 is highly expressed in germinal center B-cells, but apparently not at other stages of B-cell development. They also are expressed in scattered extrafollicular T-cells *(5–7)*.

Mice bearing homozygous disruptions of the BCL-6 locus lack germinal centers and have impaired secondary immune responses *(8,9)*, and these defects are B-cell autonomous *(10)*. Such mice also have severe Th2-mediated inflammatory disease, which suggests that BCL-6 has functions in cells other than B lymphocytes and, indeed, it has been suggested that this transcription factor is important in macrophage differentiation *(11)*.

The precise mechanism by which BCL-6 exerts its effects has been investigated using a B-cell line that undergoes plasma cell differentiation when cultured with interleukins 2 and 5 *(12)*. It was demonstrated that BCL-6 allows the continuing growth of this cell line under conditions in which there would normally be plasma cell differentiation and apoptotic cell death. BCL-6 similarly prevents the differentiation or allows prolonged growth of primary mouse splenocytes *(12,13)*.

The DNA sequence to which BCL-6 binds is similar to that of the signal transducers and activators of transcription (STAT) family of transcription factors *(14)*. This knowledge prompted the concept that BCL-6 prevents, possibly by direct competition for binding sites, the effects of STAT driven transcription. Experiments using the mouse B-cell lymphoma line BCL-1 have demonstrated that BCL-6 can suppress STAT3-driven transcription, and this transcription is largely responsible for its effects on cell growth *(12)*. Supportive evidence for the importance of STAT3 at this stage of B-cell development has been shown by functional studies in a B-cell line *(15)* and by the presence of activated STAT3 in germinal center B-cells *(16)*. However, BCL-6 may also inhibit the effects of other STATs, for example, STAT6 *(9,17)* or STAT5 (S. Wagner, unpublished observations).

Recent studies using gene expression profiling have begun to reveal the molecular targets for BCL-6 in the control of differentiation and cell growth as well as inflammation *(18)*. The ability of BCL-6 to promote cell survival suggests that it may have a role in the generation or maintenance of memory B-cells *(19)*. Memory B-cells usually are regarded as being the product of a T-dependent antibody response and bearing somatic hypermutation, although memory B-cells can be produced during responses to T-independent antigens. Indeed, memory B-cells lacking somatic hypermutations can be generated without germinal centers and without BCL-6 *(20)*.

1.2. Expression in Other Lineages

STATs have important functions in lineages other than B-cells. For example, they have been implicated in the development or growth of thymic epithelium and other epithelial tissues, including mammary epithelium, T-cells, monocytes, granulocytes, liver, and neurons *(21)*. Some of the characteristics of mice bearing disrupted BCL-6 loci support a role for BCL-6 in controlling differentiation in other lineages, particularly monocytes *(11)*. BCL-6 is expressed in various epithelial sites *(22,23)*, and one might speculate that it has the function of modulating STAT-driven transcription to control replicative potential and differentiation in these locations.

1.3. Significance of BCL-6 in Lymphomas

Studies using cytogenetics have demonstrated that BCL-6 is rearranged in between 33% *(25)* of cases of diffuse large cell lymphoma (DLCL). However, another series, in which rearrangement was analyzed by Southern blots *(26)*, found only 23% of cases had alterations to the BCL-6 locus. Evidence is increasing to suggest that BCL-6 contributes to lymphomagenesis in DLCL; dysregulation of BCL-6, possibly by somatic hypermutation within the 5' untranslated region (*see* **Subheading 1.5.2.**), is further supportive of this conclusion. However, there is some discordance between the presence of a chromosomal translocation at 3q27 and BCL-6 protein expression *(27)*. For those cases of DLCL with a translocation only, 62% have BCL-6 protein expression whereas the remainder do not. Conversely 85% of cases without cytogenetic abnormalities at 3q27 do express BCL-6 protein. There is no obvious way to interpret these findings: one possibility is that forced BCL-6 protein expression by means of a chromosomal rearrangement may be necessary to establish the malignant clone but is not necessary for its maintenance and therefore, inactivation can be allowed.

However, BCL-6 also is expressed in other lymphomas, especially follicular lymphoma ***(28)***, Burkitt's lymphoma ***(29)***, and both nodular lymphocyte-predominant Hodgkin's disease (85% of cases) and, to a lesser extent, classical Hodgkin's disease (50% of cases) ***(29)***. Translocations involving BCL-6 are not a feature of these diseases, and it is most likely that expression of this transcription factor is a reflection of the normal biology of the cell of origin of the tumors, that is, the germinal center B-cell. Although little is known of the biology of BCL-6 in T-cells, it has been demonstrated that 45% of anaplastic large cell lymphomas, but not other T-cell lymphomas, express this transcription factor ***(30)***.

An observation that was originally made on the basis of southern analysis and clinical follow-up is that rearrangement of the BCL-6 locus in DLCL is associated with a more favorable outcome than those cases in which it is not rearranged ***(26)***. This claim was substantiated in one survey of gene expression in DLCL ***(31)***, but not in another ***(32)***, possibly because of the differences in statistical analysis or selection of patients. However, that there are different patterns of gene expression within DLCL, which predict different clinical outcomes, might be anticipated, and increasingly sophisticated analyses are likely to reveal a number of patterns that are characteristic of varying clinical outcomes ***(33)***.

1.4. BCL-6 and Cytogenetics

Chromosomal translocations produce their effects in malignant disease essentially by one of two mechanisms. First, a fusion gene can be produced that commonly has a modular structure, for example, a DNA binding domain from one gene is joined to an effector domain from a different gene or, second, translocation can cause overexpression of a gene whose effects are to enhance cell growth or prevent apoptosis. It is surprising that fusion genes are found predominantly in myeloid malignancies, whereas translocations causing overexpression of an unaltered gene occur in lymphoproliferative conditions.

BCL-6 rearrangement in DLCL conforms to this paradigm. The major breakpoint region is within the 5' noncoding region of the BCL-6 gene in approximately half of all cases that have chromosomal translocations involving the BCL-6 locus at 3q27. Some of the remaining cases, between 30% and 50%, have breakpoints that are 245 to 285 kb upstream of BCL-6 ***(34)***. In both of these situations, it is presumed that BCL-6 comes under the transcriptional control of elements, which drive the gene constitutively ***(34,35)***.

In 52–58% of cases of DLCL that have translocations involving 3q27, an immunoglobulin gene locus is brought close to BCL-6 ***(36,37)***. One of these studies ***(36)*** further demonstrated that 74% (22/30) of these cases use the immunoglobulin heavy chain locus, 3% (1/30) the kappa light chain locus,

Table 1
Partner Loci Involved In BCL-6 Translocations

Translocation	Nonimmunoglobulin Locus	Gene class	Reference
t(3;16)(q27;p11)	Interleukin 21 receptor	Cytokine receptor	*38*
t(3;6)(q27;p21)	SRP20	Regulation of pre-mRNA splicing	*39*
t(3;13)(q27;q14)	L-plastin	Actin binding protein	*40*
t(3;7)(q27;p12	Ikaros	Regulator of lymphocyte differentiation	*41,42*
t(3;4)(q27;p13)	RhoH/TTF	Rho GTP binding protein	*43*
t(3;11)(q27; q23)	BOB1/OBF1	B lymphocyte transcription factor	*44*
	H4	Histone	*36*
	HSP89alpha	Heat shock protein	*36,76*
	HSP90beta	Heat shock protein	*36*
	PIM-1	Lymphocyte growth factor and proto-oncogene	*36,43*
	MHC class II transactivator	Transcription factor	*42*
	Eukaryotic initiation factor 4AII	Transcription factor	*42*
	Transferrin receptor	Surface receptor	*42*

Where no chromosomal translocation is given, the partner locus has been discovered by long-range PCR.

and 23% (7/30) the lambda light chain locus. Analysis of the heavy chain locus demonstrated that breakpoints occur within the switch region *(35)*, similar to the translocations between the same immunoglobulin locus and c-MYC in sporadic cases of Burkitt's lymphoma, and suggesting that these chromosomal events occur at a late stage in B-cell development rather than during variable-diversity-joining, that is, V-D-J, rearrangement in the bone marrow. In approx 40% of DLCL cases, translocations do not involve the immunoglobulin locus. These appear to have a worse prognosis than those with an altered immunoglobulin locus *(37)*. The nonimmunoglobulin loci that have been identified in translocations are detailed in **Table 1**.

As has been mentioned previously, diffuse lymphoma is a heterogeneous disease both histologically and molecularly *(32,33)*, and one outcome of this is that chromosomal translocations involving other genes are also found. One study *(46)* using Southern analysis found 15.3% of cases to have a BCL-1 translocation, 5.8% BCL-2 translocation, and 10.2% a c-MYC translocation. A combined cytogenetic and gene expression study *(47)* demonstrated the t(14;18)(q32;q21) translocation, that is, disrupting the BCL-2 locus, in 20% of cases of diffuse lymphoma and all of these had a germinal center B-cell gene expression signature *(31)* of which BCL-6 expression is a feature.

In a minority of cases translocations involving 3q27 are associated with other cytogenetic abnormalities. For example, one series *(48)* found 3/22 cases to also bear a disrupted BCL2 locus t(14;18) and 2/22 to bear a disrupted c-MYC locus t(8;14). Cases in which all three common translocations occur together have been reported *(49)*.

1.5. BCL-6 and Hypermutation

1.5.1. Somatic Hypermutation in Normal B-Cells

The increase in affinity of serum for antigen on repeated immunization is accounted for both by changes in immunoglobulin V gene usage and by accumulation of point mutations in the V genes *(50)*. The characteristics and requirement for cis-acting control elements are well recognized *(51)* and, more recently, an enzyme (activation induced deaminase *[52,53]*) has been found to be essential not only for this process but also for immunoglobulin class switching and gene conversion *(54–56)*. Somatic hypermutation occurs within the lymph node germinal center *(57)*, which is also the site of BCL-6 expression. The BCL-6 gene from normal germinal center B-cells has been sequenced to find out whether all actively transcribed genes in this location bear point mutations. Surprisingly, BCL-6 was found to be mutated but other genes, for example, c-MYC and alpha-fetoprotein, were not *(58,59)*. However, it has since been shown that several proto-oncogenes as well as BCL-6 can be mutated in normal B-cells *(60)*. Although calculation of the rate of mutation is complicated by the low absolute numbers of mutations, it may be that BCL-6 mutates at a lower rate than immunoglobulin genes *(58,59)* in normal B-cells.

1.5.2. BCL-6 Mutation in Lymphomas

Mutation clearly could provide a mechanism for dysregulation of BCL-6 expression, which could play a role in lymphomagenesis. Analysis of material from two patients and a B-cell line that expresses BCL-6 *(61)* revealed deletions of varying extent but with a shared common region of about 200 bp (**Fig. 1**) in the first intron of BCL-6. This study suggests that there may be negative control elements whose function is disrupted and leads to constitutive BCL-6 expression. Indirect support for this view is provided by the finding of a 184-bp region of homology between mouse and human sequence that overlaps the deleted region. Such regions of intronic homology are likely to be

```
  37695                             tcatgatca ttattttacc ttttaattct ttttttttcc

A 37741 gctcttgcca aatgctttgg ctccaagttt tctatgtgta tctattgata taaatgtata
B 37741 gctcttgcca aatgctttgg ctccaagttt tctatgtgta tctattgata taaatgtata
C 37741 gctcttgcca aatgctttgg ctccaagttt tctatgtgta tctattgata taaatgtata

          1 1  3     4  54    1
A 37801 tatttattta ttctagctgt caggtgttaa aataaatgcc gaagattagt cccacgtctc
B 37801 tatttattta ttctagctgt caggtgttaa aataaatgcc gaagattagt cccacgtctc
C 37801 tatttattta ttctagctgt caggtgttaa aataaatgcc gaagattagt cccacgtctc

  37861 tcccaccata ggatatagat TGTTATGTAT TTATTATTAT TATTGTTGTC TTTGAGTGAA

  37921 TCGGCCGGTT TGGGGAGGCT TTTGCCACCC TCCCTTGTGT TGTTTTGGTT TTTGGAAAGG

  37981 AGGTGGAGGA GAGGAAGGAG GGGAATTAGG GGGCGGCCGG AGCAGAGAGG ACGAGACAGT

A 38041 GCTTGGGGGG TGATTCGGGC TAGTCTGGGG GCTGTCTGGC CCCAGACCGC GGAGAGGACG
        1 11        1 211311      1  1   1        1 1 1           2 11 1
B 38041 GCTTGGGGGG TGATTCGGGC TAGTCTGGGG GCTGTCTGGC CCCAGACCGC GGAGAGGACG
C 38041 GCTTGGGGGG TGATTCGGGC TAGTCTGGGG GCTGTCTGGC CCCAGACCGC GGAGAGGACG

                                3 22111  4 2 2  31   2
A 38101 CGCGCTCGCG CTCTCGCTCT TTCTGCTGCT GCTTGCGTAC GGCTTGTGAT CTCTCTGGAT
            212111 11 1223112 1 2  111 1 4   11111   1  1 1 1         1 1
B 38101 CGCGCTCGCG CTCTCGCTCT TTCTGCTGCT GCTTGCGTAC GGCTTGTGAT CTCTCTGGAT
C 38101 CGCGCTCGCG CTCTCGCTCT TTCTGCTGCT GCTTGCGTAC GGCTTGTGAT CTCTCTGGAT

A 38161 TCGTGCGGCT GTGTTTTTTC CCTCTTTTCT CGCTTGCAAA CTGCTTTCCT TGCTCCG
              11     22   2 1 1 1   11                      1   11   1
B 38161 TCGTGCGGCT GTGTTTTTTC CCTCTTTTCT CGCTTGCAAA CTGCTTTCCT TGCTCCG
C 38161 TCGTGCGGCT GTGTTTTTTC CCTCTTTTCT CGCTTGCAAA CTGCTTTCCT TGCTCCG
```

Fig. 1. Compilation of data on the first intron of human BCL-6 showing the relationships between mutations and regions of interest. The nucleotide numbering is from a human BAC clone (Homo sapiens 3 BAC RP11–211G3 Roswell Park Cancer Institute Human BAC Library) accession number AC072022. A region of human and mouse homology (37702–37880) is in plain lower case. Such regions are often the site of control elements ***(54)***. The region italicized in lower case is a putative negative control or silencer region as identified by Kikuchi et al. ***(55)***. The underlined nucleotides form the core region of deletions found by Nakamura et al. ***(53)***, either in the malignant cells of patients with diffuse large cell lymphoma or in a BCL-6 expressing cell line. The mutation data are taken from three sources. Sequence A derived from Capello et al. ***(58)*** shows a 26-bp block of nucleotides (37800–37826) with numbers of mutations per nucleotide presented above. Sequence B is from Lossos et al. ***(56,60)*** and again the number of mutations found at each position is presented above the sequence. Sequence C describes two boxed stretches of nucleotides (37800–37826 and 38117–38138) which are short "mutational hotspots" discovered by Artiga et al. ***(59)***. The two areas shaded in gray show the clear correspondence between the different data sets. There is an RGYW motif at position 37815. The breakpoint cluster defined by Akasaka et al. ***(36)*** is italicized and in upper case. It is apparent that this 521-bp sequence contains regulatory elements, flanked by mutational hotspots and is also the site of breakpoint clusters.

involved in transcriptional control *(62)*. More direct evidence for the existence of negative transcriptional control elements or silencers comes from experiments in which luciferase reporter constructs were driven by sections of the first intron of BCL-6 *(63)*. Although there is a control region within the first exon, there also appear to be control elements (in the mouse/human homology and deleted in lymphoma sections) within the first intron of BCL-6.

Furthermore, gel mobility shift assays have shown the presence of specific protein binding complexes *(61,64)*, again supporting the importance of the first intron as a focus for transcription factor binding. Thus, one possibility is that disruption of the core region by hypermutation leads to loss of the normal mechanisms that "turn off" BCL-6. To pursue this concept, sequencing from cases of lymphoma has been conducted by various groups.

1.5.3. Location of Mutations in Lymphoma and Effects on BCL-6 Expression

Great consistency has been seen in results obtained from sequencing the first intron of BCL-6 in lymphomas (**Fig. 1**). There are two mutational hotspots *(65–68)*, one of which contains an RGYW motif, which is a particular focus of targeting by the mutational mechanism *(69)* and, overall, approx 50% of DLCL may bear mutations *(70)*. Thus, there are indications that the mechanism of BCL-6 hypermutation and immunoglobulin gene hypermutation are the same, but some evidence that this is not the case is provided by an analysis of chronic lymphocytic leukemia, a disease that can be divided into two subgroups depending on the presence of immunoglobulin gene hypermutation. Some of the cases of chronic lymphocytic leukemia lacking immunoglobulin gene hypermutation did have BCL-6 changes *(71)*. Others, however, have not confirmed this *(72)*, although they have demonstrated a constant association between immunoglobulin gene and BCL-6 intron mutations. Lymphocyte predominant Hodgkin's disease has recently been recognized to have a germinal center origin, and sequencing of material derived from single cells has shown that all cases bear mutations *(73)*.

An unresolved question is: can mutations indeed lead to increased BCL-6 expression? Despite the fact that lymphomas, like other malignant diseases, are clonal the expression of BCL-6 is not uniform within tissue samples, and this is a surprising result in itself. For example, one series found that 10% of cases had fewer than 20% of BCL-6-positive cells on immunohistochemistry, and 25% of cases had greater than 80% positive cells whilst most cases had intermediate numbers of positive cells *(67)*. Using the proportion of positive cells as an index of protein expression, no correlation was found with the presence of mutations. However, such an analysis has the weakness that variations in BCL-6 expression during the cell cycle are not taken into account, and nor is an assessment of how amounts of BCL-6 within individual positive cells compares to that within normal germinal center B-cells.

More recently, it has been specifically demonstrated that there are two autoregulatory BCL-6 binding sites within the first exon of the gene. Occupancy of these sites by BCL-6 causes repression of BCL-6 transcription. Not only is this autoregulatory region removed in the majority of translocations *(77)*, but a subset of point mutations of this region found in diffuse large cell lymphoma also deregulate BCL-6 expression *(75)*.

1.5.4. Correlation With Clinical Outcome

The presence of mutations may be associated with bulkier disease at presentation as assessed by lactate dehydrogenase level *(70)*. No consensus exists on the effects of intronic mutations on survival. One series of cases suggests that mutation of the second hotspot (**Fig. 1**; 38117-38138) confers a better overall and disease free survival compared with those having a wild-type sequence *(67)*. However, others *(70)* found that although there was no effect on overall survival, patients with mutated BCL-6 introns did have an improved 5-yr disease-free survival.

Acquisition of mutations during the course of evolution of follicular lymphoma has been examined *(76)*. Although relapsed follicular lymphomas did not have new intronic mutations, most transformed cases did bear mutations not seen at presentation or relapse. This association may mean that dysregulated BCL-6 has a role in the transformation of follicular lymphoma or may be a reflection of an altered pattern of gene expression in which mutation is more likely.

2. Materials

2.1. DNA Extraction

The cellularity and size of tissue biopsies influence the quality and quantity of genomic DNA obtained. Factors affecting the integrity of the genomic DNA extracted include the transit time between the tissue biopsy and the time of delivery to the laboratory and whether biopsy has been exposed to a fixative. Furthermore, exposure of tissue to fixative often precludes Southern blot analysis because the genomic DNA obtained is often of small molecular weight, that is, fragmented. These difficulties have largely been overcome by the introduction of polymerase chain reaction (PCR)-based molecular studies. High molecular weight genomic DNA is not essential for PCR, which requires small amounts of DNA. Indeed genomic DNA obtained from paraffin-embedded tissue is analyzable by PCR (*see* **Note 1**). There are a number of commercially available kits with easy-to-follow protocols for the extraction of DNA.

In the absence of kits being available, genomic DNA can be obtained using phenol/chloroform. The biopsy initially is cut finely in a plastic Petri dish using a clean sterile blade. The tissue is then immersed in 5 to 10 mL of phosphate-buffered saline (PBS) and disrupted further with the blunt end of 5-mL syringe plunger. The cell suspension is collected and centrifuged to obtain cell pellet from which DNA can be extracted (*see* below).

2.2. Stock Solutions

1. 5 *M* NaCl.
2. 1 *M* Tris-HCl, pH. 8.0.
3. 1 *M* Tris-HCl, pH 7.4.
4. 5 *M* NaOH.
5. 0.5 *M* Ethylenediamine tetraacetic acid (EDTA), pH 8.0.
6. PBS.
7. 10% Nonidet P-40 (NP40.
8. Sodium dodecyl sulfate (SDS, lauryl sulfate): 20%.
9. 10X lysis buffer: 3 *M* NaCl, 0.1 *M* EDTA, 0.1 *M* Tris-HCl, pH 7.4.

2.3. Working Solutions

1. PBS + 0.1% NP40.
2. Lysis solution. Prepared fresh when required; 7 *M* Urea, 1X lysis buffer.
3. Chloroform:isoamyl alcohol (24:1:).
4. Ethanol 70%.
5. TE: 10 m*M* Tris-HCl, pH 7.4, 1 m*M* EDTA).

2.4. TE Equilibrated Phenol

DNA is soluble in acidic water-saturated phenol and so it is necessary to equilibrate it to a neutral pH.

1. Take 500 mL of water-saturated phenol. Prepare 500 mL of 0.5 *M* Tris, pH 8.5, add 150 mL of this to the phenol, and mix by inversion for 2–3 min. Leave to stand until the aqueous and organic phases have separated.
2. Remove and discard the upper aqueous layer. Add another 125 mL of 0.5 *M* Tris, mix, let stand, and remove the aqueous layer as before and then repeat.
3. To the remaining 100 mL of 0.5 *M* Tris, add 400 mL of water to give 500 mL of 0.1 *M* Tris. Add 150 mL of this to the phenol, and then mix, allow to stand, and remove as shown in **step 2**. Repeat two more times.
4. To the remaining 50 mL of 0.1 *M*, Tris add 449 mL of water and 1 mL of 0.5 mol/ EDTA to give 500 mL of TE. Add, mix, let stand, and remove this in three stages as before. The phenol will have reduced in volume during this procedure, but is now TE equilibrated and ready for use.

3. Methods

3.1. Technique of DNA Extraction

1. Add two to three drops of lysis solution. Disrupt the cellular pellet and homogenize using a nonwettable sterile stick (for example, a plastic disposable bacterial inoculating loop) or a clean siliconized glass rod. The solution will become viscous on adding lysis solution.
2. Add successive 0.5 mL volumes of the lysis solution, mixing each time, until the viscosity is such that the solution can be pipetted up and down without difficulty. The final volume, usually 2 to 3 mL, will depend on the size, nature and quality of sample.
3. Add one-tenth volume of 20% SDS. And vortex briefly and incubate at 37°C for a minimum of 15 min. If necessary, the sample can be left overnight.
4. Transfer the sample to a polypropylene tube. Add an equal volume of chloroform/ isoamyl alcohol and an equal volume of phenol. Vortex briefly and centrifuge at 700*g* for 15 min.
5. Transfer the upper aqueous phase to a new tube. Leave behind the white protein interface and the organic phase. This may be difficult if the solution is too viscous, in which case further dilution with lysis solution maybe necessary.
6. Repeat **steps 8** and **9** at least once more and continue until the interface is clear. Add an equal volume of chloroform:isoamyl alcohol and vortex briefly and centrifuge as before and again transfer the aqueous phase to a new tube.
7. Add 2.5 volumes of absolute ethanol. Mix the solution by inverting the tube several times. The DNA should precipitate as a "cotton wool" ball. Using a micropipet tip, transfer the DNA to a microcentrifuge tube containing 1mL of 70% ethanol.
8. Centrifuge in a microcentrifuge at 14,000 rpm for 5 min. Pour off the residual ethanol and remove all of this with a micropipet.
9. Add 50–500 µL of 1X TE depending on the size of the pellet. Leave to resuspend for at least one night. Mix gently by flicking the tube; never vortex. The DNA can be stored for long periods at 4°C or frozen at –20°C.

3.2. PCR

The simplicity of PCR has revolutionized molecular biology based studies since its description by Mullis and colleagues in the mid- to late eighties. PCR enables investigators to amplify DNA region of interest flanked by two single-stranded oligonucleotides, or primers, which usually are 20 bases in length (see **Note 2**).

PCR amplification is achieved by denaturing the DNA template at 96°C to separate the complementary strands. Target-specific primers are then allowed to anneal by cooling the PCR mix to optimum annealing temperature. A suboptimum temperature can lead to a nonspecific amplification. The temperature is then raised to 72°C, which is optimal temperature for *Taq* (*Thermus aquaticus*) polymerase, to extend the primers in 5' to 3' direction. The addition of Thermostable *Taq* polymerase to the PCR mix permits the automation of PCR by eliminating the need to add fresh DNA polymerase after each denaturation step. PCR can be performed in polypropylene tubes or 96-well microtiter plates, which are subjected to heating and cooling cycles using a thermocycler.

The precise PCR conditions vary according to the template sequence, primers, and thermocycler. Commercial companies provide PCR buffer and $MgCl_2$ with *Taq* polymerase. The optimum $MgCl_2$ concentration, usually between 1.5 and 3.0 m*M*, is determined by performing a series of titration experiments.

The DNA polymerase requires primers to initiate DNA synthesis. The extension of primers requires the presence of the four deoxynucleotides (dATP, dGTP, dCTP, and dTTP) and specific buffer conditions. The specificity of the PCR and its efficiency is affected by number of factors, including $MgCl_2$ concentration, PCR buffer, and primer sequences. Optimum annealing temperature, $MgCl_2$, concentration and incubations times are dependent on the sequence to be amplified and the primers (*see* **Note 3**). Templates with high GC content may require the addition of 10% dimethyl sulfoxide. Specificity can be improved by using "hot start" *Taq* polymerase, which becomes active on incubation at 96°C. Contamination is a major concern when performing PCR; however, this can be minimized by using aerosol-resistant tips, dedicated micropipets, and different areas of the laboratory for each stage of the process. Another potential source of contamination is at the stage of overlaying the PCR mixture with mineral oil, which can be eliminated by using thermocyclers with heated lids (*see* **Note 4**).

3.3. PCR Amplifciation of Intron 1 of BCL6

Primers A (5' CCGCTGCTCATGATCATTATTT 3') and B (5' TAGACA CGATACTTCATCTCAT 3', as in *[59]*) amplify a PCR fragment 791 bp in length containing intron 1 of the BCL6 using 1.5 m*M* $MgCl_2$.

The PCR conditions are as follows:

1. 96°C for 5 min.
2. 55–60°C for 30 s.
3. 72°C, for 1 min.
4. 96°C for 30 s.
5. Repeat **steps 2** to **4** for 30 to 40 times as necessary for specific application.

4. Notes

1. Template preparation: PCR may fail if the template is degraded. The latter can arise if DNA was extracted from paraffin-embedded tissue, particularly with some fixatives used in preparation of biopsies. Degraded template can be over-

come by re-extracting from the starting material. Alternatively, PCR may fail because an inhibitor is present; this can be overcome by either diluting the template or by subjecting it to re-extraction. Because PCR requires very small quantities of DNA, the above procedure can be adjusted to enable DNA extraction in 1.5-mL microcentrifuge tubes throughout once cellular pellet has been collected after disruption of the biopsy. The 1.5-mL microcentrifuge tubes are spun at 14,000 rpm for 1 min as and when required unless stated otherwise. Also, precautions must be taken to avoid contamination during extraction of DNA and PCR itself at all stages. Two separate working areas for DNA extraction and PCR are to be recommended. Analar- or molecular biology-grade reagents and double-distilled deionized water should be used throughout. DNA extracted from paraffin-embedded tissue often requires 40 cycles of amplification for adequate amounts of product to be obtained. PCR also may fail because the target sequence is too rich in GC (>60%), the addition of 10% dimethyl sulfoxide in final PCR volume can overcome this difficulty.

2. PCR primers: The design of the primers also is critical for successful PCR. A number of software programs are freely available on the Internet to assist with designing primers. When designing primers, certain rules need to be adhered to, such as avoiding repetitive sequences and avoiding three or more G or Cs at the 3' end. Although, one or two mismatches within the primer sequence can possibly be tolerated, absolute complementary pairing to the target sequence is essential at the extension end of the primer, that is, the 3' end. The primer should not be able to form secondary structures because of internal complimentary. Sequences at the 3' end, which allow the primer to pair with another primer, should be avoided because this gives rise to primer-dimer and will diminish the PCR yield. Primer-dimers can arise through suboptimum PCR conditions or failure to perform Hot start.
3. PCR optimization: Optimum conditions when starting to amplify a new target can be determined empirically. Optimum magnesium chloride concentration and annealing temperature are the key parameters to determining optimum conditions for a new PCR target. A magnesium chloride concentration that is too high can lead to nonspecific amplification as can an annealing temperature that is too low. In addtition, PCR may fail if the magnesium chloride concentration is too low or the annealing temperature is too high. The optimum magnesium chloride concentration can be determined by performing titration experiments. Once this has been determined, the series of PCR experiments are performed at various annealing temperatures, usually ranging from 58 to 62°C, to identify optimum annealing temperature. Nonspecific amplification may also be avoided by using Hot start *Taq* polymerase and/or touchdown PCR. Touchdown PCR starts with the annealing temperature greater than the T_m for the primers and is gradually reduced in subsequent cycles to less than T_m. This ensures specific amplification during the early cycles, which act as a template for the subsequent cycles.
4. Experimental controls: There are a number of reasons why PCR may fail, once the simple error of omitting to add one of the constituents of PCR has been ex-

cluded by repeating the amplification. Inclusion of a positive control will confirm that all the necessary reagents were added and working. Having negative controls will help to ensure the reagents are free of contamination. The latter can be avoided by using dedicated automatic pipets, aerosol resistant tips and geographically separated working areas for the various PCR steps.

Acknowledgment

SDW is supported by the Royal Society Rink Research Fellowship.

References

1. Ye, B. H., Rao, P. H., Chaganti, R. S., and Dalla-Favera R. (1993) Cloning of bcl-6, the locus involved in chromosome translocations affecting band 3q27 in B-cell lymphoma. *Cancer Res.* **53,** 2732–2735.
2. Chang, C. C., Ye, B. H., Chaganti, R. S., and Dalla-Favera R. (1996) BCL-6, a POZ/zinc-finger protein, is a sequence-specific transcriptional repressor. *Proc. Natl. Acad. Sci. USA* **93,** 6947–6952.
3. Niu, H., Ye, B. H., and Dalla-Favera R. (1998) Antigen receptor signaling induces MAP kinase-mediated phosphorylation and degradation of the BCL-6 transcription factor. *Genes Dev.* **12,** 1953–1961.
4. MacLennan, I., and Gray, D. (1986) Antigen-driven selection of virgin and memory B-cells. *Immunol. Rev.* **91,** 61–85.
5. Allman, D., Jain, A., Dent, A., Maile, R. R., Selvaggi, T., Kehry, M. R., and Staudt, L. M. (1996) BCL-6 expression during B-cell activation. *Blood* **87,** 5257–5268.
6. Cattoretti, G., Chang, C. C., Cechova, K., Zhang, J., Ye, B. H., Falini, B., et al. (1995) BCL-6 protein is expressed in germinal-center B-cells. *Blood* **86,** 45–53.
7. Onizuka, T., Moriyama, M., Yamochi, T., Kuroda, T., Kazama, A., Kanazawa, N., et al. (1995) BCL-6 gene product, a 92- to 98-kD nuclear phosphoprotein, is highly expressed in germinal center B-cells and their neoplastic counterparts. *Blood* **86,** 28–37.
8. Ye, B. H., Cattoretti, G., Shen, Q., Zhang, J., Hawe, N., de Waard, R., et al. (1997) The BCL-6 proto-oncogene controls germinal-center formation and Th2-type inflammation. *Nat. Genet.* **16,** 161–170.
9. Dent, A. L., Shaffer, A. L., Yu, X., Allman, D., Staudt, L. M. (1997) Control of inflammation, cytokine expression and germinal center formation by BCL-6. *Science* **276,** 589–592.
10. Fukuda, T., Yoshida, T., Okada, S., Hatano, M., Miki, T., Ishibashi, K., et al. (1997) Disruption of the Bcl6 gene results in an impaired germinal center formation. *J. Exp. Med.* **186,** 439–448.
11. Toney, L. M., Cattoretti, G., Graf, J. A., Merghoub, T., Pandolfi, P. P., Dalla-Favera, R., et al. (2000) BCL-6 regulates chemokine gene transcription in macrophages. *Nat. Immunol.* **1,** 214–220.
12. Reljic, R., Wagner, S. D., Peakman, L. J., and Fearon, D. T. (2000) BCL-6 suppresses STAT3 dependent B-cell terminal differentiation. *J. Exp. Med.* **192,** 1841–1848.

13. Shvarts, A., Brummelkamp, T. R., Scheeren, F., Koh, E., Daley, G. Q., Spits, H., et al. (2002) A senescence rescue screen identifies BCL6 as an inhibitor of anti-proliferative p19(ARF)-p53 signaling. *Genes Dev.* **16,** 681–686.
14. Dent, A. L., Hu-Li, J., Paul, W. E., Staudt, L. M. (1998) T helper type 2 inflammatory disease in the absence of interleukin 4 and transcription factor STAT6. *Proc. Natl. Acad. Sci. USA* **95,** 13823–13828.
15. Faris, M., Kokot, N., Stahl, N., and Nel, A. E. (1997) Involvement of Stat3 in interleukin-6-induced IgM production in a human B-cell line. *Immunology* **90,** 350–357.
16. Skinnider, B. F., Elia, A. J., Gascoyne, R. D., Patterson, B., Trumper, L., Kapp, U., et al. (2002) Signal transducer and activator of transcription 6 is frequently activated in Hodgkin and Reed-Sternberg cells of Hodgkin lymphoma. *Blood* **99,** 618–626.
17. Harris, M. B., Chang, C. C., Berton, M. T., Danial, N. N., Zhang, J., Kuehner, D., et al. (1999) Transcriptional repression of Stat6-dependent interleukin-4-induced genes by BCL-6: specific regulation of iepsilon transcription and immunoglobulin E switching.. *Mol. Cell Biol.* **19,** 7264–7275.
18. Shaffer, A. L., Yu, X., He, Y., Boldrick, J., Chan, E. P., and Staudt, L. M. (2000) BCL-6 represses genes that function in lymphocyte differentiation, inflammation, and cell cycle control. *Immunity* **13,** 199–212.
19. Fearon, D. T., Manders, P., and Wagner, S. D. (2001) Arrested differentiation, the self renewing memory lymphocyte and vaccination. *Science* **293,** 248–250.
20. Toyama, H., Okada, S., Hatano, M., Takahashi, Y., Takeda, N., Ichii, H., et al.. (2002) Memory B-cells without somatic hypermutation are generated from Bcl6-deficient B-cells. *Immunity* 17, 329–339.
21. Levy, D., and Darnell, J. (2002) Signalling: STATS: transcriptional control and biological impact. *Nat. Rev. Mol. Cell Biol.* **3,** 651–662.
22. Bajalica-Lagerkrantz, S., Piehl, F., Farnebo, F., Larsson, C., and Lagerkrantz, J. (1998) Expression of the BCL-6 gene in the pre- and postnatal mouse. *Biochem. Biophys. Res. Commun.* **247,** 357–360.
23. Yoshida, T., Fukuda, T., Okabe, S., Hatano, M., Miki, T., Hirosawa, N., Isono, K., and Tokuhisa, T. (1996) The BCL6 gene is predominantly expressed in keratinocytes at their terminal differentiation stage. *Biochem. Biophys. Res. Commun.* **228,** 216–220.
24. Ye, B. H., Lista, F., Lo Coco, F., Knowles, D. M., Offit, K., Chaganti, R. S., et al. (1993) Alterations of a zinc finger-encoding gene, BCL-6, in diffuse large-cell lymphoma. *Science* **262,** 747–750.
25. Lo Coco, F., Ye, B. H., Lista, F., Corradini, P., Offit, K., Knowles, D. M., et al. (1994) Rearrangements of the BCL6 gene in diffuse large cell non-Hodgkin's lymphoma. *Blood* **83,** 1757–1759.
26. Offit, K., Coco, F. L., Louie, D., Parsa, N., Leung, D., Portlock, C., et al.. (1994) Rearrangement of the bcl-6 gene as a prognostic marker in diffuse large-cell lymphoma. *N. Engl. J. Med.* **331,** 74–80.

27. Skinnider, B. F., Horsman, D. E., Dupuis, B., and Gascoyne, R. D. (1999) Bcl-6 and Bcl-2 protein expression in diffuse large B-cell lymphoma and follicular lymphoma: correlation with 3q27 and 18q21 chromosomal abnormalities. *Hum. Pathol.* **30,** 803–808.
28. Raible, M. D., Hsi, E. D., and Alkan, S. (1999) Bcl-6 protein expression by follicle center lymphomas. A marker for differentiating follicle center lymphomas from other low-grade lymphoproliferative disorders. *Am. J. Clin. Pathol.* **112,** 101–107.
29. Dogan, A., Bagdi, E., Munson, P., and Isaacson, P. G. (2000) CD10 and BCL-6 expression in paraffin sections of normal lymphoid tissue and B-cell lymphomas. *Am. J. Surg. Pathol.* **24,** 846–852.
30. Carbone, A., Gloghini, A., Gaidano, G., Dalla-Favera, R., and Falini B. (1997) BCL-6 protein expression in human peripheral T-cell neoplasms is restricted to CD30+ anaplastic large-cell lymphomas. *Blood* **90,** 2445–2450.
31. Alizadeh, A. A., Eisen, M. B., Davis, R. E., Ma, C., Lossos, I. S., Rosenwald, A., et al. (2000) Distinct types of diffuse large B-cell lymphoma identified by gene expression profiling. *Nature* **403,** 503–511.
32. Shipp, M., Ross, K., Tamayo, P., Weng, A., Kutok, J., Aguiar, R., et al. (2002) Diffuse large B-cell lymphoma outcome prediction by gene expression profiling and supervised machine learning. *Nat. Med.* **8,** 68–74.
33. Rosenwald, A., Wright, G., Chan, W. C., Connors, J. M., Campo, E., Fisher, R. I., et al., and Lymphoma/Leukemia Molecular Profiling Project. (2002) The use of molecular profiling to predict survival after chemotherapy for diffuse large-B-cell lymphoma. *N. Engl. J. Med.* **346,** 1937–1947.
34. Butler, M. P., Iida, S., Capello, D., Rossi, D., Rao, P. H., Nallasivam, P., et al. (2002) Alternative translocation breakpoint cluster region 5' to BCL-6 in B-cell non-Hodgkin's lymphoma. *Cancer Res.* **62,** 4089–4094.
35. Ye, B., Chaganti, S., Chang, C., Niu, H., Corradini, P., Chaganti, R, et al. (1995) Chromosomal translocations cause deregulated BCL6 expression by promoter substitution in B-cell lymphoma. *EMBO J.* **14,** 6209–6217.
36. Akasaka, H., Akasaka, T., Kurata, M., Ueda, C., Shimizu, A., Uchiyama, T., et al. (2000) Molecular anatomy of BCL6 translocations revealed by long-distance polymerase chain reaction-based assays. *Cancer Res.* **60,** 2335–2341.
37. Akasaka, T., Ueda, C., Kurata, M., Akasaka, H., Yamabe, H., Uchiyama, T., and Ohno, H. (2000) Nonimmunoglobulin (non-Ig)/BCL6 gene fusion in diffuse large B-cell lymphoma results in worse prognosis than Ig/BCL6. *Blood* **96,** 2907–2909.
38. Ueda, C., Akasaka, T., Kurata, M., Maesako, Y., Nishikori, M., Ichinohasama, R., et al. (2002) The gene for interleukin-21 receptor is the partner of BCL6 in t(3;16)(q27;p11), which is recurrently observed in diffuse large B-cell lymphoma. *Oncogene* **21,** 368–376.
39. Chen, W., Itoyama, T., and Chaganti, R. (2001) Splicing factor SRP20 is a novel partner of BCL6 in a t(3;6)(q27;p21) translocation in transformed follicular lymphoma. *Genes Chromosomes Cancer* **32,** 281–284.

40. Galiegue-Zouitina, S., Quief, S., Hildebrand, M. P., Denis, C., Detourmignies, L., Lai, J. L., et al. (1999) Nonrandom fusion of L-plastin (LCP1) and LAZ3 (BCL6) genes by t(3;13)(q27;q14) chromosome translocation in two cases of B-cell non-Hodgkin lymphoma. *Genes Chromosomes Cancer* **26,** 97–105.
41. Hosokawa, Y., Maeda, Y., Ichinohasama, R., Miura, I., Taniwaki, M., and Seto, M. (2000) The Ikaros gene, a central regulator of lymphoid differentiation, fuses to the BCL6 gene as a result of t(3;7)(q27;p12) translocation in a patient with diffuse large B-cell lymphoma. *Blood* **95,** 2719–2721.
42. Yoshida, S., Y. Kaneita, Y. Aoki, M. Seto, S. Mori, and M. Moriyama. (1999) Identification of heterologous translocation partner genes fused to the BCL6 gene in diffuse large B-cell lymphomas: 5'-RACE and LA - PCR analyses of biopsy samples. *Oncogene* **18,** 7994–7999.
43. Dallery, E., Galiegue-Zouitina, S., Collyn-d'Hooghe, M., Quief, S., Denis, C., Hildebrand, M. P., et al.(1995) TTF, a gene encoding a novel small G protein, fuses to the lymphoma-associated LAZ3 gene by t(3;4) chromosomal translocation. *Oncogene* **10,** 2171–2178.
44. Galiegue-Zouitina, S., Quief, S., Hildebrand, M.,. Denis, C., Lecocq, G., Collyn-d'Hooghe, M., et al. (1995) Fusion of the LAZ3/BCL6 and BOB1/OBF1 genes by t(3; 11) (q27; q23) chromosomal translocation. *C R Acad. Sci. III* **318,** 1125–1131.
45. Xu, W. S., Liang, R. H., and Srivastava, G. (2000) Identification and characterization of BCL6 translocation partner genes in primary gastric high-grade B-cell lymphoma: heat shock protein 89 alpha is a novel fusion partner gene of BCL6. *Genes Chromosomes Cancer* **27,** 69–75.
46. Kawasaki, C., Ohshim, K., Suzumiya, J., Kanda, M., Tsuchiya, T., Tamura, K., et al. (2001) Rearrangements of bcl-1, bcl-2, bcl-6, and c-myc in diffuse large B-cell lymphomas. *Leuk. Lymphoma* **42,** 1099–1106.
47. Huang, J., Sanger, W., Greiner, T., Staudt, L. Weisenburger, D., Pickering, D., et al. (2002) The t(14;18) defines a unique subset of diffuse large B-cell lymphoma with a germinal center B-cell gene expression profile. *Blood* **99,** 2285–2290.
48. Horsman, D. E., McNeil, B. K., Anderson, M., Shenkier, T., and Gascoyne, R. D. (1995) Frequent association of t(3;14) or variant with other lymphoma-specific translocations. *Br. J. Haematol.* **89,** 569–575.
49. Au, W. Y., Gascoyne, R. D., Viswanatha, D. S., Skinnider, B. F., Connors, J. M., Klasa, R. J., et al. (1999) Concurrent chromosomal alterations at 3q27, 8q24 and 18q21 in B-cell lymphomas. *Br. J. Haematol.* **105,** 437–440.
50. Berek, C., and Milstein, C. (1987) Mutation drift and repertoire shift in the maturation of the immune response. *Immunol. Rev.* **96,** 23–41.
51. Wagner, S., and Neuberger, M. (1996) Somatic hypermutation of immunoglobulin genes. *Annu. Rev. Immunol.* **14,** 441–457.
52. Revy, P., Muto, T., Levy, Y., Geissmann, F., Plebani, A., Sanal, O., et al. (2000) Activation-induced cytidine deaminase (AID) deficiency causes the autosomal recessive form of the Hyper-IgM syndrome (HIGM2). *Cell* **102,** 565–575.

53. Muramatsu, M., Kinoshita, K., Fagarasan, S., Yamada, S., Shinkai, Y., and Honjo T. (2000) Class switch recombination and hypermutation require activation-induced cytidine deaminase (AID), a potential RNA editing enzyme. *Cell* **102,** 553–563.
54. Harris, R. S., Sale, J. E., Petersen-Mahrt, S. K., and Neuberger, M. S. (2002) AID is essential for immunoglobulin V gene conversion in a cultured B-cell line. *Curr. Biol.* **12,** 435–438.
55. Nagaoka, H., Muramatsu, M., Yamamura, N., Kinoshita, K., and Honjo T. (2002) Activation-induced deaminase (AID)-directed hypermutation in the immunoglobulin Smu region: implication of AID involvement in a common step of class switch recombination and somatic hypermutation. *J. Exp. Med.* **195,** 529–534.
56. Okazaki, I. M., Kinoshita, K., Muramatsu, M., Yoshikawa, K., and Honjo T. (2002) The AID enzyme induces class switch recombination in fibroblasts. *Nature* **416,** 340–345.
57. Jacob, J., Kelsoe, G., Rajewsky, K., and Weiss U. (1991) Intraclonal generation of antibody mutants in germinal centers. *Nature* **354,** 389–392.
58. Pasqualucci, L., Migliazza, A., Fracchiolla, N., William, C., Neri, A., Baldini, L., et al. (1998) BCL-6 mutations in normal germinal center B-cells: evidence of somatic hypermutation acting outside Ig loci. *Proc. Natl. Acad. Sci. USA* **95,** 11816–11821.
59. Shen, H. M., Peters, A., Baron, B., Zhu, X., and Storb U. (1998) Mutation of BCL-6 gene in normal B-cells by the process of somatic hypermutation of Ig genes. *Science* **280,** 1750–1752.
60. Pasqualucci, L., Neumeister, P., Goossens, T., Nanjangud, G., Chaganti, R. S., Kuppers, R., et al. (2001) Hypermutation of multiple proto-oncogenes in B-cell diffuse large-cell lymphomas. *Nature* **412,** 341–346.
61. Nakamura, Y., K. Saito, and S. Furusawa. (1999) Analysis of internal deletions within the BCL6 gene in B-cell non-Hodgkin's lymphoma. *Br. J. Haematol.* **105,** 274–277.
62. Gottgens, B., Gilbert, J. G., Barton, L. M., Grafham, D., Rogers, J., Bentley, D. R., et al. (2001) Long-range comparison of human and mouse SCL loci: localized regions of sensitivity to restriction endonucleases correspond precisely with peaks of conserved noncoding sequences. *Genome Res.* **11,** 87–97.
63. Kikuchi, M., Miki, T., Kumagai, T., Fukuda, T., Kamiyama, R., Miyasaka, N., and Hirosawa, S. (2000) Identification of negative regulatory regions within the first exon and intron of the BCL-6 gene. *Oncogene* **19,** 4941–4945.
64. Lossos, I., Jacobs, Y., Cleary, M., and Levy, R. (2001) Correspondence re: Akasaka, H. et al. Molecular anatomy of BCL6 translocations revealed by long-distance polymerase chain reaction based assays. *Cancer Res.* **60,** 2335–2341, 2000. *Cancer Res.* **61,** 7363–7364.
65. Migliazza, A., Martinotti, S., Chen, W., Fusco, C., Ye, B. H., Knowles, D. M., et al. (1995) Frequent somatic hypermutation of the 5' noncoding region of the BCL6 gene in B-cell lymphoma. *Proc. Natl. Acad. Sci. USA* **92,** 12520–12524.
66. Capello, D., Vitolo, U., Pasqualucci, L., Quattrone, S., Migliaretti, G., Fassone, L., et al. (2000) Distribution and pattern of BCL-6 mutations throughout the spectrum of B-cell neoplasia. *Blood* **95,** 651–659.

67. Artiga, M. J., Saez, A. I., Romero, C., Sanchez-Beato, M., Mateo, M. S., Navas, C., et al. (2002) A short mutational hot spot in the first intron of BCL-6 is associated with increased BCL-6 expression and with longer overall survival in large B-cell lymphomas. *Am. J. Pathol.* **160,** 1371–1380.
68. Lossos, I. S., Levy R. (2000) Mutation analysis of the 5' noncoding regulatory region of the BCL-6 gene in non-Hodgkin lymphoma: evidence for recurrent mutations and intraclonal heterogeneity. *Blood* **95,** 1400–1405.
69. Rogozin, I., and N. Kolchanov. (1992) Somatic hypermutagenesis in immunoglobulin genes. I. I. Influence of neighbouring base sequences on mutagenesis. *Biochim. Biophys. Acta.* **1171,** 11–18.
70. Vitolo, U., Botto, B., Capello, D., Vivenza, D., Zagonel, V., Gloghini, A., et al. (2002) Point mutations of the BCL-6 gene: clinical and prognostic correlation in B-diffuse large cell lymphoma. *Leukemia* **16,** 268–275.
71. Sahota, S., Davis, Z., Hamblin, T., and Stevenson, F. (2000) Somatic mutation of bcl-6 genes can occur in the absence of V(H) mutations in chronic lymphocytic leukemia. *Blood* **95,** 3534–3540.
72. Pasqualucci, L., Neri, A., Baldini, L., Dalla-Favera, R., and Migliazza A. (2000) BCL-6 mutations are associated with immunoglobulin variable heavy chain mutations in B-cell chronic lymphocytic leukemia. *Cancer Res.* **60,** 5644–5648.
73. Seitz, V., Hummel, M., Anagnostopoulos, I., and Stein, H. (2001) Analysis of BCL-6 mutations in classic Hodgkin disease of the B- and T-cell type. *Blood* **97,** 2401–2405.
74. Wang, X., Li, Z., Naganuma, A., and Ye, B. (2002) Negative autoregulation of BCL-6 is bypassed by genetic alterations in diffuse large B-cell lymphomas. *Proc. Natl. Acad. Sci. USA* **99,** 15018–15023.
75. Pasqualucci, L., Migliazza, A., Basso, K., Houldsworth, J., Chaganti, R., and Dalla-Favera, R. (2003) Mutations of the BCL-6 proto-oncogene disrupt its negative autoregulation in diffuse large cell lymphoma. *Blood* **101,** 2914–2923.
76. Lossos, I., and Levy, R. (2000) Higher-grade transformation of follicle center lymphoma is associated withsomatic mutation of the 5' noncoding regulatory region of the BCL-6 gene. *Blood* **96,** 635–639.

14

Antibody Techniques Used in the Study of Anaplastic Lymphoma Kinase-Positive ALCL

Karen Pulford, Helen M. Roberton, and Margaret Jones

Summary

Antibodies enable relatively simple, rapid, and reproducible studies to be performed on protein expression in both normal and neoplastic cells. The availability of suitable reagents for routine diagnostic use has revolutionized the study of leukemia and lymphoma pathology. The use of antibodies specific for anaplastic lymphoma kinase (ALK) protein has permitted the identification of the tumor entity ALK-positive from the poorly defined morphological category of anaplastic large cell lymphoma. Antibody techniques have also provided major new insights into the biology of these tumors. This chapter describes the use of antibodies in both immunolabeling (immunocytochemical and immunofluorescence) procedures and in biochemical procedures in the study of ALK-positive ALCL.

Key Words: Lymphoma; ALCL; ALK; receptor tyrosine kinase; fusion proteins; immunohistochemistry; SDS-PAGE; Western blotting; immunoprecipitation.

1. Introduction

Antibodies are invaluable tools for use in relatively simple, rapid, and reproducible techniques to investigate protein expression in both normal and neoplastic cells. In addition to the subcellular localization of proteins, antibodies provide important information concerning changes in protein levels and distribution that occur within the cell during normal cellular differentiation or as part of an oncogenic process. This chapter describes techniques using antibodies that can be used for the study of ALK-positive ALCL.

1.1. ALK-Positive ALCL

Anaplastic large cell lymphoma (ALCL) accounts for approx 3% of adult non-Hodgkin's lymphomas but for 10 to 30% of pediatric lymphomas *(1)*. The t(2;5)(p23;q35) chromosomal abnormality is associated with ALCL. The genes involved are the *nucleophosmin* (*NPM*) gene at 5q35, which encodes

From: *Methods in Molecular Medicine, Vol. 115: Lymphoma: Methods and Protocols*
Edited by: T. Illidge and P. W. M. Johnson © Humana Press Inc., Totowa, NJ

the 38-kDa cell cycle-regulated NPM protein and the *anaplastic lymphoma kinase* (*ALK*) gene at 2p23, which encodes the 200-kDa ALK receptor tyrosine kinase. The resulting oncogenic 80-kDa NPM-ALK protein consists of 40% of the amino region of NPM and the entire intracytoplasmic region (including the tyrosine kinase domain) of ALK *(2,3)*. The restricted distribution of ALK in normal cells (present only in scattered cells in the brain) means that ALK protein expression in lymphoid cells constitutes a tumour-specific marker *(4)*.

The production of antibodies (monoclonal antibodies in particular) specific for ALK protein permitted the direct visualization of ALK protein in both fresh and routinely fixed tissue biopsies and revolutionized the study of ALCL *(4–6)*. Sixty to 85% of ALCLs were found to express ALK proteins and comprise the tumor entity ALK-positive ALCL or "Alkoma." The neoplastic cells, which are characterized by the expression of T-cell markers and/or cytotoxic granule proteins CD30 and EMA, are present in all morphological subtypes of ALCL *(6,7)*. Variable numbers of the "hallmark cell" containing an eccentric horseshoe-shaped nucleus with an eosinophilic region frequently observed at or near the Golgi region are found in all cases of this lymphoma *(7)*. ALK-positive ALCL has an improved prognosis compared to ALK-negative ALCL *(8,9)*. ALK-positive ALCL can easily be distinguished from the rare cases of B-cell CD30-negative lymphoma *(10)*, and from other CD30-positive tumors, such as primary cutaneous lymphoma, Hodgkin's disease and Hodgkin's disease-like ALCL *(1)*.

Antibody techniques have also provided major new insights into the biology of ALK-positive ALCL. Although as many as 80% of these tumors show the nuclear and cytoplasmic immunolabeling for ALK protein that is typical of NPM-ALK expression, variations in ALK distribution have been described in the remaining 20% of ALK-positive ALCL *(7)*. These observations, when combined with molecular, karyotyping, and biochemical studies, have confirmed the presence of oncogenic variant ALK proteins, other than NPM-ALK, in ALK-positive ALCL (**Table 1**).

1.2. Outline of the Immunolabeling Techniques Used in the Diagnosis of ALK-Positive ALCL

Immunolabeling techniques have superseded the use of molecular biological techniques in the diagnosis of ALK-positive ALCL. The simplest method of immunolabeling used for diagnostic purposes is the indirect labeling technique, in which the first step consists of incubating the tissue with a primary monoclonal or polyclonal antibody specific for the protein of interest, for example, CD30 or ALK. This antibody is then linked to a secondary antibody tagged with either an enzyme or a fluorochrome. The specific protein can then be visualized by developing the enzyme substrate followed by light

Table 1
Examples of ALK Fusion Proteins Expressed in ALK-Positive ALCL

Chromosomal abnormality	Fusion protein[a]	Distribution pattern[b]	Frequency (%)	MW (kDa)	Ref.
t(2;5)(p23;q35)	NPM-ALK	Nuclear/cytoplasm	70–80	80	*4*
t(1;2)(p25;p23)	TPM3-ALK	Cytoplasm	10–20	104	*11*
t(2;3)(p23;q35)	TFG-ALK_L	Cytoplasm	2.5	97	*12*
	TFG-ALK_S	Cytoplasm		85	*12*
	TFG-ALK_{XL}	Cytoplasm		113	*13*
inv(2)(p23;q35)	ATIC-ALK	Cytoplasm	2–5	96	*14,15*
t(2;17)(p23;q11-qter)	CLTC-ALK	Granules in the cytoplasm	2–5	250	*16,17*
t(2;11)(p23;q11–12)	MSN-ALK	Membrane	1–2	126	*18*

[a]All of the partner proteins contain motifs which permit dimerization of the fusion protein mimicking ligand binding. This results in the constitutive activation of the ALK kinase domain.

[b]The distribution of ALK is dependent upon the normal cellular distribution of the partner protein present in the fusion protein.

microscopy *(19)* or, in the case of a fluorochrome, by using a fluorescence microscope *(20)*. This basic labeling technique can be modified by the inclusion of additional steps in the staining procedure, such as those used in the streptavidin-biotin system or in the soluble enzyme immune complex APAAP technique *(21)*. These latter techniques rely on the formation of stable immune complexes, which contain larger numbers of substrate molecules thus increasing the sensitivity of the labeling procedure. Double labeling procedures using a combination of two different primary antibodies and secondary antibodies tagged with different enzyme substrates *(22)* or fluorochromes can also be used to study the simultaneous expression of more than one protein in the same tissue preparation *(20)*.

1.3. Outline of the Biochemical Techniques Used in the Study of ALK-Positive ALCL

Biochemical analyses using antibodies have provided valuable additional information on NPM-ALK and variant ALK proteins, their functional activity in vivo, and the identity of interacting proteins, such as PLC-g and PI-3 kinase *(23,24)*. The first step is the solubilization of the proteins from cells under study. Once the proteins have been extracted, they are available for analysis with antibodies using either Western blotting or immunoprecipitation techniques. In Western blotting studies, the proteins are separated on the basis of size by sodium dodecyl sulfate polyacrylamide gel electrophoresis (SDS-

PAGE). They are then transferred to a membrane, where they can be stained using antibodies in an indirect labeling technique, for example, antibodies to ALK will permit the molecular weight of any ALK proteins to be found and provide evidence of the identity of the ALK fusion protein (**Table 1**) (**25**). Immunoprecipitation techniques permit the purification and concentration of specific proteins of interest through the use of antibodies directed against specific proteins being linked onto solid immunoadsorbent beads, for example, Protein G:Gammabind Plus Sepharose. Relevant proteins in solution bind to the specific antibody on the beads and can then be removed from solution by brief centrifugation. The resulting antigen:antibody complexes present in the immunoadsorbent pellet are then separated by SDS-PAGE and identified by Western blotting *(26)*. In an in vitro kinase assay, radiolabeled immunoprecipitated proteins are detected and identified by autoradiography after SDS-PAGE *(25)*.

2. Materials

2.1. Preparation of Tissue Sections and Slides

1. Cryostat (e.g., Leica CM 3050S).
2. Cytocentrifuge (e.g., Cytospin 2, Shandon International, Pittsburgh, PA.).
3. Microtome (e.g., Leica RM2135).
4. Microwave.
5. SnowCoat X-tra slides for use with paraffin embedded sections (SurgiPath Europe Ltd., St. Neots, UK).
7. Citroclear (HD Supplies, Aylesbury, UK).
8. PAP pen: S-2002 (DakoCytomation, Glostrup, Denmark).
9. Phosphate-buffered saline (PBS) tablets (OXOID Ltd., Basingstoke, UK).
10. TBS: 0.5 *M* Tris HCl, pH 7.6, diluted 1:10 with 1.5 *M* NaCl. Store at room temperature.
11. Tris/ethylene diamine tetraacetic acid (EDTA), pH 9.0, buffer: 0.006 *M* Tris, 0.016 *M* Na_2EDTA. Store at room temperature.
12. Acetone.
13. Ethanol.
14. H_2O_2 block: 0.3% H_2O_2 in methanol.
15. SU-DHL-1 cells (DSMZ-German Collection of Micro-organisms and Cell Cultures, Braunchsweig, Germany; *see* **Note 1**).
16. Tissue culture medium: RPMI 1640 containing 10% fetal calf serum, glutamine and penicillin and streptomycin (Gibco Life Technologies (Paisley, Scotland, UK).
17. SaranWrap (Fahrenheit Lab. Supplies, Milton Keynes, UK).

2.2. Single Immunolabeling Procedures

1. Staining tray and trough (Raymond Lamb, London, UK).
2. Monoclonal antibodies and rabbit polyclonal primary antibodies (*see* **Table 2**).

Table 2
Primary Antibodies for Use in Immunolabeling and Biochemical Studies of ALK-Positive ALCL

Target protein	Antibody name	Isotype and species	Application[a]	Source/Reference
ALK	ALK1	Mouse IgG3	IHC (CS, PS), IF, WB, IP	DakoCytomation
ALK	ALKc	Mouse IgG1	IHC (CS, PS), IF, WB, IP	Pharmingen
EMA, epithelial membrane antigen	E29	Mouse IgG2a	IHC (CS, PS), IF,WB,IP	DakoCytomation
CD2	CD2	Mouse IgG1	IHC (CS, PS), IF	DakoCytomation
CD4	MT310	Mouse IgG1	IHC (CS, PS),	DakoCytomation
CD8	C8/144B	Mouse IgG1	IHC (CS, PS),	DakoCytomation
CD15	C3D-1	Mouse IgGM	IHC (CS, PS), IF, WB, IP	DakoCytomation
CD20	L26	Mouse IgG2a	IHC (CS, PS), IF, WB?	DakoCytomation
CD30	Ber-H2	Mouse IgG1	IHC (CS, PS), IF, IP, WB	DakoCytomation
Leucocyte common antigen	CD45	Mouse IgG1	IHC (CS, PS), IF, IP, WB	DakoCytomation
CD68	KP1 or PGM1	Mouse IgG1	IHC (CS, PS), IF, IP, WB	DakoCytomation
Cytokeratin	LP34	Mouse IgG1	IHC (CS, PS), IF	DakoCytomation
NPM (amino-terminus)	NA24	Mouse IgM	IHC (PS), WB	***(26)***
Phosphotyrosine	4G10	Mouse IgG2b	IHC (CS, PS), IF, WB, IP	Upstate Biotechnology Inc, New York
TIA	Anti-TIA	Mouse IgG1	IHC (CS, PS), IF	Coulter,
Granzyme B	CLB-GB7	Mouse IgG2a	IHC (CS, PS), IF	Research Diagnostics,
Perforin	NCL-Perforin	Mouse IgG1	IHC (CS, PS), IF	Novacastra, Newcastle, UK
CD3	CD3	Rabbit	IHC (CS, PS), IF	DakoCytomation

[a]Suitable for IHC, immunohistochemistry; CS, cryostat sections; PS, routinely fixed sections; IF,immunofluorescence studies; WB, Western blotting; IP, immunoprecipitation studies.

3. Horseradish peroxidase conjugated (HRP) goat anti-mouse Ig: P0447 (DakoCytomation). Store at 4°C.
4. HRP conjugated goat anti-rabbit Ig: P0448 (DakoCytomation). Store at 4°C.
5. Rabbit anti-mouse Ig: Z259 (DakoCytomation). Store at 4°C.
6. Mouse anti-rabbit Ig: M0737 (DakoCytomation). Store at 4°C.
7. Dako StreptABComplex/HRP Duet (Mouse/Rabbit) kit: K492 (DakoCytomation). Store at 4°C.
8. Diaminobenzidine substrate kit: SigmaFast 3,3'-diaminobenzidine tablet set: D-4293 (Sigma-Aldrich Company Ltd., Poole, U.K). Store at –20°C.
9. Hematoxylin counterstain: Gill No 3 (Sigma-Aldrich Company Ltd.).
10. Aquamount (BDH Merck Ltd., Poole, UK).
11. Alkaline phosphatase: anti-alkaline phosphatase complexes, D-0651 (Dako Cytomation).
12. Fast Red substrate buffer: 0.1 *M* Tris-HCl, pH 8.2. Store at 4°C.
13. Fast Red TR salt: F-2768 (Sigma Aldrich Company Ltd.). Store at –20°C.
14. Napthol-phosphate AS-MX salt: N-5000 (Sigma Aldrich Company Ltd.). Store at –20°C.
15. 1 *M* Levamisole: L-9756 (Sigma Aldrich Company Ltd.). Can be made up in advance and stored at 4°C.

2.3. Double Immunolabeling Studies

1. Reagents 1–15 from **Subheading 2.2.**
2. Fluorescein-isothiocyanate (FITC)-conjugated goat anti-rabbit Ig: 4050-02.
3. Texas Red™-conjugated goat anti-rabbit Ig: 4050-07.
4. FITC-conjugated goat anti-mouse IgG1: 1070-02.
5. Texas Red™-conjugated goat anti-rabbit Ig: 1070-07.
6. FITC-conjugated goat anti-mouse IgG2a: 1080-02.
7. Texas Red™-conjugated goat anti-mouse IgG2a: 1080-07.
8. FITC-conjugated goat anti-mouse IgG2b:1090-02.
9. Texas Red™-conjugated goat anti-mouse IgG2b: 1090-07.
10. FITC-conjugated goat antimouse IgG3: 1100-02.
11. Texas Red™-conjugated goat anti-mouse IgG3: 1100-07.
12. FITC-conjugated goat anti-mouse IgM: 1020-02.
13. Texas Red™-conjugated goat anti-mouse IgM: 1020-07. (All fluorochrome conjugates are obtained from Cambridge Biosciences, Cambridge, UK). Store in the dark at 4°C.
14. Fast Blue substrate for APAAP technique: SK5300 (Vector Laboratories, Burlingame, CA). Store at –20°C.
15. 4'6-Diamine-2'-phenylindole dihydrochloride (DAPI; Boehringer Mannheim, Lewes, Sussex, UK). Store in 250-mL aliquots at 4°C.
16. Fluorescence Mounting Medium: S-3025 (DakoCytomation).

2.4. Western Blotting

1. Gel apparatus (e.g., ATTA system, Genetic Research Instrumentation, London, UK).
2. Western blotter (e.g., Semi-Phor by Hoeffer, Amersham Pharmacia Biotech, Amersham, Bucks, UK).

Table 3
Composition of SDS-PAGE Gels

Reagent	10% Resolving gel	7.5% Resolving gel	6% Resolving gel	Stacking gel
Acrylamide: bisacrylamide 29:1	5 mL	3.75 mL	3.25 mL	1.5 mL
0.75 *M* Tris, pH 8.8	7.5 mL	7.5 mL	7.5 mL	–
10% SDS	150 µL	150 µL	150 µL	80 µL
1% Ammonium persulphate (stored at 4°C)	1.5 mL	1.5 mL	1.5 mL	0.8 mL
Double distilled water	0.8 mL	2.1 mL	2.6 mL	5.0 µL
TEMED	50 µL	50 µL	50 µL	50 µL
1 *M* Tris, pH 6.8	–	–	–	1.0 mL

With exception of acrylamide: bisacrylamide from Bio-Rad Laboratories all of the other reagents are from Sigma-Aldrich. Store all reagents except SDS at 4°C.

3. Laemmli sample buffer: 0.2 *M* Tris, pH 6.8; 2% SDS; 8 *M* urea, and a small amount bromophenol blue. This solution should be stored at room temperature. The reducing agent dithiothreitol should be added at 6 mg/mL immediately before use.
4. Metabolic inhibitors: Complete Mini-EDTA free Protease Inhibitor Cocktail (Roche Diagnostics Ltd., Lewes, UK). Make up as directed and store in aliquots at –20°C.
5. Lysis buffer A (extraction of cytoplasmic proteins): 0.5% Nonidet P-40 (NP-40), 20 m*M* sodium phosphate, pH 7.5; 50 m*M* NaF, 5 m*M* tetra sodium pyrophosphate, and 10 m*M* b-glycerophosphate. Store at 4°C. Add the metabolic inhibitor cocktail immediately prior to use (*see* **Note 2**).
6. Lysis buffer B (extraction of nuclear proteins): Lysis buffer A containing 425 m*M* NaCl.
7. SDS-PAGE running buffer (10X): 2.5 *M* Tris, 1.92 *M* glycine.
8. Composition of SDS-PAGE gels is given in **Table 3**. The quantities given are for use with the ATTA gel system.
9. CAPS buffer (10X): 100 m*M* CAPS (3-cyclohexylamino-1-propanesulfonic acid) pH 11.0. Store at room temperature.
10. CAPS transfer buffer: 25 mL methanol, 25 mL CAPS 10X buffer, 200 mL distilled water.
11. Polyvinylidene difluoride (PVDF) membrane: (Immobilon P, Millipore Corp. Bedford, MA).
12. Blotting paper: Whatman 3MM (LabSales Co., Cambridge, UK).
13. ECL Chemiluminescent peroxidase substrate kit: RPN 2106 (Amersham Pharmacia Biotech). Store at 4°C.

14. PBST: PBS containing 0.05% Tween-20.
15. Stripping buffer: 60 m*M* Tris, pH 6.8; 2% SDS, 100 m*M* β-mercaptoethanol. Make up using a fume cupboard and use when required.
16. Prestained molecular weight markers of 14- to 220-kDa molecular weight range: RPN756 (Amersham Pharmacia Biotech). Store at –20°C.
17. Bradford's reagent (Bio-Rad Laboratories Ltd).
18. Glogos 2 autoradiographic markers (Stratagene Europe, Amsterdam, Netherlands).

2.5. Immunoprecipitation Studies

1. Gel drier (e.g., SpeediGel, Savant, Holbrook, NY).
2. Immunoprecipitation buffer: 50 m*M* Tris, pH 7.4; 150 m*M* NaCl; 1.0% NP-40; and 1 mg/mL bovine serum albumin (BSA; fraction V). Store at 4°C. Add the metabolic inhibitor cocktail, 1 m*M* $Na_2(VO)_4$ and 1 m*M* NaF immediately prior to use (*see* **Note 2**).
3. Protein G:Gammabind Plus Sepharose (Amersham Pharmacia Biotech, Amersham, Bucks, UK). Store at 4°C.
4. Kinase assay buffer: 25 m*M* HEPES, pH 7.5, and 0.1 % NP-40. Store at 4°C.
5. Redivue [γ-^{32}P]ATP – 3000 Ci.mmol (Amersham Pharmacia Biotech). ^{32}P is a strong beta emitter, and all of the relevant safety procedures for working with this isotope should be followed. Fresh isotope should be ordered after 1 mo (*see* **Note 3**).
6. Kinase substrate buffer: 25 m*M* HEPES, pH 7.5; 0.1 % NP-40; 10 m*M* sodium fluoride; 10 m*M* $MgCL_2$; and 1 m*M* $Na_2(VO)_4$ and 5 mCi [γ-^{32}P]ATP per sample. Make up immediately before use.
7. SDS-PAGE gel fixative: 7% glacial acetic acid, 10% methanol in water. Store at room temperature.

3. Methods

3.1. Preparation of Tissue Sections and Cells for Immunolabeling Techniques

3.1.1. Cryostat Tissue Sections

1. Snap freeze tissue by immersing small pieces of the biopsy (no more than 1 cm^3) in liquid nitrogen and store at –70°C.
2. Cut cryostat sections of 8 µm thickness.
3. Air dry the sections overnight and fix in acetone for 10 min at room temperature (*see* **Note 4**).
4. Allow the acetone to evaporate and circle around sections with a PAP pen (*see* **Note 5**).
5. Place pairs of slides back to back, wrap in foil and store at –20°C until required.

3.1.2. Paraffin-Embedded Tissue Sections

Most tissue samples used for immunolabeling studies are subjected to a routine histological fixative, for example, buffered formol saline, before being embedded in paraffin.

1. Store paraffin-embedded tissue blocks face down in ice at 4°C overnight before cutting the sections (*see* **Note 6**).
2. Place blocks on the microtome and cut sections of 4 m*M* thickness onto Snowcoat X-tra slides (*see* **Note 7**).
3. Allow slides to air-dry and incubate at 37°C overnight (*see* **Note 7**).
4. Store cut sections in a container at 4°C before use (*see* **Note 8**).
5. Dewax and hydrate the tissue sections before use by placing slides in a slide rack and leave in each of the following solutions for 5 min.
   a. Citroclear (*see* **Note 9**).
   b. Citroclear.
   c. 100% ethanol.
   d. 100% ethanol.
   e. 50:50 ethanol:water.
   f. Tap water.
   g. PBS.

3.1.3. Cytocentrifuge Preparations of SU-DHL-1 Cells (Positive Control; see ***Note 1****)*

1. Resuspend suspension of cultured SU-DHL-1 cells at 0.5–1 million cells per milliliter in tissue culture medium and use to prepare cytocentrifuge preparations.
2. Circle cell spots with the PAP pen.
3. Air-dry for at least 1 h at room temperature or overnight.
4. Fix and store as described for cryostat tissue sections in Subheading **3.1.1.**

3.1.4. Microwave Antigen Retrieval Technique

Only a minority of antibodies recognize their epitopes after the use of routine fixatives such as buffered formol saline. Early methods to unmask antigenic epitopes involved the use of enzymes such as trypsin, but these methods were dependent upon the purity of the enzyme preparation. Recent techniques, using heating of the tissue sections without enzyme treatment, permit the retrieval of many more antigenic epitopes. The microwave pretreatment described below can be used for all of the antibodies described in this chapter.

1. Place slides in Tris/EDTA, pH 9.0, in a glass rack in a microwave proof container. Make sure that the slides are fully immersed. Cover with Saran wrap.
2. Microwave at 700 watts equivalent for 10 min. Do this in two lots of 5-min cycles, checking each time that the slides are covered by buffer.
3. Remove slides from the Tris:EDTA and place directly into PBS or TBS.
4. Dry around each section one slide at a time and encircle the tissue with the PAP pen. Replace in PBS. The slides are now ready for staining.

3.2. Single Immunolabeling Procedures for Tissue Sections

The incubation steps in the immunolabeling procedures are all performed at room temperature in a humidified staining tray (*see* **Note 10**).

3.2.1. Two-Stage Immunoperoxidase Labeling Technique

1. Remove cryostat sections and cytocentrifuge preparations from the freezer and allow to reach room temperature before unwrapping from the foil (*see* **Note 11**). These slides are now ready for use.
2. Incubate dewaxed and hydrated routinely fixed tissue sections in hydrogen peroxide block for 30 minutes to block endogenous peroxidase present in cells such as granulocytes.
3. Place these slides in a staining trough containing PBS and leave for 5 min. The routinely fixed slides are now ready for staining.
4. Remove these slides one at a time, wipe around the sections/cells, and incubate with 100–200 µL of primary antibody for 30 min in a humidified staining tray (*see* **Notes 12**). In the case of cryostat sections or cytocentrifuge preparations then antibody is added directly to the dry slide. One slide should be used as a negative control where an istotope matched irrelevant antibody is used.
5. Wash for 5 min in fresh PBS.
6. Remove slides and incubate with 100 µL of HRP-conjugated goat-anti-mouse Ig (diluted 1:50 for mouse primary antibodies) or HRP-conjugated swine anti-rabbit Ig (diluted 1:100 for rabbit primary antibodies) for 30 min (*see* **Note 13**).
7. Wash in fresh PBS for 5 min.
8. Add 100 µL of DAB substrate to each section and leave for 8 min. Gloves must be worn (*see* **Note 14**).
9. Wash slides in tap water.
10. Counterstain the nuclei in hematoxylin for 5–15 s (check intensity of nuclear labeling using a microscope).
11. Wash the slides in tap water until the hematoxylin has turned blue.
12. Mount in Aquamount (*see* **Note 15**).
13. A brown precipitate shows the distribution of the protein of interest.

Examples of the immunocytochemical labeling of ALK-positive ALCL using the immunoperoxidase technique are illustrated in **Fig. 1A,B.**

3.2.2. Streptavidin-Biotin-Peroxidase Three-Stage Labeling Technique (see **Note 16**)

This method, which relies on the high affinity of biotin for streptavidin, should be used in situations in which weak staining results are obtained from the indirect immunoperoxidase method. The incorporation of a biotinylated secondary antibody and streptavidin-biotin HRP complexes results in a greater number of HRP enzyme molecules being available per antigenic epitope thus increasing the intensity of the labeling procedure.

The StreptABComplex/HRP Duet (Mouse/Rabbit) kit suggested for use here contains only one set of reagents that can be used to recognize both mouse and rabbit primary antibodies. The detailed instructions supplied with the kit should be carefully followed. Once the substrate reaction has been completed the slides should be washed, counterstained and mounted in Aquamount as described in **Subheading 3.2.1.**

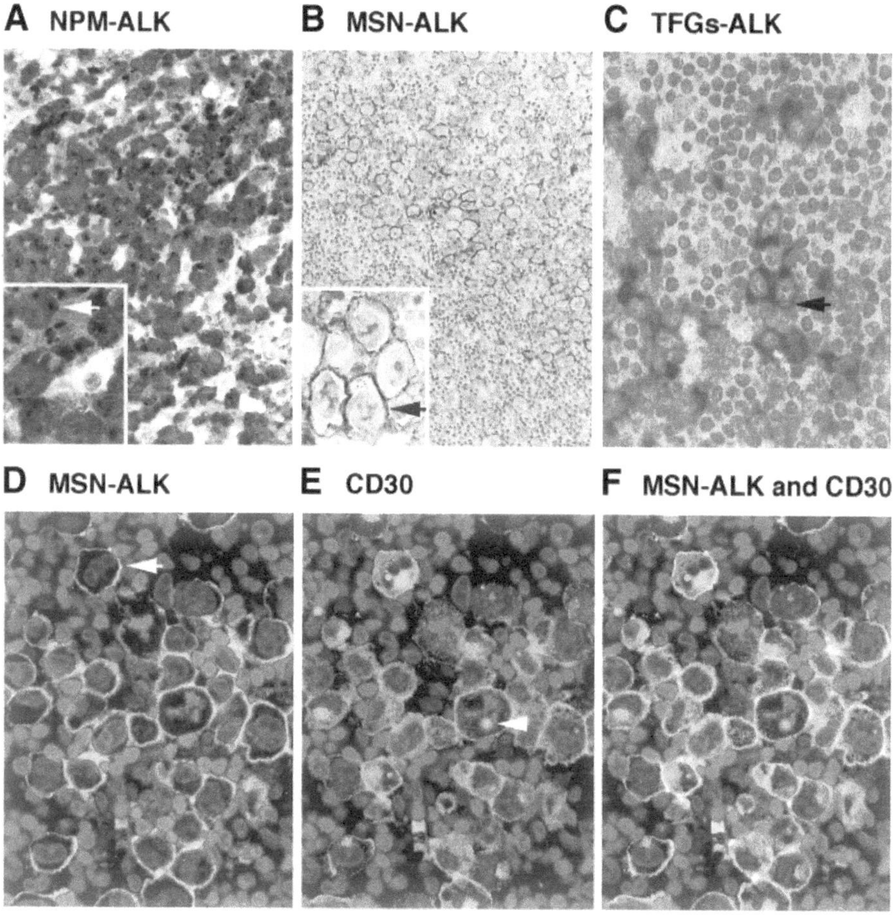

Fig. 1. Immunolabeling studies on ALK-positive ALCL. (**A**) and (**B**) show immunoperoxidase labeling (with the brown DAB substrate) obtained with anti-ALK on two cases of ALK-positive ALCL. The typical nuclear and cytoplasmic distribution of NPM-ALK is shown in (**A**). The inset allows the nuclear and nucleolar distribution of NPM-ALK to be seen in more detail (arrow). In (**B**), the MSN-ALK protein is detected only at the cell membrane (arrow). In (**C**), APAAP labeling (with the Fast Red: Napthol AS MX red substrate) of a third case of ALK-positive ALCL shows the TFGs-ALK fusion protein only in the cytoplasm (arrow). Note the presence of hematoxylin stained nuclei in the tumor cells in (**B**) and (**C**). The results of double immunofluorescence labeling of a case of ALK-positive ALCL using antibodies specific for ALK (isotype IgG3) and CD30 (isotype IgG1) are shown in (**D**) to (**F**). The distribution of MSN-ALK (red) at the cell membrane (arrow) can be seen in (**D**) whereas (**E**) shows CD30 (green) present at the cell membrane and also in the Golgi apparatus (arrowhead). In (**F**) superimposition of these two pictures confirms the present of CD30 and ALK protein in the tumor cells. The cell nuclei are blue as a result of the DAPI staining step. *See* **Color Plate 10**, following page 270.

3.2.3. Alkaline Phosphatase:Antialkaline Phosphatase (APAAP) Labeling Technique

The antigen–antibody complexes in this method are detected using a red substrate. (It should be noted at this point that there is also a commercially available StreptABComplex/AP Duet [Mouse/Rabbit] kit, which uses alkaline phosphatase rather than HRP as a substrate). The APAAP technique is particularly suitable for staining slides of bone marrow or tissue samples containing cells with high levels of endogenous peroxidase, and the blocking step for endogenous peroxidase can be omitted ***(21)***.

For mouse monoclonal primary antibodies, use the following procedure.

1. Incubate sections in 100–200 µL of primary antibody for 30 min using a humidified staining tray at room temperature. Include a negative control.
2. Wash for 5 min in TBS (*see* **Note 17**).
3. Incubate for 30 min in rabbit anti-mouse Ig (note this antibody is not conjugated to an enzyme).
4. Wash for 5 min in TBS.
5. Incubate for 30 min with the alkaline phosphatase: anti-alkaline complexes for 30 min.
6. Wash in TBS.
7. **Steps 4–6** can be repeated using 10-min incubation intervals if additional sensitivity is required.
8. Prepare the Fast Red substrate as follows: Weigh 2 mg of Napthol AS-MX phosphate and 10 mg of Fast Red TR salt into a glass universal. Dissolve in 10 mL of Tris Fast Red Substrate buffer, pH 8.2. Add 30 µL of levamisole (*see* **Note 18**).
9. Filter substrate directly onto slides and incubate for 15–20 min. This substrate should be made immediately before use.
10. Counterstain and mount slides as previously described in **Subheading 3.2.1.**

For rabbit polyclonal primary antibodies then the following additional steps must be performed.

11. Incubate sections or cytocentrifuge preparations in primary antibody for 30 min (*see* **step 2**).
12. Wash for 5 min in TBS.
13. Incubate with mouse anti-rabbit Ig monoclonal antibody (MR12) for 30 min at room temperature.
14. Follow **steps 2–10** as described above.

Examples of APAAP labeling of a case of ALK-positive ALCL are illustrated in **Fig. 1C**.

3.3. Double Immunolabeling Procedures

3.3.1. Enzymatic Techniques

This technique can be used to study the expression of two proteins present in different cell populations on the same section or when the relevant proteins are present in different subcellular compartments, for example, the nucleus and the cytoplasm *(22)*.

1. It is recommended that the antigen present in the smallest amount should be visualized first using an immunoperoxidase labeling technique (*see* **Note 19**).
2. The counterstain step should be omitted.
3. Perform the APAAP labeling technique as described in **Subheading 3.2.3.**
4. Wash, counterstain and mount in Aquamount as described in **Subheading 3.2.1.**

3.3.2. Immunofluorescence Technique

Although the staining technique described here can be used for cryostat and paraffin-embedded fixed sections, cellular morphology is better preserved in paraffin-embedded sections. Routinely fixed tissues also exhibit less autofluorescence, the presence of which can make interpretation of the results difficult. The availability of species-specific and isotype-specific secondary antibodies conjugated to fluorochromes means that immunofluorescence is a relatively simple, quick, and effective technique to label pairs of proteins in contrasting colors in the same cell *(20)*.

1. There is no need to block endogenous peroxidase.
2. Incubate the slides with mixtures of two primary antibodies: these can be from different species (in the case of a mouse and rabbit combination) or two mouse monoclonal antibodies of different subtypes (*see* **Note 12**). One slide should be used as a negative control.
3. Incubate for 30 min.
4. Wash in PBS for 5 min.
5. Incubate the washed slides for 30 min with a mixture of relevant fluorochrome conjugated antibodies at correct dilutions in the dark. An example of suitable pairs are FITC-goat anti-rabbit Ig and Texas Red™ goat anti-mouse IgG1 diluted 1:25.
6. Wash in PBS.
7. Mount in Fluorescence Mounting Medium containing 1 µL of DAPI added to each mL of mounting medium (*see* **Note 20**).
8. Place slides in a slide tray wrapped in foil and view with a fluorescence microscope (*see* **Note 21**).
9. The slides can be stored in slide trays wrapped in foil in the dark at 4°C for several weeks.

Examples of immunofluorescent labeling of ALK-positive ALCL techniques are illustrated in lymphoma are illustrated in **Fig. 1D–F**.

3.4. Western Blotting Studies

The biochemical techniques described here can be applied to minimal amounts of tissue and provide information on protein expression that would not be available from molecular biological analysis. The use of such small amounts of tissue means that valuable biopsy material is used sparingly *(25)*.

3.4.1. Preparation of Cryostat Sections and Cytocentrifuge Preparations

1. Prepare as described in **Subheadings 3.1.1.** and **3.1.3.**
2. Fix slides immediately in acetone for 10 min at room temperature (*see* **Note 22**).
3. Air-dry for 10 min.
4. Circle tissue sections/cells with the PAP pen.
5. Wrap slides in foil and store at –70°C.

3.4.2. Simultaneous Preparation of Nuclear and Cytoplasmic Antigens

1. Add 50-μL aliquots of Laemmli sample buffer to each tissue section or cytocentrifuge preparation on its removal from storage at –70°C (*see* **Note 23**).
2. Leave for 5 min.
3. Remove the sample buffer, taking care to "scrape off" the tissue fragments and cells into clean Eppendorf tubes.
4. Dilute the pre-stained molecular weight markers 1:1 with Laemmli sample buffer.
5. Heat the samples for 4 min at 95°C.
6. Microfuge for 1 min at 20,000*g*.
7. The supernatant is now ready for study using SDS-PAGE and Western blotting.

3.4.3. Sequential Solubilization of Nuclear and Cytoplasmic Extracts

1. Add 50- to 100-μL aliquots of lysis buffer A to each tissue section or cytocentrifuge preparation (*see* **Notes 2**, **24**, and **25**).
2. Incubate slides on ice for 10 min.
3. Move cells, tissue sections, and lysis buffer into prechilled clean tubes.
4. Vortex each sample at high speed for 1 min.
5. Microfuge samples at 6000*g* for 3 min to pellet the cell nuclei.
6. Place the supernatant containing the solubilized cytoplasmic proteins into prechilled clean tubes.
7. Add 50 μL of lysis buffer B to each nuclear pellet.
8. Incubate on ice for 15 min, vortexing for 15 s at 15-min intervals.
9. Spin all samples at 20,000*g* for 10 min.
10. Remove the supernatant containing the solubilized nuclear proteins into prechilled clean tubes.
11. Check protein concentrations of nuclear and cytoplasmic proteins using Bradford's reagent following the manufacturer's instructions. Protein concentrations can range from 0.1 to 1 μg/μL.

12. The samples should be aliquoted and stored at –70°C (*see* **Note 26**).
13. If the samples are to be studied immediately than add Laemmli sample buffer at a ratio of 1:1 and treat the samples as described in **steps 4–7** of **Subheading 3.4.2.**

3.4.4. Western Blotting Technique

During this procedure, solubilized proteins extracted from the tissue sections are transferred from SDS-PAGE gels on to an Immobilon membrane. This membrane can then be stained with a variety of antibodies, for example, anti-ALK, anti-phosphotyrosine and anti-NPM (amino-region) using an indirect HRP labeling technique *(25)*.

1. Make up 7.5% SDS-PAGE gel using values given in **Table 2** (*see* **Note 27**).
2. Add 10–20 µL of protein in sample buffer to each well of the SDS-PAGE gel.
3. Run gel at 20 mA per gel until the leading front enters the resolving gel. Turn up the current to 30 mA until the leading front reaches the end of the gel.
4. Switch off power, dismantle the gel apparatus and perform the Western blotting procedure as follows:
   a. Cut a piece of Immobilon membrane and two sheets of Whatman 3MM paper to a suitable size to accommodate the SDS-PAGE gel(s) (*see* **Note 28**).
   b. Soak the Immobilon membrane in methanol.
   c. Pour off methanol and add CAPS transfer buffer.
   d. Soak two pieces of blotting paper in CAPS transfer buffer.
   e. Place one piece of blotting paper on the base of the Western blotting apparatus, making sure that no air bubbles are present.
   f. Place the Immobilon membrane on top of the blotting paper.
   g. Dip the SDS-PAGE gel(s) into the transfer buffer (*see* **Note 29**).
   h. Place the gel(s) on top of the Immobilon.
   i. Cover with the second sheet of blotting paper (*see* **Note 30**).
   j. Close blotter and transfer the proteins from the gel to the membrane for 50 min at 9 volts/cm^2.
5. Undo the apparatus, and annotate the Immobilon membrane.
6. Soak the membrane in 3% BSA in PBS for 1 h at room temperature or at 4°C overnight (*see* **Note 31**). The Immobilon is now ready to be used but may be stored in a plastic envelope at –20°C at this stage.
7. Incubate the membrane in primary antibody for 30 min at room temperature. Make sure that the membrane does not dry out during this time (*see* **Note 32**).
8. Wash for 30 min in three changes of PBST on a shaking platform.
9. Incubate with HRP-conjugated goat anti-mouse Ig diluted 1:1000 (or anti-rabbit Ig if a primary rabbit antibody was used (*see* **Note 33**).
10. Wash for at least 2 h with frequent changes of PBST (*see* **Note 34**).
11. The antigen-antibody complexes bound to the membrane are visualized using the ECL chemiluminescent substrate (*see* **Note 35**) as follows:
    a. Make up a fresh solution substrate containing equal amounts of the two solutions in the ECL kit.

b. Place the membrane with the antigen-antibody complexes face up on a flat surface. Pipet the substrate over the membrane, blotting off the excess solution.
c. Place the membrane inside a plastic sleeve, add a Glogos 2 marker, and expose the sleeve to X-ray film in an X-ray cassette for 1 min (*see* **Note 36**).
d. Develop this film. If necessary then another film can be placed over the membrane for longer periods of time e.g., 5- to 30-min intervals.
e. If the signal is still weak after 30 min of exposure, then wash the membrane in fresh PBST, add more ECL substrate, and cover with an X-ray film and expose overnight before developing. If background levels are high then wash the blots for a longer period of time.
f. The stained blots can be dried and stored at –20°C for future stripping and re-probing with other antibodies if necessary.

Examples of results obtained from Western blotting of cases of ALK-positive ALCL are illustrated in **Fig. 2A,B**.

3.4.5. Stripping Western Blots

1. Incubate the stained membrane in stripping buffer (**Subheading 2.4.**) for 30 min at 70°C.
2. Wash the membrane extensively for at least 5 h in multiple changes of PBST.
3. Block in 3% BSA in PBS before use as before.
4. Test the efficiency of the stripping procedure by incubating the membrane in the ECL substrate and expose to X-ray film for 5 min. If no signal is detected then the membrane is ready for re-probing with additional antibodies (*see* **Note 37**).

3.5. Immunoprecipitation Technique

A combination of immunoprecipitation and Western blotting techniques enables the functional status of ALK and the identity of interacting proteins to be studied *(23,27)*.

3.5.1. Immunoprecipitation Followed by Western Blotting

1. Prepare Protein G:GammaBind Plus Sepharose pre-bound to antibody as follows:
   a. Wash Protein G:GammaBind Plus Sepharose three times in PBS.
   b. Add 2 mL of purified antibody in 1.25 mL PBS or 1.25 mL monoclonal antibody supernatant to 0.5 mL 10% (vol/vol) Protein G:GammaBind.
   c. Rotate overnight at 4°C.
   d. Wash Protein G:GammaBind three times to remove unbound antibody and resuspend pellet to 10% vol/vol in PBS. This is now ready for use.

Fig. 2. (*opposite page*) Biochemical studies on four (1–4) cases of ALK-positive ALCL. Immunolabeling studies had previously shown that case 1 had the typical nuclear and cytoplasmic expression pattern associated with NPM-ALK whereas cases 2–4 showed only a cytoplasmic distribution of ALK suggesting the presence

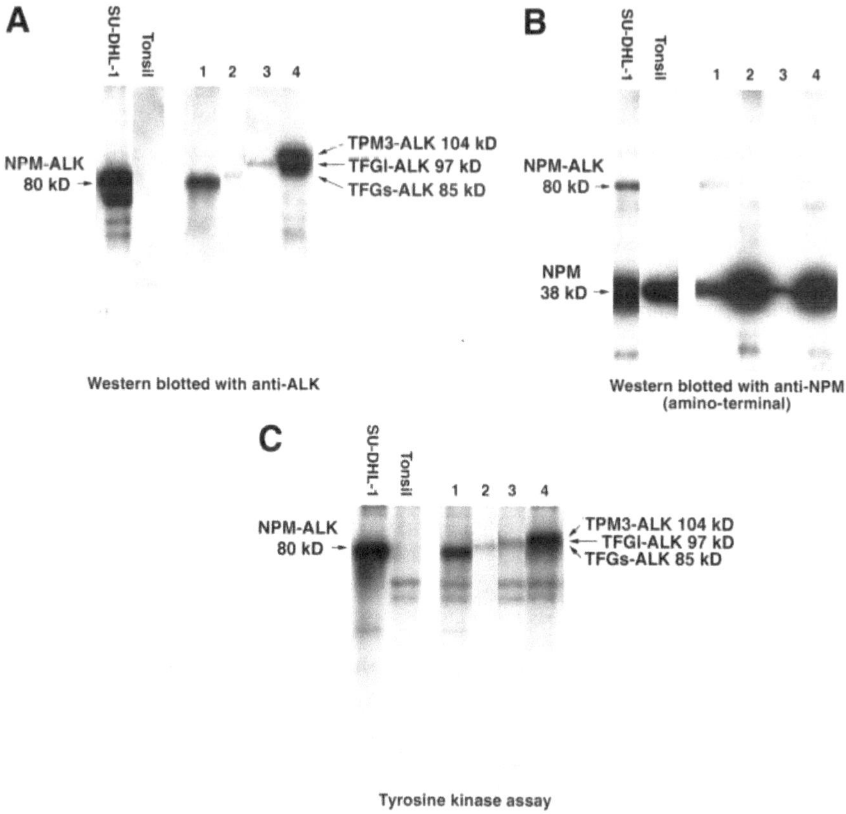

Fig. 2. (*continued*) of variant ALK proteins. **(A)** and **(B)** demonstrate the results obtained by Western blotting proteins extracted from tissue sections of these four cases of ALK-positive ALCL. SU-DHL-1 cells and tonsil extracts were used as the positive and negative controls, respectively. In **(A)**, blotting with anti-ALK demonstrates the presence of 80-kDa NPM-ALK in the SU-DHL-1 cell line. A protein of similar size was detected in case 1 in keeping with the predicted presence of NPM-ALK in this tumor. However, ALK proteins of differing molecular weights, namely 85, 97, and 104 kD, were found in the other three cases. No ALK proteins were detected in normal tonsil. **(B)** Blotting with anti-NPM (amino-terminus) confirmed the presence of an 80-kDa protein in case 1 that was comparable in size to the NPM-ALK detected in the SU-DHL-1 cell line. In contrast, only 38-kDa wild-type NPM was present in cases 2–4 (and in the tonsil), providing further evidence for the presence of ALK proteins other than NPM-ALK in these lymphomas. These variant ALK proteins were later identified using 5'-RACE (*see* **Table 1**) as TFG-ALK_S (85 kDa), TFG-ALK_L (97 kDa), and TPM3-ALK (104 kDa). **(C)** shows the results of an in vitro kinase assay performed on ALK-positive ALCL cases 1–4 and confirms that NPM-ALK TFG-ALK_S (85 kDa), TFG-ALK_L (97 kDa), and TPM3-ALK (104 kDa) proteins present in cases 1–4 are functional tyrosine kinases capable of autophosphorylation.

2. Add 50–100 μL of immunoprecipitation lysis buffer to each cytocentrifuge preparation or cryostat tissue section.
3. Leave at 4°C for 30 min.
4. Remove cells, tissue sections, and lysis buffer into pre-chilled clean tubes.
5. Microfuge all samples at 20,000*g* for 10 min.
6. Place supernatants in a clean prechilled tubes.
7. Preclear the supernatant by rotating with 50 μL of washed unbound 20% (vol/vol) Protein G:GammaBind Plus Sepharose for 30 min at 4°C.
8. Microfuge at 20,000*g* for 1 min.
9. Place supernatants in clean tubes and repeat **steps 7** to **9**.
10. Add 50-μL aliquots of Protein G:GammaBind Plus Sepharose prebound to antibody to 50-mL aliquots of precleared lysate.
11. Leave rotating overnight at 4°C.
12. Wash the pellet five times with ice-cold lysis buffer discarding the supernatant each time.
13. Add an equal volume of Laemmli sample buffer to the pellet. These samples can investigated immediately by SDS-PAGE and Western blotting as described above or stored at –70°C.

3.5.2. In Vitro Tyrosine Kinase Assay

1. Perform **steps 1** to **11** as described in **Subheading 3.5.1.**
2. Wash the pellet three times in lysis buffer and then twice in kinase buffer.
3. After the final wash, resuspend the Protein G:GammaBind pellets in 20 μL of freshly prepared kinase buffer containing 5 μCi [γ-^{32}P]ATP. Seal the tubes with parafilm (*see* **Notes 38** and **39**).
4. Incubate at 26°C for 15 min.
5. Stop the reaction by adding 25 μL of Laemmli sample buffer to each tube. Seal the tubes.
6. Heat proteins at 95°C for 4 min (*see* **Note 39**).
7. Separate the proteins by SDS-PAGE on a 10% gel (*see* **Note 27**).
8. Allow the leading front to run off the bottom of the gel (*see* **Note 40**).
9. Place the gels in SDS-PAGE fixative for at least 2 h.
10. Dry down the gels.
11. Place in cassette and expose to X-ray film for a minimum of 4 h.
12. Develop film. Fresh X-ray films can be added to the dried gel if longer exposure times are necessary.

Examples of results obtained from in vitro tyrosine kinase assays of cases of ALK-positive ALCL illustrated in **Fig. 2C**.

4. Notes

1. Control slides should be cut to test the reactivity of the antibodies used. Tonsil is an example of a good control tissue because it is relatively easy to obtain and contains proteins (with the exception of ALK) recognized by the antibodies un-

der study. The ALCL-derived SU-DHL-1 cell line has the t(2;5) and contains high levels of NPM-ALK and is, therefore, recommended as the positive control for ALK.

2. The inclusion of the protease inhibitors prevents the degradation of proteins of interest, whereas the addition of phosphatase inhibitors (NaF and $Na_2(VO)_4$) prevents the dephosphorylation of the ALK and other tyrosine phosphorylated proteins.
3. The use of the Redivue form of [γ-^{32}P]ATP means that the isotope can be stored at 4°C rather than being subjected to repeated freezing/thawing. Any accidental spillage can be easily detected. This isotope has a relatively short half-life, and unused stock should be discarded after a month. A sterile tip should always be used to aliquot out from the stock solution.
4. Acetone is a very gentle fixative and is the fixation method of choice for cryostat sections. Although its use has the advantage that most epitopes recognized by antibodies are conserved, the morphology of the cells may not be optimal. Because prolonged incubation in buffers may result in the additional loss of morphological detail, the authors recommend that the incubation intervals given in the staining procedures should be followed. The same solution of acetone should be used no more than twice.
5. The PAP pen draws a wax-based boundary around the tissue section/cell preparation under investigation thus preventing the spread of solutions added to the slide.
6. Keeping the paraffin-embedded block on ice hardens the wax facilitating the cutting of good sections.
7. The vigorous movement of air bubbles that occurs during the antigen retrieval step can cause routinely processed tissue sections to fall off the slides. This problem is alleviated by using Snowcoat X-tra slides and by incubating the dried sections overnight at 37°C before staining.
8. Storage of paraffin-embedded sections at 4°C prior to use improves the stability of the antigens.
9. The use of Citroclear for de-waxing the paraffin embedded sections avoids the safety hazards associated with xylene.
10. The use of an humidified staining tray (just add a few milliliters of water to the base of a staining tray) will prevent tissue and cell preparations drying out which can result in the development of staining artefacts
11. Unwrapping slides before they have reached room temperature will result in condensation on the tissue, which will have a deleterious effect on cell morphology in immunolabeling studies.
12. The dilutions of relevant antibodies must be determined before their use on tissue sections. Do not store diluted antibody (i.e., less than 10–100 µg/mL) for long periods of time. All antibodies should be stored as recommended by the supplier. Antibodies in current use should be stored at 4°C. Repeated freeze/thawing cycles of the antibodies should be avoided.
13. The polyclonal antibodies used in this chapter have all been preabsorbed with immunoglobulin from the species under investigation, thus reducing the problem of cross-reactivity of these reagents

14. DAB is carcinogenic and so gloves should be worn. The use of the Sigma-Fast tablet kit for developing the peroxidase substrate is a safer and more reliable alternative to that the method previously described (6 mg of diaminobenzidine tetrahydrochloride in water containing 3% (vol/vol) H_2O_2).
15. The water-based Aquamount mounting medium is used since the DAB precipitate is water insoluble while that of the APAAP technique is soluble in alcohol-based mountants. Aquamount has the additional advantage in that coverslips can be removed easily after soaking the finished slides in water for re-counterstaining or for performing additional staining procedures if required.
16. Certain tissues such as liver and kidney contain high levels of endogenous biotin. The use of these tissues may therefore result in a high background being obtained using this staining procedure. Biotin blocking kits are commercially available, for example, Biotin-Blocking System, X0590 (DakoCytomation).
17. TBS and not PBS must be used in the APAAP technique. The phosphates in PBS will inhibit the alkaline phosphatase reaction.
18. Levamisole blocks endogenous alkaline phosphatase, which may be present in the cells, and its addition to the substrate buffer is essential. The absence of labeling for alkaline phosphatase in neutrophils in the control slide is a good internal control to test the efficacy of this blocking step.
19. Nickel chloride (1 mg/mL) can be added to the DAB substrate for a more intense blue/brown color of the staining reaction.
20. The use of DAPI during the immunofluorescence labeling enables cell nuclei to be visualized as well as the immunolabeled cells.
21. The authors used a Zeiss Axioskop microscope fitted for epifluorescence. The filter wheel (Ludl, Hawthorne, NY) contained single wavelength filters for each fluorochrome (365HT25; 485DF15; 575DF25) and a triple DAP/FITC/Texas red (XF56) all from Omega (Brattleboro, VT). Images were taken with a cooled CCD camera (Model C5985, Hamamatsu Photonics, Billerica, MA). The filterwheel and image were controlled using Openlab software (Improvision, Coventry, UK). Image adjustment was performed using Photoshop software (Adobe, San Jose, CA) on an Apple Macintosh computer ***(20)***.
22. Pilot experiments demonstrated that optimal results were obtained using an acetone fixation step for tissue sections and cytocentrifuge preparations.
23. The addition of 50–100 µL of sample buffer/lysis solution to each tissue section/cytocentrifuge preparation provides enough material for three tracks in an SDS-PAGE gel thus permitting the reactivity of three different antibodies to be studied using a particular tissue section. The sensitivity of the technique is dependent to a large extent upon the number of tumor cells in the tissue biopsy but studies from the SU-DHL-1 cells show that $1–4 \times 10^4$ cells per SDS-PAGE well is sufficient for the biochemical studies here.
24. All reagents and cell extracts must be kept at 4°C to prevent protein degradation.
25. The original work performed by the authors utilized the detergent Brij 96. This reagent, soluble at 4°C, is no longer available from Sigma. Although Brij 96 can

be purchased from BDH, the authors have not found this detergent to be soluble at low temperatures.

26. Laemmli sample buffer should be added to aliquots of solubilized protein extracts on their removal from storage at –70°C before they have thawed.
27. The authors recommend the use of a 7.5 % SDS-PAGE gel for preliminary experiments. If the proteins of interest are larger than 150 kDa, then lower percentage gels should be used whereas 10% gels should be used for smaller proteins. For in vitro kinase assays, however, the use of a 10% gel will provide improved resolution of the radiolabeled proteins.
28. Great care must be taken when handling the Immobilon. Gloves and clean plastic ware must always be used. Only the edges of the membrane should be handled.
29. Wetting the SDS-PAGE gels with CAPS transfer buffer allows them to be easily positioned on the Immobilon membrane thus reducing the risk of the gel tearing.
30. It is essential to ensure that there are no air bubbles in any part of the Western blotting "sandwich" because their presence will prevent the passage of current at that site stopping transfer of proteins from the gel to the Immobilon membrane.
31. The use of 3% BSA (or 3% powdered milk) blocks any spare protein binding sites on the membrane thus preventing nonspecific binding by antibodies used in the staining procedures
32. Drying out of the membrane will result in a high background on staining.
33. Western blotting is a more sensitive procedure than immunostaining of tissue sections and the HRP-conjugated polyclonal secondary antibodies can therefore be used at higher dilutions.
34. An adequate washing stage using Tween-20 is extremely important in removing nonspecifically bound HRP-conjugated antibodies, thus reducing the background staining of the membrane.
35. The chemiluminescent substrate, ECL, is the authors' method of choice for detecting antigen:antibody complexes in Western blotting. In addition to its sensitivity, the use of ECL permits permanent records of the results in the form of autoradiographs to be obtained. An alternative is the DAB substrate, with the inclusion of 5 mg of cobalt chloride. The substrate is added to the membrane, and the reaction is left to develop until blue/black bands can be visualized. After washing with tap water, these stained membranes can be dried and stored but the protein bands will fade with time.
36. Glogos 2 markers are luminescent and will expose the X-ray film allowing the X-ray film and Immobilon membrane to be accurately compared for the analysis of results.
37. Stripping Western blots to permit reprobing with other antibodies has the advantage that the results of labeling experiment can be directly compared with another on the same membrane. However, protein will be lost from the Immobilon membrane during the stripping procedure, and the authors recommend that the membrane not be stripped more than once.
38. $MnCl_2$ is a catalyst for tyrosine kinases and its inclusion is essential for the in vitro kinase assay.

39. All tubes which contain isotope and which are heated must be sealed shut with parafilm to ensure that no radioactive solution is released if a lid opens unexpectedly.
40. All of the unassociated radioactivity in the in vitro kinase assays will be present in the leading front. Therefore, allowing the leading front to run off the gel and enter the tank buffer will result in minimal background radioactivity remaining in the gel. The use of the gel system suggested here allows the radioactivity released into the tank buffer to be safely contained improving the safety aspect of this technique.

References

1. Delsol, G., Ralfkaier, E., Stein, H., Wright, D., Jaffe, E. S., Harris, N. L., et al. (2001) Anaplastic large cell lymphoma, in *World Health Organisation Classification of Tumours. Pathology and Genetics, Tumours of Haematopoietic and Lymphoid Tissues*. (Jaffe, E. S. et al., eds.), IARC Press, Lyon, France, pp. 230–235.
2. Morris, S. W., Kirstein, M. N., Valentine, M. B., Dittmer, K. G., Shapiro, D. N., Saltman, D. I., et al. (1994) Fusion of a kinase gene, ALK, to a nucleolar protein gene, NPM, in non-Hodgkin's lymphoma. *Science* **263,** 1281–1284.
3. Shiota, M., Fujimoto, J., Semba, T., Satoh, H., Yamamoto, T., and Mori, S. (1994) Hyperphosphorylation of a novel 80 kDa protein tyrosine kinase similar to Ltk in a human Ki-1 lymphoma cell line, AMS3. *Oncogene* **9,** 1567–1574.
4. Pulford, K., Lamant, L., Morris, S. W., Butler, L. H., Wood, K. M., Stroud, D., et al. (1997) Detection of anaplastic lymphoma kinase (ALK) and nucleolar protein nucleophosmin (NPM)-ALK proteins in normal and neoplastic cells with the monoclonal antibody ALK1. *Blood* **89,** 1394–1404.
5. Shiota, M., Fujimoto, J., Taneka, M., Satoh, H,. Ichinohasama, R., Abe, M., et al. (1994) Diagnosis of t(2;5)(p23;q35)-Associated Ki-1 lymphoma with immunohistochemistry. *Blood* **84,** 3684.
6. Falini, B., Fizzotti, M., Pulford, K., Pileri, S. A., Delsol, G., Carbone, A., et al. (1998) ALK expression defines a distinct group of T/null lymphomas ("ALK lymphomas") with a wide morphological spectrum. *Am. J. Pathol.* **153,** 875–886.
7. Benharroch, D., Meguerian-Bedoyan, Z., Lamant, L., Amin, C., Brugieres, L., Terier-Lacombe, M. J., et al. (1998) ALK-positive lymphoma: a single disease with a broad spectrum of morphology. *Blood* **96,** 2076–2084.
8. Falini, B., Pileri, S., Zinzanim, P. L., Carbone, A., Zagonalm, V., Wolf-Peeters, C., et al. (1999) ALK+ Lymphoma: Clinico-pathological findings and outcome. *Blood* **93,** 2697–2706.
9. Gascoyne, R. D., Aoun, P., Wu, D., Chhanabhai, M., Skinnider, B. F., Greiner, T. C., et al. (1999) Prognostic significance of anaplastic lymphoma kinase (ALK) protein expression in adults with anaplastic large cell lymphoma. *Blood* **93,** 3913–3921.
10. Delsol, G., Lamant, L., Mariame, B., Pulford, K., Dastague, N., Brousset, P., et al. (1997) A new subtype of large B-cell lymphoma expressing the ALK kinase and lacking the 2;5 translocation. *Blood* **89,** 1483–1490.

11. Lamant, L., Dastugue, N., Pulford, K., Delsol, G., and Mariame, B, (1999) A new fusion gene TPM3-ALK in anaplastic large cell lymphoma created by a (1;2)(q25;p23) translocation. *Blood* **93,** 3088–3095.
12. Hernandez, L., Pinyol, M., Hernandez, S., Bea, S., Pulford, K., Rosenwald, A., et al. (1999) TRK-fused gene (TFG) is a new partner of ALK in anaplastic large cell lymphoma producing two structurally different TFG-ALK translocations. *Blood* **94,** 3265–3268.
13. Hernandez, L., Bea, S., Bellosillo, B., Pinyol, M., Falini, B., Carbone, A., et al. (2000) Diversity of genomic breakpoints in TFG-ALK translocations in anaplastic large cell lymphomas. Identification of a new TFG-ALKXL chimeric gene with transforming activity. *Am. J. Pathol.* **160,** 1487–1494.
14. Trinei, M., Lanfrancone, L., Campo, E., Pulford, K., Mason, D. Y., Pelicci, P. G., et al. (2000) A new variant anaplastic lymphoma kinase (ALK)-fusion protein (ATIC- ALK) in a case of ALK-positive anaplastic large cell lymphoma. *Cancer Res.* **60,** 793–798.
15. Colleoni, G. W., Bridge, J. A., Garicochea, B., Liu, J., Filippa, D. A., and Ladanyi, M. (2000) ATIC-ALK: A novel variant ALK gene fusion in anaplastic large cell lymphoma resulting from the recurrent cryptic chromosomal inversion, inv(2)(p23q35). *Am. J. Pathol.* **156,** 781–789.
16. Touriol, C., Greenland, C., Lamant, L., Pulford, K., Bernard, F., Rousset, T., et al. (2000) Further demonstration of the diversity of chromosomal changes involving 2p23 in ALK-positive lymphoma: 2 cases expressing ALK kinase fused to CLTCL (clathrin chain polypeptide-like). *Blood.* **95,** 3204–3207.
17. Morris, S. W., Xue, L., Ma, Z., and Kinney, M. C. (2001). ALK+CD30+ lymphomas: a distinct molecular genetic subtype of non-Hodgkin's lymphoma. *Br. J. Haematol.* **113,** 275–295.
18. Tort, F., Pinyol, M., Pulford, K., Roncador, G., Hernandez, L., Nayacg, I., et al. (2001) Molecular characterization of a new *ALK* translocation involving moesin *(MSN-ALK)* in anaplastic large cell lymphoma. *Lab. Invest.* **81,** 419–426.
19. Naeim, M. J., Gerdes, J., Abdulaziz, Z. A., Sunderland, C. A., Allington, M. J., Stein, H., et al. (1984). The value of immunohistological screening in the production of monoclonal antibodies. *J. Immunol. Methods* **50,** 145.
20. Mason, D. Y., Micklem, K., and Jones, M. (2000). Double immunofluorescence labelling of routinely processed paraffin sections. *J. Pathol.* **191,** 452–461.
21. Cordell, J. L., Falini, B., Erber, W. N., Ghosh, A. K., Abdulaziz, Z., MacDonald, S., et al. (1984) Immunoenzymatic labelling of monoclonal antibodies using immune complexes of alkaline phosphatase and monoclonal anti-alkaline phosphatase (APAAP complexes). *J. Histochem. Cytochem.* **32,** 219–229.
22. Mason, D. Y., Abdulaziz, Z., Falini, B., and Stein, H. (1983) Single and double immunoenzymatic techniques for labelling tissue sections with monoclonal antibodies. *Ann. NY Acad. Sci.* **420,** 127–133.
23. Bischof, D., Pulford, K., Mason, D. Y., and Morris, S. W. (1997) Role of the nucleophosmin (NPM) portion of the Non-Hodgkin's lymphoma-associated

NPM-Anaplastic Lymphoma Kinase fusion protein in oncogenesis. *Mol. Cell Biol.* **17,** 2312–2325.

24. Bai, R. Y., Ouyang, T., Miething, C., Morris, S. W., Peschel, C., and Duyster, J. (2000) Nucleophosmin-anaplastic lymphoma kinase associated with anaplastic large-cell lymphoma activates the phosphatidylinositol 3-kinase/Akt antiapoptotic signaling pathway. *Blood* **96,** 4319–4327.
25. Pulford, K., Falini, B., Cordell, J., Rosenwald, A., Ott, G., Muller-Hermelink, H. K., et al. (1999) Biochemical detection of novel anaplastic lymphoma kinase proteins in tissue sections of anaplastic large cell lymphoma. *Am. J. Pathol.* **154,** 1657–1663.
26. Cordell, J. L., Pulford, K. A.F., Bigerna, B., Roncador, G., Banham, A., Colomba, E., et al. (1998) Detection of normal and chimaeric nucleophosmin in human cells. *Blood.* **93,** 632–642.
27. Lamant, L., Pulford, K., Bischof, D., Morris, S. W., Mason, D. Y., Delsol, G., and Mariame, B. (2000) Expression of the ALK tyrosine kinase gene in neuroblastoma. *Am. J. Pathol.* **156,** 1711–1721.

15

Identification of Anaplastic Lymphoma Kinase Variant Translocations Using 5'RACE

Luis Hernández and Elias Campo

Summary

Anaplastic lymphoma kinase (ALK) is abnormally expressed in anaplastic large cell lymphoma (ALCL) and its expression associated with chromosomal translocations involving the *ALK* gene at 2p23. These translocations lead to the synthesis of novel chimeric proteins that retain the C-terminal portion of ALK, where the tyrosine kinase domain is located. In most of these tumors, the t(2;5)(p23;q35) translocation causes fusion of the *ALK* gene to the 5' region of the nucleophosmin (*NPM*) gene, but other different *ALK* partners have been identified, including nonmuscle tropomyosin (*TPM3*), TRK-fused gene (*TFG*), 5' aminoimidazole-4-carboxamide ribonucleotide formyltranferase/IMP cyclohydrolase (*ATIC*), clathrin heavy chain gene (*CLTC*), and moesin (*MSN*). The characterization of these *ALK* partners has been performed using different molecular methods, including the 5' Rapid Amplification of complementary deoxyribonucleic acid (cDNA) Ends (5'RACE) polymerase chain reaction (PCR)-based technique. This approach allows the potential amplification and identification of either 5' or 3' mRNA ends from an internal known sequence. In ALK translocations, identification of the 5' gene involved has been performed using primers designed within the known 3' catalytic domain of the *ALK*. Initial reaction consists in a first-strand cDNA synthesis primed using a gene-specific antisense primer (ALK1), performing the cDNA conversion of specific messenger ribonucleic acids, and maximizing the potential for complete extension to the 5'-end of the message. After cDNA synthesis, the first-strand product is purified from unincorporated dNTPs and ALK1. Terminal deoxynucleotidyl transferase is used to add homopolymeric tails to the 3' ends of the cDNA. Tailed cDNA is then amplified by PCR using a nested gene-specific primer (ALK2), which anneals 3' to ALK1, and a complementary homopolymer containing an anchor primer (i.e., AAP), which permits amplification from the homopolymeric tail. This allows amplification of unknown sequences between the ALK2 and the 5' end of the mRNA. Further, nested PCRs usually are required to confer an adequate level of specificity to the process to permit the characterization of RACE products. The reamplification is achieved by using a nested gene-specific primer (ALK3), which anneals 3' to ALK2, and a universal amplification primer, which anneals to the 5' sequence previously introduced by the AAP primer. The result of the 5' amplification yields a product that corresponds to a fragment of the fusion gene,

From: *Methods in Molecular Medicine, Vol. 115: Lymphoma: Methods and Protocols*
Edited by: T. Illidge and P. W. M. Johnson © Humana Press Inc., Totowa, NJ

including a partial fragment of the unknown *ALK* partner. Hybridization with an internal *ALK* primer is needed to confirm the specificity of the PCR fragments obtained because unspecific bands frequently are generated in these amplifications. The confirmed specific PCR product is subsequently purified and sequenced. Once this gene is identified, terminal primers could be designed to amplify the entire coding region of the fusion gene to be cloned for a complete sequencing analysis, thus allowing further functional studies of the new chimeric *ALK* gene.

Key Words: Translocation; ALK; RACE; ALCL; RT-PCR; Southern hybridization.

1. Introduction

Anaplastic large cell lymphoma (ALCL) expressing anaplastic lymphoma kinase (ALK; also referred to as ALK-positive ALCL or ALKoma) is a distinct clinicopathological and molecular entity characterized by a proliferation of T/null lymphoid cells that show a diverse immunostaining pattern for ALK protein ***(1–3)***. This aberrant ALK expression is associated with chromosomal translocations involving the *ALK* gene at 2p23 ***(4)***. These translocations lead to the synthesis of novel chimeric proteins that retain the C-terminal portion of ALK, where the tyrosine kinase domain is located. In most of these tumors, the t(2;5)(p23;q35) translocation causes fusion of the *ALK* gene to the 5' region of the nucleophosmin *(NPM)* gene ***(5)***. Several cytogenetic and molecular studies also have demonstrated that chromosomal aberrations other than the t(2;5)(p23;q35) may give rise to novel *ALK* fusion genes in ALCL. So far, five different genes, nonmuscle tropomyosin (*TPM3*), TRK-fused gene (*TFG*), 5' aminoimidazole-4-carboxamide ribonucleotide formyltranferase/IMP cyclohydrolase (*ATIC*), clathrin heavy chain gene (*CLTC*), and moesin (*MSN*), have been cloned as alternative partners to *NPM* in ALCL (*see* **Fig. 1**) ***(6–13)***.

The characterization of these *ALK* partners has been performed using different molecular methods, including the 5' Rapid Amplification of complementary deoxyribonucleic acid (cDNA) Ends (5' RACE) technique. This approach allows the potential amplification and identification of either 5' or 3' messenger ribonucleic acids (mRNA) ends from an internal known sequence. In the present work, the goal of the polymerase chain reaction (PCR)-based 5' RACE technique is to identify the 5' gene involved in new *ALK* translocations using primers designed within the known 3' catalytic domain of the *ALK*. Although the precise protocol varies among different users, the general strategy remains consistent (*see* **Fig. 2**) ***(14)***. First-strand cDNA synthesis is primed using a gene-specific antisense primer (GSP1), performing the cDNA conversion of specific mRNAs and maximizing the potential for complete extension to the 5'-end of the message. For 5'RACE of ALK chimeric variants, a common GSP1 primer (ALK1 in **Fig. 2**) is used and this primer anneals in a sequence near the ALK 5' region that is juxtaposed with the NPM gene in the classic rearrangement of NPM-ALK. After the synthesis of cDNA, the first-strand product is

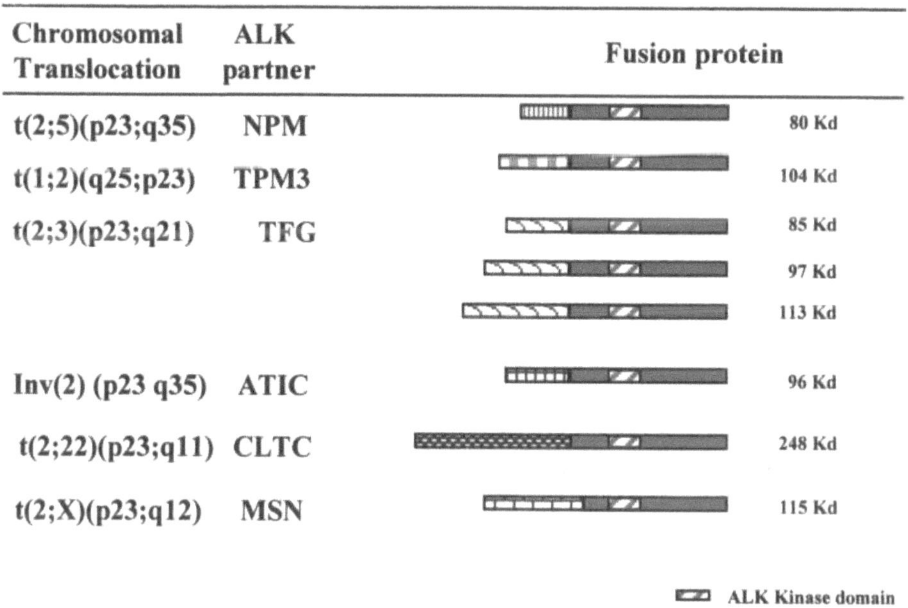

Fig. 1. ALK translocation variants in ALCL. ALK portion is showed in solid gray (retaining the marked kinase domain).

purified from unincorporated dNTPs and GSP1. Terminal deoxynucleotidyl transferase (TdT) is used to add homopolymeric tails to the 3' ends of the cDNA. Tailed cDNA is then amplified by PCR using a nested gene-specific primer (GSP2; ALK 2 in the **Fig. 2**), which anneals 3' to GSP1, and a complementary homopolymer containing an anchor primer (AAP), which permits amplification from the homopolymeric tail. This allows amplification of unknown sequences between the GSP2 and the 5'-end of the mRNA. Further, nested PCRs usually are required to confer an adequate level of specificity to the process to permit the characterization of RACE products. The reamplification is achieved using a nested gene-specific primer (GSP3; ALK 3 in the **Fig. 2**), which anneals 3' to GSP2, and a universal amplification primer (UAP), which anneals to the 5' sequence previously introduced by the APP primer.

The result of the 5' amplification yields a product corresponding to a fragment of the fusion gene, including a partial fragment of the unknown *ALK* partner. Hybridization with an internal *ALK* primer is needed to confirm the specificity of the obtained PCR fragments because unspecific bands frequently are generated in these amplifications (*see* **Fig. 3**). The confirmed specific PCR

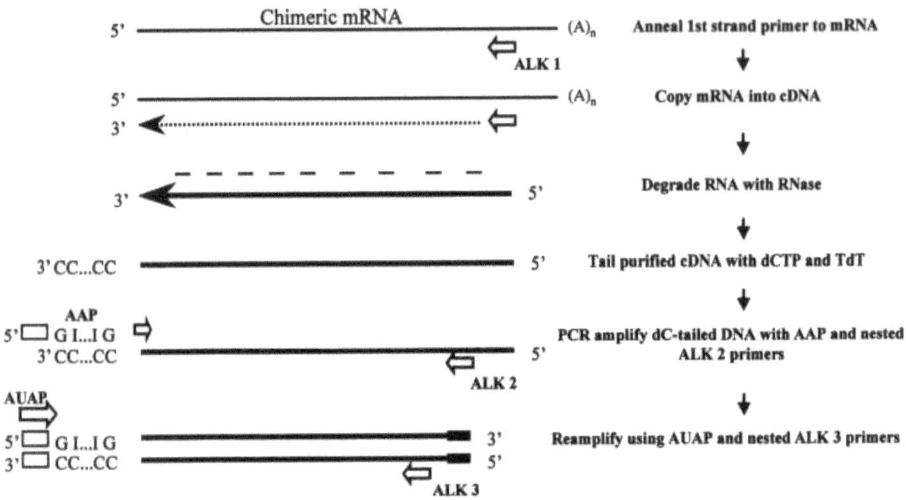

Fig. 2. 5'RACE *ALK* strategy showing the localization of the primers used.

product subsequently is purified and sequenced. The obtained sequence can now be compared with the GenBank sequences to identify the corresponding ALK partner. If the new sequence were not known, further rounds of 5'RACE using 3' primers of the obtained new sequence eventually would lead to the characterization of the whole 5' sequence of the chimeric gene. In any case, once this gene is identified, terminal primers could be designed to amplify the entire coding region of the fusion gene to be cloned for a complete sequencing analysis, thus allowing further functional studies of the new chimeric ALK gene.

2. Materials

There are many methods in which to perform RACE experiments. We have extensively used the "5' RACE system for rapid amplification of cDNA Ends, Version 2.0" (Life Technologies Inc, Paisley, UK). This kit contains the reagents listed in **Subheadings 2.1.–2.3.**, and the UAP, AAP, and control GSP1, GSP2, and GSP3 primers. All the reagents must be stored at –20°C, with the exception of the components of the DNA isolation system (*see* **Subheading 2.2.**), which must be stored at 4°C.

2.1. First-Strand cDNA Synthesis

Although different reverse transcription systems currently are available and most of them are probably suitable for the first-strand synthesis of the 5'RACE technique, we performed this reaction using the system here described because

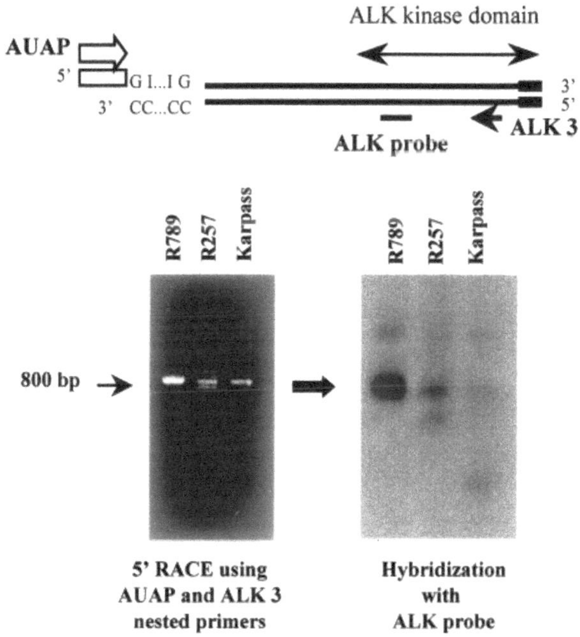

Fig. 3. Southern hybridization of an example of 5'RACE products obtained from *ALK* gene. Top, Probe localization. Bottom, The hybridization demonstrates the specificity of the intense band obtained in the case R789. The other cases are controls with the *NPM-ALK* rearrangement. Although all samples showed similar size bands, in the following sequence analysis *TFG* gene was the *ALK* partner in case R789 (TFG-ALK_S).

most of the reagents are included in the 5'RACE kit and the performance of the final product has been optimized using this reverse transcription system. The use of control RNA with the corresponding control primers is strongly recommended for monitoring the possible pitfalls of the technique. In addition to the reactives here described, a tabletop microcentrifuge, wet ice, a thermocycler and the corresponding thin-walled polypropylene tubes are also needed.

1. Diethylpyrocarbonate (DEPC)-treated water, which is included in the kit. Alternatively, add 200 µL of DEPC (Sigma, St. Louis, MO) to 1 L of distilled water. Shake well, then loosen cap and incubate for 2 h at 37ºC and autoclave.
2. 10X PCR buffer: 200 m*M* Tris HCl, pH 8.4, 500 m*M* KCl.
3. 25 m*M* $MgCl_2$.
4. 10 m*M* each dATP, dCTP, dGTP, and dTTP .
5. 0.1 *M* DTT.
6. SuperScript^{TM} II Reverse Transcriptase (200 U/µL).

7. RNAse mix (mixture of RNAse H and RNAse T1).
8. 1 m*M* ALK1 (5'-TTGTTCGCTGCATTGGGGT-3').
9. 1 m*M* control GSP1 (for the control RNA).
10. 1-5 mg total RNA from the sample.
11. 1 µL of control RNA.

2.2. GlassMax DNA Isolation Spin Cartridge Purification of cDNA

In addition to the reactives here described, a tabletop microcentrifuge, wet ice, 1.6-mL polypropylene Eppendorf tubes, and a thermal bath equilibrated at 65°C also are needed.

1. 1.6 *M* NaI.
2. GlassMAX spin cartridges (also included in the kit).
3. 1X Wash buffer. Before using the system for the first time, the wash buffer must be prepared from the buffer concentrate supplied in the kit: Pipet 1 mL of the concentrate into a 50-mL Falcon tube, and then add 18 mL of deionized water and 21 mL of absolute ethanol, mixing thoroughly.
4. 70% ethanol.

2.3. TdT Tailing of cDNA

The reaction can be performed in a thermocycler using the corresponding polypropylene Eppendorf tubes.

1. DEPC-treated water.
2. 5X tailing buffer: 50 m*M* Tris-HCl, pH 8.4, 125 m*M* KCl, 7.5 m*M* $MgCl_2$.
3. 2 m*M* dCTP.
4. TdT.

2.4. PCR of dC-Tailed cDNA

The described precautions against DNA contamination must be followed when setting up this and the following PCR ***(15)***. Pre- and post-PCR procedures and equipment are separated geographically; all solutions are stored as aliquots and only used once. Thus, in addition of a thermocycler, a flow cabinet is strongly recommended for setting up the PCR reaction. Use the corresponding thin-walled polypropylene tubes and keep them in wet ice.

1. Sterilized, deionized water.
2. 10X PCR buffer: 200 m*M* Tris HCl, pH 8.4, 500 m*M* KCl.
3. 25 m*M* $MgCl_2$.
4. 100 m*M* each of dATP, dCTP, dGTP, and dTTP.
5. 10 m*M* ALK2 (5'-ATCAGCAAATTCAACCACCAG-3') or control GSP2 (for control reaction).
6. 10 m*M* Abridged Anchor Primer AAP (5'-GGCCACGCGTCGACTAGTAC GGGIIGGGIIGGGIIG-3').
7. 5 U/µL of Taq DNA pol (Boehringer Mannheim, Mannheim, Germany).

2.5. Nested PCR Amplification

The dilution of the first PCR products obtained in the previous step must be performed in a different room and using a different set of material (tips, micropipets, Eppendorf tubes) than was used for setting up the PCR.

1. Sterilized, deionized water.
2. 10X PCR buffer: 200 m*M* Tris HCl, pH 8.4, 500 m*M* KCl.
3. 25 m*M* $MgCl_2$.
4. 100 m*M* each of dATP, dCTP, dGTP, and dTTP.
5. 10 m*M* ALK3 (5'-GAATGCCCAACGACCCAAG-3') or control GSP3 (for control reaction).
6. 10 m*M* UAP.
7. UAP (5'-GGCCACGCGTCGACTAGTACGGGIIGGGIIGGGIIG-3').
8. 5 U/μL of Taq DNA pol (Boehringer Mannheim, Mannheim, Germany).
9. TE buffer: 200 m*M* Tris-HCl, pH 8.0, 1 m*M* ethylene diamine tetraacetic (EDTA).

2.6. Gel Electrophoresis and Southern Blot Analysis

Because ethidium bromide is carcinogenic, the use of gloves, in addition to careful handling, is recommended. A microwave oven can be used to melt the agarose in TBE buffer. An appropriate volume of agarose gel must be made depending on the specific electrophoresis cubette that will be used. Use a long-wavelength ultraviolet (UV) light font to visualize the DNA bands. A shaking water bath or a hybridization oven must be used in the hybridization steps. A UV cross-linker (like Stratalinker™, Stratagene, La Jolla, CA) must be used for DNA fixation to the nylon membrane after the transference step.

1. Agarose. Store at room temperature.
2. Ethidium bromide. Stock 10 mg/mL, final concentration of the working solution 10 mg/mL in TBE 1X. Store at 4°C.
3. TBE (5X): Tris base (54 g), boric acid (27.5 g), 0.5 *M* EDTA (20 mL). Add deionized water up to 1 L. Store at room temperature. A dilution to 1X must be used to dilute the agarose and to use as an electrophoresis buffer.
4. Loading buffer, 5X. Bromophenol blue (104 mg), xyleneyanol (104 mg), and glycerol (12.5 mL). Add deionized water to 50 mL. Store at 4°C in aliquots of 1.5 mL.
5. DNA ladder (size standard) like 1-kb ladder (Life Technologies Inc., Paisley, UK).
6. Nylon membrane (Hybond-N, Amersham, Buckinghamshire, UK).
7. Base solution, pH 11.0–12.0: NaOH (20 g), NaCl (87.5 g), and deionized water (1 L), stable for several weeks at room temperature.
8. Neutralizing solution, pH 7.0–8.0: Tris base (60.5 g), NaCl (87.5 g), HCl pure (35 mL), and deionized water (1 L), stable for several weeks at room temperature.

9. ALK probe 5'-GTCGAGGTGCGGAGCTTGCTCAGC-3'. Store aliquoted at –20°C.
10. 20X standard saline citrate (SSC): 0.3 *M* citrate 3X Na (44.1 g), 3 *M* NaCl, pH 7.0, (87.66 g). Store at room temperature.
11. Hybridization buffer: mix the following components and incubate at 55°C for 30 min. Divide into 20-mL aliquots and store at –20°C:

5X SSC	125 mL
0.1% (w/v) Hybridization component (see below)	0.5 g
0.02% (w/v) SDS	0.1 g
0.5% (w/v) Blocking agent (see below)	2.5 g
Deionized water	to 500 mL final volume

12. All the following reagents are from ECL™ 3'- oligolabeling and detection system (Amersham, Buckinghamshire, UK):
13. Blocking agent. Store at –20°C until required. For prolonged storage aliquoting is recommended. Small aliquots may be stored at 4°C up to a month if required.
14. Anti-fluorescein HRP conjugate.
15. Hybridization component. Store at room temperature.
16. Fluorescein-11-dUTP. Store at –20°C.
17. Terminal transferase (2 U/µL), pH 7.0. Store at –20°C.
18. Cacodylate buffer, pH 7.2 (Warning: highly toxic substance). Store at –20°C.
19. ECL detection reagent 1 and 2. Store at 4°C.
20. Solution A: 20X SSC (225 mL), 10% SDS (9 mL), and deionized water to 900 mL final volume. Use only as fresh solution
21. Solution B: 20X SSC (22.5 mL), 10% SDS (9 mL), deionized water to 900 mL final volume. Use only as fresh solution.
22. Buffer 1, pH 7.5: 0.15 *M* NaCl (4.38 g) and 0.1 *M* Trizma base (6.05 g). Adjust pH to 7.5 with HCl then add deionized water to 500 mL of final volume. May be stored for a week at 4°C.
23. Buffer 2, pH 7.5: 0.4 *M* NaCl (11.5 g) and 0.1 *M* Trizma base (6.05 g). Adjust pH to 7.5 with HCl then add deionized water to 500 mL final volume. May be stored for a week at 4°C.

2.7. DNA Extraction From Agarose Gel

All the reagents are included in commercial kits as CONCERT™ Gel extraction system (Life Technologies, Inc. Paisley, UK). Store at room temperature. Other materials needed in this step are 1.6-mL polypropylene Eppendorf tubes, sterile surgical blades (to cut the desired bands from the gel), and a precision scale.

1. Gel solubilization buffer (L1).
2. Wash Buffer (L2). Add pure ethanol to wash buffer before first use following the instructions on the label.
3. TE buffer: 10 m*M* Tris-HCl, pH 8.0, 0.1 m*M* EDTA.
4. Spin cartridges, wash tubes, and recovery tubes.

5. 50°C water bath or heat block.
6. 70°C water bath or heat block.

2.8. RACE Product Direct Sequencing

The sequencing reaction will be performed using a thermocycler with the corresponding thin-walled polypropylene tubes, and the sequence analysis must be performed in an ABI Prism sequencer.

1. ABI Prism BigDye™ Terminator Cycle Sequencing Ready Reaction Kit 2.0. (Applied Biosystems, Warrington, UK). Terminator ready reaction mix composition (included in the kit) is:

   A-dye terminator labeled with dichloro (R6G).
   C-dye terminator labeled with dichloro (ROX).
   G-dye terminator labeled with dichloro (R110).
   T-dye terminator labeled with dichloro (TAMRA).
   Deoxynucleoside triphosphates (dATP, dCTP, dITP, dUTP).
   AmpliTaq DNA polymerase.
   $MgCl_2$.
   Tris-HCl buffer, pH 9.0.
2. 10 μ*M* Sequencing primer ALK probe (*see* **Subheading 2.6**).
3. 95% and 70% ethanol.

2.9. Full-Length ALK Fusion Gene PCR Amplification

Follow the recommendations in the previous subheadings for PCRs.

1. Sterilized deionized water.
2. 10X PCR buffer: 200 m*M* Tris HCl, pH 8.4, 500 m*M* KCl.
3. 25 m*M* $MgCl_2$.
4. 100 m*M* each dATP, dCTP, dGTP, and dTTP.
5. 10 m*M* each forward and reverse primer.
6. 5 U/μL Taq DNA pol (Boehringer Mannheim, Mannheim, Germany).

3. Methods

3.1. First-Strand cDNA Synthesis

In this first step, we use a gene-specific primer of ALK to obtain a 5' extended cDNA. Work on wet ice while setting up the reaction and use sterile gloves and RNAse free materials. Supersript™ II RT is not inhibited significantly by ribosomal and transfer RNA, and may be used effectively to synthesize first strand cDNA from a total RNA preparation.

1. Add the following to a thin-walled PCR tube

1 mM GSP1 primer (*see* **Note 1**)	2.5 μL
Sample RNA (*see* **Note 2**)	1–5 μg
DEPC-treated water	to a final volume of 15.5 μL

2. Incubate the mixture 10 min at 70°C to denature RNA. Chill 1 min on ice. Collect the contents of the tube by brief centrifugation and add the following in the given order:

10X PCR buffer	2.5 µL
25 m*M* $MgCl_2$	2.5 µL
10 m*M* dNTP mix	1 µL
0.1 *M* DTT	2.5 µL
Final volume	8.5 µL

3. Mix gently and collect by brief centrifugation. Incubate for 1 min at 42°C.
4. Add 1 µL of Superscript™ II RT. Mix gently and incubate for 50 min at 42°C. (*see* **Note 3**).
5. Incubate at 70°C for 15 min to terminate the reaction.
6. Centrifuge 10–20 s and place reaction at 37°C.
7. Add 1 µL of RNAse mix, mix gently but thoroughly and incubate for 30 min at 37°C.
8. Collect the reaction by brief centrifugation and place on ice. The procedure may be stopped at this point.

3.2. GlassMAX DNA Isolation Spin Cartridge Purification of cDNA

This step is needed to remove the excess of nucleotides and GSP1 from the first strand product. In presence of a chaotropic agent (sodium iodide), cDNAs with a minimal length of 200 bases are bound to the silica-based membrane. Buffer components, dNTPs, enzymes, and oligonucleotides remain in solution and are removed by centrifugation. Residual impurities and sodium iodide are removed by passing several volumes of 1X wash buffer followed by a 70% through the GlassMAX cartridge. Purified cDNA is recovered in deionized water.

1. Equilibrate the binding solution to room temperature.
2. For each sample to be purified, equilibrate 100 µL of sterilized, deionized water at 65°C for use in **step 9**.
3. Add 120 µL of binding solution (6 *M* NaI) to the first strand reaction (*see* **Note 4**).
4. Transfer the cDNA/NaI solution to a GlassMAX spin cartridge. Centrifuge at 13,000*g* for 20 s.
5. Remove the cartridge insert from the tube and transfer the flowthrough to a microcentrifuge tube (*see* **Note 5**). Place the cartridge insert back into the tube.
6. Add 0.4 mL of cold (4°C) 1X wash buffer to the spin cartridge. Centrifuge at 13,000*g* for 20 s. Discard the flowthrough. Repeat this wash step three additional times (*see* **Note 6**).
7. Wash the cartridge twice with 400 µL of cold (4°C) 70% ethanol as described in **step 6.**
8. After removing the final 70% ethanol wash from the tube, centrifuge at 13,000*g* for 1 min.

9. Transfer the spin cartridge insert into a fresh sample recovery tube. Add 50 µL of sterilized, deionized, previously preheated water to the spin cartridge (*see* **Note 7**). Centrifuge at 13,000*g* for 20 s to elute the cDNA. The procedure may be stopped at this point and the reactions stored at –20°C.

3.3. TdT Tailing of cDNA

TdT tailing creates the bridged anchor primer binding site on the 3'-end of the cDNA.

1. Add the following components to each tube and mix gently:

DEPC-treated water	6.5 µL
5X tailing buffer	5 µL
2 m*M* dCTP	2.5 µL
GlassMAX purified cDNA sample	10 µL
Final volume	24 µL

2. Incubate for 3 min at 94°C. Chill 1 min on ice. Collect the contents of the tube by brief centrifugation and place on ice.
3. Add 1 µL of TdT (*see* **Note 8**), mix gently, and incubate for 10 min at 37°C.
4. Heat inactivate the TdT for 10 min at 65°C. Collect the contents of the reaction by brief centrifugation and place on ice. The procedure may be stopped at this point and the reactions stored at –20°C.

3.4. PCR of dC-Tailed cDNA

The first and following nested (*see* **Subheading 3.5.**) PCR amplifications must be set up with the tubes in wet ice to avoid non-specific extension of the primers. The cycling protocol and annealing/extension temperatures used in this protocol correspond to those used in the TFG 5'RACE *(7)*, but these conditions must be optimized for RACE extensions of other genes.

1. Equilibrate the thermal cycler to 94°C.
2. Label the thin-wall PCR tubes sitting on ice with appropriate nomenclature.
3. Add the following to a 1.5-mL Eppendorf tube sitting on ice (reaction mix, composition/sample):

Sterilized, deionized water	31.5 µL
10X PCR buffer	5 µL
25 m*M* $MgCl_2$	3 µL
10 m*M* dNTP mix	1 µL
10 m*M* ALK2 primer (*see* **Note 9**)	2 µL
10 m*M* AAP primer	2 µL

4. Add 0.5 µL of Taq polymerase/sample and gently mix all the components by up and down pipetting.
5. Dispense 45 µL of the reaction mix in each of the corresponding PCR tubes.
6. Add 5 µL of the dC-tailed cDNA to the corresponding tubes except for the negative control, where 5 µL of sterilized water must be added.

7. Transfer the tubes directly from the ice to the pre-equilibrated thermal cycler.
8. Perform 35 cycles of PCR. A typical cycling protocol for cDNA with <1 kb amplified region is as follows:

Pre-amplification denaturation	94°C for 2 min
Cycle:	
Denaturation	94°C for 1 min
Annealing	55°C for 1 min
Extension	72°C for 1 min, 30 s
Followed by:	
Final extension	72°C for 7 min
Indefinite hold	4°C, until samples are removed

3.5. Nested PCR Amplification

A single PCR with 35 cycles will not often generate enough specific product to be detectable by ethidium bromide staining. A second nested PCR is strongly recommended in order to enhance the product yield and the specificity of the amplification.

1. Dilute a 5-μL aliquot of the primary PCR into 495 μL of TE buffer.
2. Equilibrate the thermal cycler to 94°C.
3. Label with appropriate nomenclature the thin-wall PCR tubes sitting on ice.
4. Add the following to a 1.5-mL Eppendorf tube sitting on ice (reaction mix, composition/sample):

Sterilized, deionized water	31.5 μL
10X PCR buffer	5 μL
25 m*M* $MgCl_2$	3 μL
10 m*M* dNTP mix	1 μL
10 m*M* ALK3 primer (*see* **Note 10**)	2 μL
10 m*M* AAP primer	2 μL

5. Add 0.5 μL of Taq polymerase/sample and gently mix all the components by up and down pipetting.
6. Dispense 45 μL of the reaction mix in each of the corresponding PCR tubes.
7. Add 5 μL of the dC-tailed cDNA to the corresponding tubes except for the negative control where 5 μL of sterilized water must be added.
8. Transfer the tubes directly from the ice to the pre-equilibrated thermocycler at 94°C.
9. Perform 35 cycles of PCR:

Pre-amplification denaturation	94°C for 2 min
Cycle:	
Denaturation	94°C for 1 min
Annealing	64°C for 1 min
Extension	72°C for 1 min, 30 s
Followed by:	
Final extension	72°C for 7 min
Indefinite hold	4°C, until samples are removed

3.6. Gel Electrophoresis and Southern Blot Analysis

This protocol is similar to a classical southern blot analysis, but no fragmentation of the DNA product is needed because the technique is performed on short PCR products.

3.6.1. Gel Electrophoresis

1. Prepare a 1% agarose gel in TBE 1X using a microwave oven for melting. 4.5 μL of ethidium bromide working solution must be added to the melted agarose immediately before pouring the solution in the previously sealed mould.
2. Load 10 μL of the PCR product mixed with 3 μL of loading dye.
3. In a diffferent well, load 5 μL of the molecular weight marker.
4. Electrophorese at 100 V until the first dye front reaches the end of the gel.
5. Remove the gel from the cubette and visualize/photograph under long-wavelength UV light (360 nm).

3.6.2. Southern Blotting of PCR Products

1. After the electrophoresis, the agarose gel must be washed sequentially, following this order:

   Base solution 20 min (three times).
   Deionized water (twice).
   Neutralizing solution 30 min (three times).
2. Wash briefly with 20X SSC.
3. DNA transference to the nylon Hybond membrane must be performed using a currently standard Southern's protocol.

3.6.3. DNA Fixation to the Membrane

1. Use a Cross-linker to irradiate the membrane with UV for 1 min to fix the transferred DNA to the membrane.

3.6.4. Oligonucleotide Labeling

1. Place the required tubes from the labeling components, excluding the enzyme, on ice to thaw.
2. To a 1.5-mL Eppendorf tube, on ice, add the labeling reaction components in the following order (*see* **Note 11**):

Oligonucleotide (100 pmol)	X μL
Fluorescein-11-dUTP	10 μL
Cacodylate buffer	16 μL
Water from the kit	Y μL
Terminal transferase	16 μL
Total volume	160 μL

3. Mix gently by pipetting up and down in the pipet tip.
4. Incubate the reaction mixture at 37°C for 60–90 min. Keep away the tube from light.

5. Store labeled probe on ice for immediate use or place at –20°C for long term storage.

3.6.5. Hybridization

1. Place the blot into the hybridization buffer and prehybridize at the required temperature, for a minimum of 30 min at 42°C in a shaking water bath or hybridization oven, using a volume of buffer of about 0.25 mL/cm^2 of membrane, and with constant agitation.
2. A small aliquot of the hybridization buffer must be removed and mixed with the labeled oligonucleotide probe (final concentration (5–10 ng/mL) and then return the mixture to the bulk of the hybridization buffer (*see* **Note 12**).
3. Hybridize at 42°C for 1–2 h in a shaking water bath or hybridization oven protected from the light (*see* **Note 13**).

3.6.6. Washing the Membrane

1. Remove the blot from the hybridization solution and place in a clear container. Cover with an excess of wash solution A, equivalent to 2 mL/cm^2 of membrane.
2. Incubate at room temperature for 5 min and with constant agitation.
3. Repeat **steps 1** and **2**.
4. Discard the wash solution. Place blot in a clean container and cover with an excess of appropriate pre-warmed stringency wash buffer (*see* **Note 14**).
5. Incubate at appropriate temperature (*see* **Note 14**) for 15 min with prewarmed wash solution B, and with constant agitation.
6. Replace the stringency wash buffer with fresh wash solution B and incubate for a further 15 minutes at the same temperature as in **step 5**.

3.6.7. Membrane Blocking, Antibody Incubations, and Washes

1. Place the filter in a clean container and rinse with buffer 1 for 1 min.
2. Discard buffer 1 and replace with block solution. Incubate for 30 min.
3. Rinse blot for 1 min in buffer 1.
4. Dilute the antifluorescein HRP conjugate 1000-fold in buffer 2.
5. Incubate the blot with the diluted conjugate antibody solution for 30 min.
6. Place filter in a clean container and rinse with an excess of buffer 2 for 5 min.
7. Repeat **step 6** a further three times to ensure complete removal of nonspecifically bound antibodies.

3.6.8. Signal Generation and Detection

1. Mix equal volumes of detection solution 1 and detection solution 2 to give sufficient reagent to cover the blot (0.125 mL/cm^2 is recommended).
2. Drain the excess buffer and place the blot on a sheet of SaranWrap DNA side up. Add the detection buffer directly to the blot on the side carrying the DNA.
3. Incubate for precisely 1 min at room temperature.
4. Drain off the excess detection buffer and wrap the blot in SaranWrap. Gently smooth out air pockets.

5. Place the blot DNA side up, in a film cassette. Work as quickly as possible, minimizing the delay between incubating the blots in substrate and exposing them to film (next step).
6. Switch off the lights and place a sheet of autoradiography film on top of the blots. Close the cassette.
7. Expose the film for the required length of time and develop as recommended for the film type.

3.7. DNA Extraction From Agarose Gel

Once a positive band has been identified using ALK probe hybridization, the DNA band must be recovered from a new gel electrophoresis of the same RACE reaction products (*see* **Note 15**). Before beginning: Preheat an aliquot of TE buffer to 70°C. Equilibrate a water bath or heat block to 50°C. Verify that ethanol has been added to wash buffer L2.

1. Gel slice excision: Cut the area of gel containing the DNA fragment using a clean, sharp blade. Minimize the amount of surrounding agarose excised with the fragment.
2. Gel slice weighting: Weight the gel slice. Place up to 400 mg of gel into a 1.5-mL polypropylene tube. Divide gel slices exceeding 400 mg among additional tubes. Add 30 µL of gel solubilization buffer L1 for every 10 mg of gel.
3. Gel solubilizaton and DNA binding: Incubate at 50°C for 15 min. Mix every 3 min to ensure gel dissolution. After gel slice appears dissolved, incubate for 5 min longer.
4. Cartridge loading: Place a spin cartridge into a 2-mL wash tube. Pipet the mixture from **step 3** into the spin cartridge. Centrifuge the mixture in a microcentrifuge at 12,000*g* for 1 min. Discard the flow-through.
5. Place the spin cartridge back into the 2-mL wash tube. Add 500 µL of gel solubilization buffer L1 to the spin cartridge. Incubate at room temperature for 1 min, then centrifuge at 12,000*g* for 1 min. Discard the flow-through.
6. Cartridge wash: Place the spin cartridge back into the 2-mL wash tube. Add 700 µL of wash buffer L2 to the spin cartridge and incubate for 5 min at room temperature. Centrifuge at 12,000*g* for 1 min. Discard the flow-through. Centrifuge again for 1 min to remove residual wash buffer.
7. DNA elution: Place the spin cartridge into a 1.5-mL recovery tube. Add 50 µL of warm TE buffer directly to the center of the spin cartridge. Incubate for 1 min at room temperature, then centrifuge at 12,000*g* for 2 min.

3.8. RACE Product Direct Sequencing

1. For each reaction add the following components to a separate 0.2-mL thin-walled PCR tube:

Terminator ready reaction mix	3 µL
Primer (*see* **Note 16**)	0.32 µL (3.2 pmol)
PCR product (*see* **Note 17**)	X µL
Sterilized, deionized water	to 20 µL

2. Mix well and close the tubes.
3. Place the tubes in a thermocycler and set the volume to 20 µL.
4. Repeat the following for 25 cycles:

   96°C for 10 s.
   50°C for 5 s.
   60°C for 4 min.
   To 4°C until ready to purify.
5. Start the purification of extension products by ethanol precipitation by mixing the extension product with 16 µL of deionized water and 64 µL of nondenatured 95% ethanol (*see* **Note 18**).
6. Leave the tubes at room temperature for 1 h to precipitate the extension products.
7. Place the tubes in a microcentrifuge and mark their orientations. Spin the tubes for 20 min at maximum speed.
8. Carefully aspirate the supernatants with a separate pipet tip for each sample and discard. Pellets may or may not be visible.
9. Add 250 µL of 70% ethanol to the tubes and vortex them briefly.
10. Place the tubes in the microcentrifuge in the same orientation as in **step 7** and spin for 10 min at maximum speed.
11. Aspirate the supernatants carefully as in **step 8**.
12. Place the tubes with the lids open in a heat block or thermal cycler at 90°C for 1 min.
13. The dried samples can now be analyzed in an appropriate ABI Prism sequencer.

3.9. Full-Length ALK Fusion Gene PCR Amplification

The previous sequence analysis leads to the identification of the corresponding ALK partner. Then, you can design primers spanning the whole coding region of the fusion gene to obtain a full cDNA sequence for later functional characterization.

1. Perform the PCR following the steps of **Subheading 3.4.** but using appropriate primers that must be designed according to the ALK partner identified in the RACE reaction (*see* **Note 19**).
2. PCR program must be adapted to the annealing temperature of the primers. Extension time must also be set according to the putative length of the cDNA to be amplified.
3. Direct sequencing of this PCR product must be performed using the same protocol as for RACE product sequencing but using appropriate internal primers depending on the particular sequences implicated.

4. Notes

1. A control GSP1 primer is provided with the kit to perform the first strand cDNA synthesis from the control RNA, which is also included in the kit.
2. Total RNA can be isolated with any of the standard methods currently used. Control RNA is included in the 5'RACE reagents, and 1 µL must be used in the first strand cDNA synthesis.

3. Thirty-minute incubation is usually sufficient for short (<4 kb) mRNAs. Longer transcripts require at least 50 min to synthesize enough cDNA for a consistent signal in long PCR. If you have more than 5 µg of total RNA, increase reaction volume and amount of SuperScript II RT proportionately. If you have less than 1 µg of total RNA, no changes to the protocol are necessary.
4. The binding solution must be at room temperature for efficient binding of the DNA.
5. Save the solution until recovery of the cDNA is confirmed.
6. Failure to remove all the ethanol can result in poor recovery of DNA.
7. It is very important for the deionized water to be at 65°C to maximize recovery of DNA.
8. To evaluate the specificity of the subsequent amplification reaction from the oligo-dC tail, inclusion of a control reaction that omits TdT is recommended.
9. A control GSP2 primer is provided with the kit to perform a control PCR amplification from the 5'RACE reaction previously performed on the control RNA. The predicted size of the amplified band is 711 pb.
10. The role of the GSP3 primer from the 3' gene (ALK in our case) is different from the control GSP3 primer provided with the kit. The former is used together with AAP primer but the later is used together with control GSP2 primer (use 1 µL of each primer/sample) to perform a control PCR amplification from the 5'RACE reaction on the control RNA or from control DNA (also included in the 5'RACE kit, use 5 µL in a total reaction volume of 50 µL). The predicted size of the amplified band is 500 pb. This amplification can be used to check the appropriate performance of the PCR for each step of the 5'RACE protocol (from control RNA) or to ensure a positive control in the PCR amplifications (from control DNA).
11. The volumes corresponding to X and Y should be adjusted to complete the total reaction volume. The molecular weight corresponding to 100 pmol of an oligonucleotide is dependent on the length of the sequence.
12. Avoid placing the probe directly on the blot to perform a uniform labeling in all the blot surface.
13. Hybridization time can be increased up to 17 h without any significant change in sensitivity.
14. This temperature should be 3–5°C less than the Tm of the probe (for ALK the recommended final temperature is 45°C).
15. To obtain a consistent band and thus enough DNA from the gel purification, it may be necessary to merge some gel wells to load three to four RACE products.
16. The first sequencing reaction must be performed using ALK 3 probe primer but other primers must be used as necessary in the sequencing reactions of the full-length ALK fusion transcript.
17. Depending on the length of the PCR product to be sequenced, different quantities (X) must be used according to the following relations:

100–200 bp	1–3 ng
200–500 bp	3–10 ng
500–1000 bp	5–20 ng

1000–2000 bp	10–40 ng
>2000 bp	40–100 ng

18. Final ethanol concentration must be 60% ± 3%. Avoid use of absolute (100%) ethanol as starting solution because absolute ethanol absorbs water from the atmosphere, gradually decreasing its concentration.
19. Forward and reverse primers must be designed by annealing upstream of the translation start codon (for the forward primer) and downstream of the translation stop codon (for the reverse primer).

Acknowledgments

The work performed by the authors is supported by the Instituto de Salud Carlos III (FIS 01/3046, G03/179, and C03/10) and Comisión Interministerial de Ciencia y Tecnología (CICYT, SAF 92/3261).

References

1. Falini, B., Bigerna, B., Fizzotti, M., Pulford, K., Pileri, S. A., Delsol, G., et al. (1998) ALK expression defines a distinct group of T/null lymphomas ("ALK lymphomas") with a wide morphological spectrum. *Am.J.Pathol.* **153**, 875–886
2. Benharroch, D., Meguerian-Bedoyan, Z., Lamant, L., Amin, C., Brugieres, L., Terrier-Lacombe, M. J., et al. (1998) ALK-positive lymphoma: a single disease with a broad spectrum of morphology. *Blood* **91**, 2076–2084
3. Morris, S. W., Xue, L., Ma, Z., and Kinney, M. C. (2001) Alk+ CD30+ lymphomas: a distinct molecular genetic subtype of non-Hodgkin's lymphoma. *Br. J. Haematol.* **113**, 275–295
4. Drexler, H. G., Gignac, S. M., von Wasielewski, R., Werner, M., and Dirks, W. G. (2000) Pathobiology of NPM-ALK and variant fusion genes in anaplastic large cell lymphoma and other lymphomas. *Leukemia* **14**, 1533–1559
5. Morris, S. W., Kirstein, M. N., Valentine, M. B., Dittmer, K., Shapiro, D. N., Look, A. T., et al. (1995) Fusion of a kinase gene, ALK, to a nucleolar protein gene, NPM, in Non-Hodgkin's lymphoma. *Science* **267**, 316–317
6. Lamant, L., Dastugue, N., Pulford, K., Delsol, G., and Mariame, B. (1999) A new fusion gene TPM3-ALK in Anaplastic Large Cell Lymphoma created by a (1;2)(q25;p23) translocation. *Blood* **93**, 3088–3095
7. Hernandez, L., Pinyol, M., Hernandez, S., Bea, S., Pulford, K., Rosenwald, A., et al. (1999) TRK-fused gene (TFG) is a new partner of ALK in Anaplastic Large Cell Lymphoma producing two structurally different TFG-ALK translocations. *Blood* **94**, 3265–3268
8. Colleoni, G. W., Bridge, J. A., Garicochea, B., Liu, J., Filippa, D. A., and Ladanyi, M. (2000) ATIC-ALK: A novel variant ALK gene fusion in Anaplastic Large Cell Lymphoma resulting from the recurrent cryptic chromosomal inversion, inv(2)(p23q35). *Am. J. Pathol.* **156**, 781–789
9. Trinei, M., Lanfrancone, L., Campo, E., Pulford, K., Mason, D. Y., Pelicci, P. G., and Falini, B. (2000) A new variant anaplastic lymphoma kinase (ALK)-fusion

protein (ATIC-ALK) in a case of ALK-positive Anaplastic Large Cell Lymphoma. *Cancer Res.* **60**, 793–798

10. Ma, Z., Cools, J., Marynen, P., Cui, X., Siebert, R., Gesk, S., et al. (2000) Inv(2)(p23q35) in Anaplastic Large-Cell Lymphoma induces constitutive anaplastic lymphoma kinase (ALK) tyrosine kinase activation by fusion to ATIC, an enzyme involved in purine nucleotide biosynthesis. *Blood* **95**, 2144–2149
11. Tort, F., Pinyol, M., Pulford, K., Roncador, G., Hernandez, L., Nayach, I., et al. Molecular characterization of a new ALK translocation involving moesin (MSN-ALK) in anaplastic large cell lymphoma. *Lab. Invest.* **81,** 419–426.
12. Touriol, C., Greenland, C., Lamant, L., Pulford, K., Bernard, F., Rousset, T., et al. (2000) Further demonstration of the diversity of chromosomal changes involving 2p23 in ALK-positive lymphoma: 2 cases expressing ALK kinase fused to CLTCL (clathrin chain polypeptide-like). *Blood* **95**, 3204–3207
13. Hernandez, L., Bea, S., Bellosillo, B., Pinyol, M., Falini, B., Carbone, A., et al. (2002) Diversity of genomic breakpoints in TFG-ALK translocations in anaplastic large cell lymphomas: identification of a new TFG-ALK(XL) chimeric gene with transforming activity. *Am.J.Pathol.* **160**, 1487–1494
14. Frohman, M. A., Dush, M. K., and Martin, G. R. (1988) Rapid production of full-length cDNAs from rare transcripts: amplification using a single gene-specific oligonucleotide primer. *Proc. Natl. Acad. Sci. USA* **85**, 8998–9002
15. Kwok, S. and Higuchi, R. (1989) Avoiding false positives with PCR. *Nature* **339**, 237–238.

16

Follicular Lymphoma

Quantitation of Minimal Residual Disease by PCR of the t(14;18) Translocation

Angela Darby and John G. Gribben

Summary

During the past decade, considerable advances have been made in the sensitivity of detection of residual lymphoma and leukemia cells. In particular, polymerase chain reaction (PCR)-based assays are capable of detecting one tumor cell in as many as 10^6 normal cells. The applicability of these techniques has been made possible by the identification and cloning of the breakpoints associated with specific chromosomal translocations associated with particular subtypes of lymphoma, best studied for the t(14;18), which occurs in most cases of follicular lymphoma. Although we are approaching the time when PCR-based methods of detection of minimal residual lymphoma detection become a routine part of staging, both at diagnosis and after therapy, it is not yet possible to determine whether the detection of residual lymphoma cells by PCR is an indication to continue therapy. Therefore, although these techniques provide a useful adjunct to standard methods of detection and diagnosis, their role in staging of disease outcome remains investigational.

Key Words: Follicular lymphoma, Bcl-2 gene, minimal residual disease, bone marrow purging, t(14;18) translocation.

1. Introduction

Follicular lymphoma remains incurable despite advances made in treatment. Although these patients often achieve complete remission (CR), they almost invariably relapse. The source of relapse is from persistence of minimal residual disease (MRD): residual lymphoma cells that are below the limit of detection using standard diagnostic techniques. It would seem obvious that if residual malignant cells can be detected in a patient, then additional therapy would be necessary for cure. This has never been established conclusively for the minimal residual numbers of neoplastic cells that can now be detected in patients after achievement of a clinical CR. The critical issue now is to determine

From: *Methods in Molecular Medicine, Vol. 115: Lymphoma: Methods and Protocols*
Edited by: T. Illidge and P. W. M. Johnson © Humana Press Inc., Totowa, NJ

whether such sensitive detection of residual detectable lymphoma cells by polymerase chain reaction (PCR) will identify which patients will relapse. If this proves to be the case, then molecular biologic techniques will become a routine part of staging and follow up of patients and redefine our concept of CR, so that the goal of therapy should be achievement of a "molecular CR."

1.1. PCR Amplification of t(14;18)

One of the most widely studied chromosomal translocations is t(14;18)(q32;q21), which occurs in as many as 85% of patients with follicular lymphoma and 30% of patients with diffuse lymphoma ***(1–4)***. In the t(14;18) the *bcl-2* proto-oncogene on chromosome 18 is juxtaposed with the immunoglobulin heavy chain (IgH) locus on chromosome 14 (**Fig. 1**). The breakpoints have been cloned and sequenced and have been shown to cluster at two main regions 3' to the bcl-2 coding region ***(5–8)***. The major breakpoint region (MBR) occurs within the 3' untranslated region of the bcl-2 gene ***(5–8)***, and the minor cluster region (mcr) is located some 20 kb downstream ***(9)***. Juxtaposition of the transcriptionally active IgH with the bcl-2 gene results in upregulation of bcl-2 gene product and subsequent resistance to cell death by apoptosis ***(10–13)***.

The clustering of the breakpoints at these two main regions at the bcl-2 gene and the availability of consensus regions of the IgH J regions ***(14)*** make this gene an ideal candidate for PCR amplification to detect lymphoma cells containing this translocation ***(15–18)***. This extremely sensitive technique is capable of detecting one lymphoma cell in as many as 10^6 normal cells. A major advantage in the detection of lymphoma cells bearing the bcl-2/IgH translocation is that deoxyribonucleic acid (DNA) can be used to detect the translocation. In addition, because there is a variation at the site of the breakpoint at the bcl-2 gene and because the translocation occurs into the IgH variable region, the PCR products are of different sizes and have unique sequences. The size of the PCR product can be assessed by gel electrophoresis and used as confirmation that the expected size fragment is amplified from a specific patient. Of note, this translocation also has been detected in the peripheral blood of normal individuals, and care must be taken evaluating residual disease since normal lymphocytes can also have this rearrangement ***(19–23)***.

1.2. PCR Detection of Antigen Receptor Gene Rearrangements

Although most follicular lymphomas exhibit t(14;18) and other lymphomas have characteristic chromosomal translocations, for patients with follicular lymphoma who do have a PCR amplifiable t(14;18), alternative strategies must be developed to detect MRD. Follicular lymphomas rearrange their Ig genes, providing a clonal marker that also can be amplified by PCR. The most

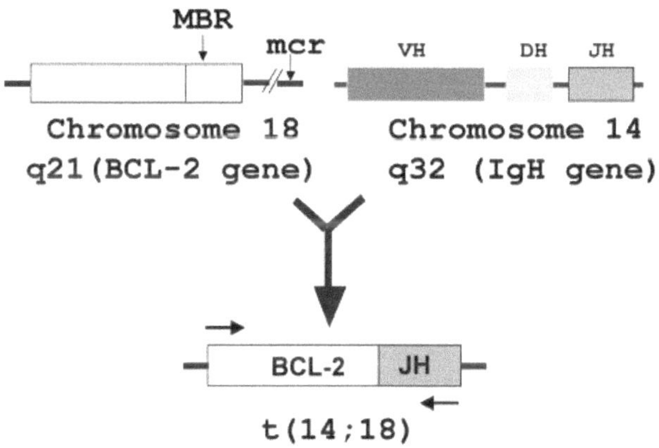

Fig. 1. The bcl-2/IgH rearrangement results from the translocation of the bcl-2 proto-oncogene from chromosome 18 to the IgH locus on chromosome 14. Most breaks occur within the MBR within the 3' untranslated region. An mcr occurs some 15 kb downstream. PCR amplification of the derivative chromosome can be performed using primers 5' to the breakpoint and consensus J_H primers.

hypervariable region of the Ig molecule is the third complementarity-determining region (CDRIII). The CDRIII is generated by the rearrangement of germline variable (V), diversity (D), and joining (J) region elements ***(24–26)***. The enzyme terminal deoxynucleotidyl transferase (TdT) inserts random nucleotides at both the V-D and D-J junctions, and further diversity is generated by random excision of nucleotides by exonucleases ***(27)***. The final V-N-D-N-J sequence that comprises the CDRIII region is unique to that cell and acts as a unique marker for that leukemic clone. PCR amplification of the CDR III region is possible due to the presence of highly conserved sequences within the Variable (V_H) and Joining (J_H) regions. The large number of V regions makes the design of single oligonucleotide primer pairs capable of amplifying all Ig rearrangements difficult. At the time of initial presentation, deoxyribonucleic acid (DNA) from patients with lymphoma can be PCR amplified using consensus V_H and J_H region primers. Although these techniques have the advantage of being applicable to a greater number of patients, they are less sensitive than the detection of chromosomal translocations. More highly sensitive tumor detection can be achieved using primers directed against the unique junctional region sequences within the rearranged antigen receptor genes ***(28)***. The clonal product can then be directly sequenced and patient-specific probes constructed using N region nucleotide sequences. This strategy successfully amplifies and allows sequencing of the CDRIII to design patient allele-specific oligonucleotide to be used as oligonucleotide probes for the subsequent detec-

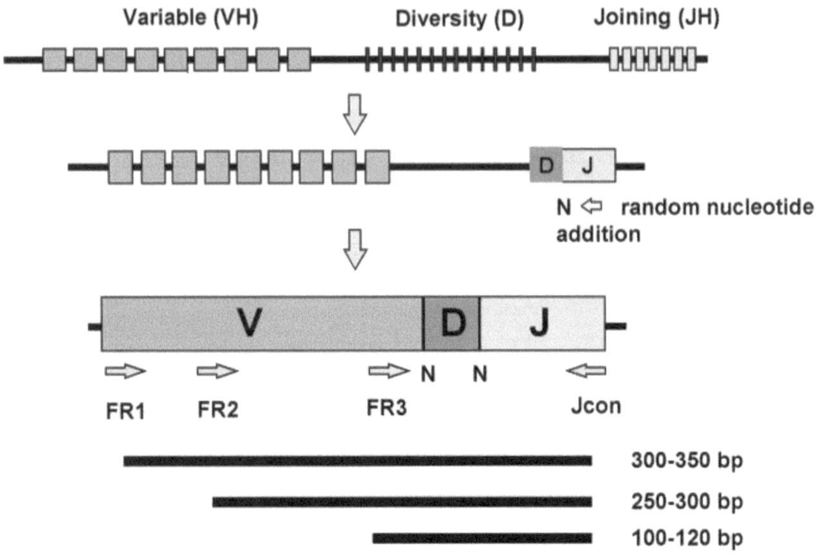

Fig. 2. PCR amplification of the complementarity determining region (CDR) III region of the IgH locus. PCR amplification can be performed using consensus primers to the FR3, resulting in a PCR product of 100–120 bp, or by using a series of family specific primers to the FR1, resulting in a PCR product of 300–350 bp.

tion of MRD or as primers for second round or nested PCR amplification *(29–32)*. The strategies used to PCR amplify the CDRIII region is shown in **Fig. 2** and use a variety of consensus primers from the framework regions (FR) of the V and J regions. The utility of PCR amplification of the CDR III region in B-cell malignancies, including anaplastic lymphocytic leukemia, myeloma, and chronic lymphocytic leukemia, has been demonstrated by many studies *(32–36)*. However, fewer studies have examined the clinical significance of MRD detection using Ig rearrangements in non-Hodgkin's lymphoma *(32,36)*. Analysis of the IgH V genes in follicular lymphoma cells demonstrates that they have acquired somatic hypermutations and frequently demonstrate clonal variation, presumably resulting from ongoing activity of the mechanism of somatic hypermutation *(37)*, making the use of consensus region primers more difficult.

1.3. Clinical Utility of Minimal Disease Detection in Lymphoma

1.3.1. PCR Detection of Bone Marrow Infiltration as a Staging Procedure

A number of studies have examined the use of PCR detection of t(14;18) as a staging procedure to detect lymphoma cells in the bone marrow (BM) and peripheral blood (PB) at the time of initial presentation. These PCR studies have all detected lymphoma cells in the BM in a number of patients who had no evidence of marrow infiltration by morphology in patients with advanced stage disease ***(18,38–42)***. However, PCR analysis cannot replace morphologic assessment of BM because not all patients have translocation that is detectable by PCR; therefore, techniques should be viewed as complementary ***(18,39)***.

1.3.2. PCR Detection of MRD After Therapy

After combination chemotherapy, PCR-detectable lymphoma cells bearing the t(14;18) remain detectable in the BM ***(18,43)***. Long-term analysis after completion of conventional-dose chemotherapy also has suggested that conventional-dose chemotherapy does not eradicate PCR-detectable disease, but that this might not be associated with poor outcome because there was no association between the presence or absence of PCR-detectable lymphoma cells and clinical outcome ***(42)***. This result confirms the previous observation that some patients can indeed remain in long-term continuous complete remission despite the presence of PCR-detectable lymphoma cells ***(44)***. Larger studies have suggested that some subsets of patients may achieve "molecular CR" after completion of chemotherapy and that this is associated with improved outcome ***(45)***. However, often studies have examined MRD in PB rather than BM. PB is less frequently involved than BM at presentation but is a more frequent finding as disease progresses ***(46,47)***. Several studies of patients at the time of presentation have suggested a high level of concordance between the detection of lymphoma cells in the PB and BM when assessed by PCR ***(39,41,48)***. However, other studies have found that the BM is more likely than PB to contain infiltrating lymphoma cells in previously untreated patients ***(40)*** and after therapy ***(49)***.

1.3.3. Contribution of Reinfused Lymphoma Cells to Relapse After Autologous Stem Cell Transplantation

There has been increasing interest in the use of high-dose therapy as salvage therapy for patients who have failed conventional-dose chemotherapy regimens. The resulting myeloablation after high-dose therapy can be rescued by the infusion of allogeneic or autologous BM. The major obstacle to the use of autologous bone marrow transplantation (ABMT) is that the reinfusion of occult tumor cells harbored within the marrow may result in more rapid relapse of disease. To minimize the effects of the infusion of significant numbers of malignant cells, most centers obtain marrow for ABMT when the patient is either in CR or when there is no evidence by histologic examination of BM infiltration of disease. As discussed previously, more sensitive techniques have clearly demonstrated that patients with histologically normal BM often harbor minimal numbers of cancer cells. A variety of methods have therefore been developed to "purge" malignant cells from the stem cell collections. Because of their specificity, monoclonal antibodies are ideal agents for selective elimination of malignant cells. Studies have demonstrated that those patients whose BM contain PCR-detectable lymphoma cells after immunologic purging had an increased incidence of relapse after autologous stem cell transplantation in non-Hodgkin's lymphoma ***(43,50)***.

1.3.4. Detection of Residual Lymphoma Cells After Autologous Stem Cell Transplantation

In a series of studies at Dana-Farber Cancer Institute, PCR analysis was performed on serial BM samples obtained after stem cell transplantation (SCT) to assess whether high-dose therapy might be capable of depleting PCR-detectable lymphoma cells ***(32,35,36,51)***. The disease-free survival of patients in these studies was greatly adversely influenced by the persistence or reappearance of residual detectable lymphoma cells after high-dose therapy. The failure to achieve or maintain a CR as assessed by PCR analysis of BM was predictive of which patients would subsequently relapse. These findings have been confirmed in other studies ***(52–55)***. The results of these studies are supportive of the notion that detection of MRD by PCR identifies those patients who require additional treatment for cure and also suggest that our therapeutic goal should be to eradicate all PCR-detectable lymphoma cells. Of note, novel treatment approaches, including immunological approaches, also are capable of eradicating PCR-detectable disease and are in these cases also associated with improved outcome ***(45,56,57)***. The results of studies performed on patients who have undergone autologous SCT at Dana-Farber Cancer Institute are shown in **Fig. 3** and demonstrate that those patient who have no PCR-detectable MRD after SCT have improved outcome compared to those patients who have PCR-detachable disease at all time points after SCT.

1.4. Quantitation Using PCR

The prognostic significance of PCR-detectable MRD is not always clear. Patients with a variety of malignancies can have a long-term persistence of PCR-detectable MRD without relapse ***(44,58,59)***. Under these circumstances, more information may be available by quantification of MRD levels rather than just their presence or absence. Real-time quantitative PCR exploits the 5'–3' nuclease activity that is associated with *Taq* polymerase and a target specific fluorogenically labeled DNA probe (*see* **Note 1**). This probe is designed to anneal between the forward and reverse oligonucleotide primers used for PCR amplification. The nuclease activity of Taq polymerase cleaves the labeled probe during the extension phase of PCR amplification, producing a fluores-

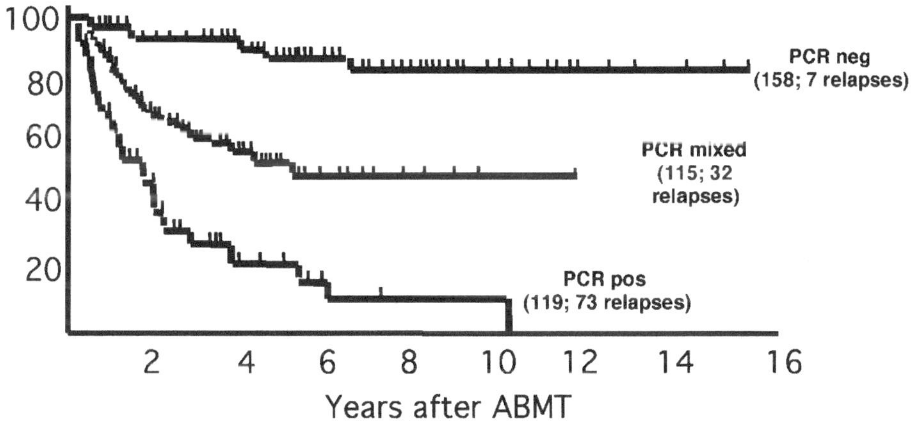

Fig. 3. Eradication of PCR-detectable disease is associated with improved outcome after ABMT. Those patients in whom no PCR-detectable tumor cells are found after ABMT (PCR neg.) have greatly improved outcome after ABMT than those patients in whom there is persistence of PCR- detectable disease (PCR pos.). Those patients who have PCR-detectable disease that is found intermittently (PCR mixed) have an intermediate prognosis.

cent signal that can be detected in solution. The amount of fluorescence produced in a reaction by this method is proportional to the starting DNA target number during early phases of amplification as shown in **Fig. 4** (*see* **Note 2**). The target number of cells within an unknown sample is then compared to known amounts of target, which are used to construct a standard curve (*see* **Note 3**). When this reaction is performed on a combined thermal cycler/sequence detector, a quantitative assessment of input target DNA copy number is made in the tube as the reaction proceeds. This method eliminates the need for post-PCR sample processing, thereby greatly increasing throughput. It also greatly reduces the potential for false-positive results by adding the additional level of specificity provided by the hybridization of a probe to sequences internal to amplification primers. Significant for purposes of MRD studies, real-time PCR has a relatively wide dynamic range. It is possible to accurately quantitate samples with greatly differing levels of tumor contamination.

Real-time quantitative PCR has been applied to the assessment of MRD levels for follicular lymphoma ***(60–62)***. Its application to MRD quantitation, in which IgH rearrangements are the targeted marker, however, is not as simple. Although the use of patient-specific probes is possible ***(63)***, this approach appears to be prohibitively expensive for large studies because of the high cost of producing a fluorogenically labeled probe specific for every patient. Techniques have been developed that use consensus IgH probes ***(64)***, but their

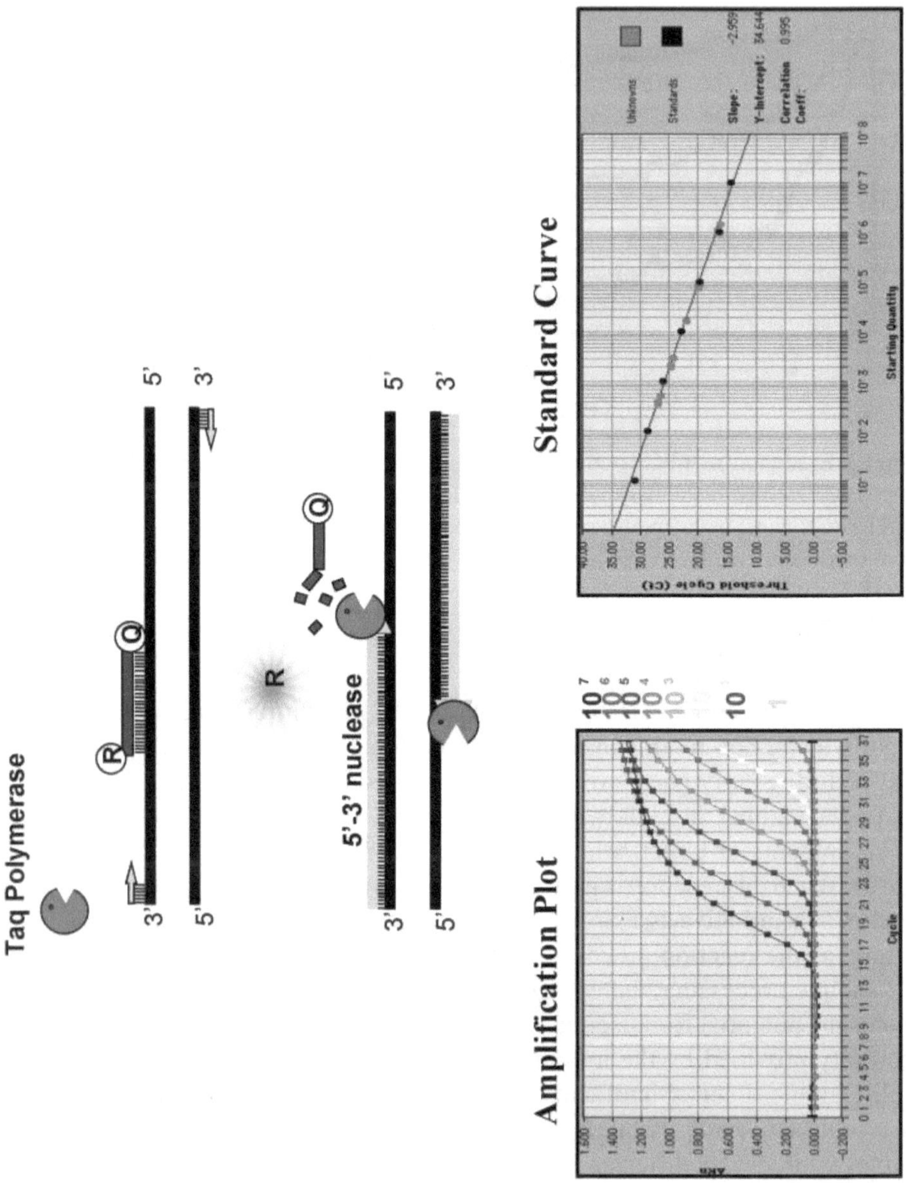
Taq Polymerase
R
Q
3'
5'
5'-3' nuclease
Amplification Plot
Cycle
Standard Curve
Threshold Cycle (Ct)
Starting Quantity
Unknowns
Standards
Slope: -2.959
Y-Intercept: 34.644
Correlation Coeff: 0.995

application is made even more difficult by the presence of somatic mutations in post-germinal center malignancies ***(61)***. *See* **Notes 4–6** for details on probe and primer selection.

2. Materials

2.1. Biological Material for Study

PCR can be carried out for the *MBR Bcl-2/IgH* rearrangement at both diagnosis and follow-up. At presentation, this is likely to be the diagnostic lymph node, bone marrow, and peripheral blood, whilst at follow-up, the tissue used is usually restricted to the bone marrow and/or peripheral blood. Blood samples and bone marrow aspirates are prepared by density gradient centrifugation to isolate the mononuclear cell fraction prior to DNA extraction.

2.2. Reagents and Solutions

2.2.1. DNA Extraction

Puregene (Flowgen Bioscience, Nottingham) kits yield good quality genomic DNA and are used by a number of laboratories which carry out this process regularly. Standard Phenol/Chloroform extraction is a cheaper alternative.

2.2.2. PCR Reaction Mixture

A 25 µL reaction mix is used containing:

1. 10X TaqMan Universal PCR Master Mix (PE Applied Biosystems).
2. 2.5 m*M* $MgCl_2$.
3. 200 µmol/L dATP, dCTP, and dGTP.
4. 400 µmol/L dUTP.
5. 0.5 U Uracil-*N*-glycosylase (UNG).
6. 1.25 U Amplitaq Gold DNA polymerase.
7. 900 nmol/L primers.
8. 200 nmol/L probe.
9. 500 ng of DNA
10. Sterile water to final volume of 25 µL.

Fig. 4. (*opposite page*) Quantitative real-time PCR analysis. The exonuclease activity of *Taq* polymerase can be used to cleave a quencher (Q) from a reporter (R) that will fluoresce in response to laser activation. The fluoresce will be proportional to the amount of starting target numbers as can be seen in the amplification plot of serial dilutions of a cell line within normal PB mononuclear cells. The target number in an unknown sample can then be quantified by comparison of the patient sample compared to a standard curve. *See* **Color Plate 12**, following page 270.

2.2.3. Oligonucleotide Sequences

Bcl-2 and Ig heavy chains:

Forward primer	tggtggtttgacctttagaga
Reverse primer	acctgaggagacggtgac

Probe (5'–3'):

Probe sequence ctgtttcaacacagacccacccagat

Reference gene:

Manufacturers supply standard housekeeping gene sets to act as a reference. β2-microglobulin is widely used.

2.3. Equipment

The ABI PRISM 7700 Sequence Detection System (PE Applied Biosystems, Foster City, CA) is most commonly used in published papers quantifying the *Bcl-2/IgH* translocation ***(65,66)***.

3. Methods

3.1. Sample Preparation

Mononculear cell suspensions are prepared by density gradient centrifugation, followed by washing in PBS, and extraction of genomic DNA using standard methods.

3.2 Amplification Conditions

1. Contamination elimination step: 60°C for 2 min (*see* **Note 7**).
2. Denaturation: 95°C for 10 min.

And then for 50 cycles:

1. Denaturation: 95°C for 15 s.
2. Combined annealing and extension: 60°C for 1 min.

Three replicates of each sample are routinely determined.

4. Notes

1. Real-time PCR is based on the detection and quantification of a fluorescent reporter whose signal increases in direct proportion to the amount of PCR product in the reaction ***(67)***. This is achieved using a fluorescent probe containing a fluorescent reporter dye [FAM (6-carboxy-fluoroscein)] at its 5' end and a quencher dye [TAMRA (6-carboxy-tetramethylrhodamine)] at the 3' end ***(68)***. The reporter and quencher are in close proximity, and, on irradiation, the excited fluorescent dye transfers energy to the nearby quencher rather than fluorescing. This is called fluorescence resonance energy transfer (FRET). During the exten-

sion phase of the PCR the probe binds to the template and the 5'–3' exonuclease activity of Taq polymerase cleaves the probe. The quencher is no longer in close proximity to the reporter dye, which can then fluoresce, with the amount of fluorescence being directly proportional to the rate of probe cleavage. Cleavage will only occur when the probe binds to the target thus fluorescence is proportional to the amount of product generated in each cycle of the PCR *(66)*. Fluorogenic probes must not have a G at the 5' end as this would position it adjacent to the reporter dye and continue to quench it even after cleavage *(67)*.

2. During the PCR reaction fluorescence is measured continuously. The increase in fluorescence above background (ΔRn) is plotted against PCR cycle number. The C_T value, or threshold cycle, is the cycle at which a significant increase in ΔRn is first observed (**Fig. 4**). This is the point when increase in fluorescence is associated with an exponential increase in PCR product during the log-linear phase. As shown in **Fig. 4**, a higher amount of initial DNA, gives an earlier detection of PCR product by fluorescence and, therefore, a lower C_T value. The C_T values for the samples containing known amounts of target are used to generate the standard curve and the amount of target in an unknown sample can then be quantified by comparison of the patient sample to the standard curve.
3. The standard curve is constructed using known amounts of target. Standard curves are prepared using a cell-line containing the bcl-2/IgH translocation. Tenfold dilutions are prepared in water producing standards ranging from 10^1 to 10^5 translocation-bearing t(14;18) cells. These standards are used to generate standard curves for both the Bcl-2/IgH gene rearrangement and the endogenous reference gene (β-2 microglobulin).
4. The selection of probes and primers *(69)* is standardized by the use of specific software for primer-probe design. The Primer Express software (Applied Biosystems) designs oligonucleotide triplets (two primers and a corresponding Taqman probe) that can all be amplified with the same protocol for reaction conditions and a universal master mix.
5. Initially the probe should be selected. Certain criteria should be fulfilled:-
   a. The G-C content should be in the range 30 to 80%.
   b. Runs of identical nucleotides should be avoided. In particular, probes should not contain four or more guanines.
   c. Guanine should not be on the 5' end of the probe.
   d. The probe should be less than 30 bp in length.
   e. The strand should be selected that gives the probe more Cs than Gs. If the software only displays probes that do not have more Cs than Gs then the complementary probe can be selected. In this case, it needs to be ensured that there is no C at the 3' end of the probe, otherwise the complement will have a G at the 5' end which is not permitted.
   f. For single probe assays the melting temperature (T_m) should be 68 to 70°C when using Primer Express Software.
6. Once the probe is selected it should be highlighted on the software and compatible primers can be selected. They should be designed so they are as close to the

probe as possible without overlapping it. The criteria for selecting a primer should be similar to the criteria for selecting a probe as outlined in **steps 1–3** in **Note 5**. If using Primer Express Software, the T_m should be 58 to 60°C. The five nucleotides at the 3' end should be no more than 2 G and/or C bases. Once the probe and primers are selected, reporter and quencher dyes can be added to the probe sequence.

7. Contamination from previous PCR reactions is eliminated via the action of uracil-*N*-glycosylase.

References

1. Yunis, J. J., Oken, M. M., Kaplan, M. E., Theologides, R. R., and Howe, A. (1982) Distinctive chromosomal abnormalities in histological subtypes of non-Hodgkin's lymphoma. *N. Engl. J. Med.* **307,** 1231–1236.
2. Weiss, L. M., Warnke, R. A., Sklar, J., and Cleary, M. L. (1987) Molecular analysis of the t(14;18) chromosomal translocation in malignant lymphomas. *N. Engl. J. Med.* **317,** 1185–1189.
3. Lee, M. S., Blick, M. B., Pathak, S., Trujillo, J. M., Butler, J. J., Katz, R. L., et al. (1987) The gene located at chromosome 18 band q21 is rearranged in uncultured diffuse lymphomas as well as follicular lymphomas. *Blood* **70,** 90–95.
4. Aisenberg, A. C. (1993) Utility of gene rearrangements in lymphoid malignancies [review]. *Ann. Rev. Med.* **44,** 75–84.
5. Bakshi, A., Jensen, J. P., Goldman, P., Wright, J. J., McBride, O. W., Epstein, A. L., et al. (1985) Cloning the chromosomal breakpoint of t(14;18) human lymphomas: clustering around J_H on chromosome 14 and near a transcriptional unit on 18. *Cell* **41,** 899–906.
6. Cleary, M. L., and Sklar, J. (1985) Nucleotide sequence of a t(14;18) chromosomal breakpoint in follicular lymphoma and demonstration of a breakpoint cluster region near a transcriptionally active locus on chromosome 18. *Proc. Natl. Acad. Sci. USA.* **82,** 7439–7443.
7. Tsujimoto, Y., Gorman, J., Jaffe, E., and Croce, C. M. (1985) The t(14;18) chromosome translocations involved in B-cell neoplasms result from mistakes in VDJ joining. *Science* **229,** 1390–1393.
8. Cleary, M. L., Smith, S. D., and Sklar, J. (1986) Cloning and structural analysis of cDNAs for bcl-2 and a hybrid bcl-2/immunoglobulin transcript resulting from the t(14;18) translocation. *Cell* **47,** 19–28.
9. Cleary, M. L., Galili, N., and Sklar, J. (1986) Detection of a second t(14;18) breakpoint cluster region in human follicular lymphomas. *J. Exp. Med.* **164,** 315–320.
10. Miyashita, T., and Reed, J. C. (1992) bcl-2 gene transfer increases relative resistance of S49.1 and WEHI7.2 lymphoid cells to cell death and DNA fragmentation induced by glucocorticoids and multiple chemotherapeutic drugs. *Cancer Res.* **52,** 5407–5411.
11. Miyashita, T., and Reed, J. C. (1993) Bcl-2 oncoprotein blocks chemotherapy-induced apoptosis in a human leukemia cell line. *Blood* **81,** 151–157.

12. Korsmeyer, S. J. (1992) Bcl-2 initiates a new category of oncogenes: regulators of cell death. *Blood* **80,** 879–886.
13. Korsmeyer, S. J., Shutter, J. R., Veis, D. J., Merry, D. E., and Oltvai, Z. N. (1993) Bcl-2/Bax: a rheostat that regulates an anti-oxidant pathway and cell death. *Semin. Cancer Biol.* **4,** 327–332.
14 Ravetch, J. V., Siebenlist, U., Korsmeyer, S., Waldman, T., and Leder, P. (1981) Structure of the human immunoglobulin m locus: characterization of embryonic and rearranged J and D genes. *Cell* **27,** 583–591.
15. Lee, M. S., Chang, K. S., Cabanillas, F., Freireich, E. J., Trujillo, J. M., and Stass, S. A. (1987) Detection of minimal residual disease carrying the t(14;18) by DNA sequence amplification. *Science* **237,** 175–178.
16. Crescenzi, M., Seto, M., Herzig, G. P., Weiss, P. D., Griffith, R. C., and Korsmeyer, S. J. (1988) Thermostable DNA polymerase chain amplification of t(14;18) chromosome breakpoints and detection of minimal residual disease. *Proc. Natl. Acad. Sci. USA* **85,** 4869–4873.
17. Ngan, B. Y., Nourse, J., and Cleary, M. L. (1989) Detection of chromosomal translocation t(14;18) within the minor cluster region of bcl-2 by polymerase chain reaction and direct genomic sequencing of the enzymatically amplified DNA in follicular lymphomas. *Blood* **73,** 1759–1762.
18. Gribben, J. G., Freedman, A., Woo, S. D., Blake, K., Shu, R. S., Freeman, G., et al. (1991) All advanced stage non-Hodgkin's lymphomas with a polymerase chain reaction amplifiable breakpoint of bcl-2 have residual cells containing the bcl-2 rearrangement at evaluation and after treatment. *Blood* **78,** 3275–3280.
19. Limpens, J., de Jong, D., Voetdijk, A. M. H., Price, C., Young, B. D., van Ommen, G. J. B., et al. (1990) Translocation t(14;18) in benign B lymphocytes. *Blood* **76,** Suppl 1, 237a.
20. Limpens, J., de Jong, D., van Krieken, J. H., Price, C. G., Young, B. D., van Ommen, G. J., et al.. (1991) Bcl-2/JH rearrangements in benign lymphoid tissues with follicular hyperplasia. *Oncogene* **6,** 2271–2276.
21. Limpens, J., Stad, R., Vos, C., de Vlaam, C., de Jong, D., van Ommen, G. J., et al. (1995) Lymphoma-associated translocation t(14; 18) in blood B-cells of normal individuals. *Blood* **85,** 2528–2536.
22. Aster, J. C., Kobayashi, Y., Shiota, M., Mori, S., and Sklar, J. (1992) Detection of the t(14; 18) at similar frequencies in hyperplastic lymphoid tissues from American and Japanese patients. *Am. J. Pathol.* **141,** 291–299.
23. Summers, K. E., Goff, L. K., Wilson, A. G., Gupta, R. K., Lister, T. A., and Fitzgibbon, J. (2001) Frequency of the Bcl-2/IgH rearrangement in normal individuals: implications for the monitoring of disease in patients with follicular lymphoma. *J. Clin. Oncol.* **19,** 420–424.
24. Seidman, J. G., Max, E. E., and Leder, P. (1979) A K-immunoglobulin gene is formed by site specific recombination without further somatic mutation. *Nature* **280,** 280.
25. Early, P., Huang, H., Davis, M., Calame, K., and Hood, L. (1980) An immunoglobulin heavy chain variable region gene is generated from three segments of DNA. *Cell* **19,** 281.

26. Sakano, H., Kurosawa, Y., Weigert, M., and Tonegawa, S. (1981) Identification and nucleotide sequence of a diversity DNA segment (D) of immunoglobulin heavy chain genes. *Nature* **290,** 562.
27. Tonegawa, S. (1983) Somatic generation of antibody diversity. *Nature* **302,** 575–581.
28. Billadeau, D., Blackstadt, M., Greipp, P., Kyle, R. A., Oken, M. M., Kay, N., et al. (1991) Analysis of B-lymphoid malignancies using allele-specific polymerase chain reaction: a technique for sequential quantitation of residual disease. *Blood* **78,** 3021–3029.
29. Deane, M., McCarthy, K. P., Wiedemann, L. M., and Norton, J. D. (1991) An improved method for detection of B-lymphoid clonality by polymerase chain reaction. *Leukemia* **5,** 726–730.
30. Wan, J. H., Sykes, P. J., Orell, S. R., and Morley, A. A. (1992) Rapid method for detecting monoclonality in B-cell lymphoma in lymph node aspirates using the polymerase chain reaction. *J Clin Pathol* **45,** 420–423.
31. Diss, T. C., Peng, H., Wotherspoon, A. C., Isaacson, P. G., and Pan, L. (1993) Detection of monoclonality in low-grade B-cell lymphomas using the polymerase chain reaction is dependent on primer selection and lymphoma type. *J Pathol* **169,** 291–295.
32. Andersen, N. S., Donovan, J. W., Borus, J. S., Poor, C. M., Neuberg, D., Aster, J. C., et al. (1997) Failure of immunologic purging in mantle cell lymphoma assessed by PCR detection of minimla residual disease. *Blood* **90,** 4212–4221.
33. Steward, C. G., Potter, M. N., and Oakhill, A. (1992) Third complementarity determining region (CDR III) sequence analysis in childhood B-lineage acute lymphoblastic leukemia: implications for the design of oligonucleotide probes for use in monitoring minimal residual disease. *Leukemia* **6,** 1213–1219.
34. Bakkus, M. H., Heirman, C., Van, R. I., Van, C. B., and Thielemans, K. (1992) Evidence that multiple myeloma Ig heavy chain VDJ genes contain somatic mutations but show no intraclonal variation. *Blood* **80,** 2326–2335.
35. Provan, D., Zwicky, C., Bartlett-Pandite, L., Maddocks, A., Corradini, P., Soiffer, R., Ritz, J., et al. (1996) Eradication of PCR detectable chronic lymphocytic leukemia cells is associated with improved outcome after bone marrow transplantation. *Blood* **88,** 2228–2235.
36. Zwicky, C. S., Maddocks, A. B., Andersen, N., and Gribben, J. G. (1996) Eradication of polymerase chain reaction immunoglobulin gene rearrangement in non-Hodgkin's lymphoma as associated with decreased relapse after autologous bone marrow transplantation. *Blood* **88,** 3314–3322.
37. Bahler, D. W., and Levy, R. (1992) Clonal evolution of a follicular lymphoma: evidence for antigen selection. *Proc. Natl. Acad. Sci. USA* **89,** 6770–6774.
38. Hickish, T. F., Purvies, H., Mansi, J., Soukop, M., and Cunningham, D. (1991) Molecular monitoring of low grade non-Hodgkin's lymphoma by gene amplification. *Br. J. Cancer* **64,** 1161–1163.
39. Berinstein, N. L., Reis, M. D., Ngan, B. Y., Sawka, C. A., Jamal, H. H., and Kuzniar, B. (1993) Detection of occult lymphoma in the peripheral blood and

bone marrow of patients with untreated early stage and advanced stage follicular lymphoma. *J. Clin. Oncol.* **11,** 1344–1352.

40. Berinstein, N. L., Jamal, H. H., Kuzniar, B., Klock, R. J., and Reis, M. D. (1993) Sensitive and reproducible detection of occult disease in patients with follicular lymphoma by PCR amplification of t(14; 18) both pre- and post-treatment. *Leukemia* **7,** 113–119.
41. Yuan, R., Dowling, P., Zucca, E., Diggelmann, H., and Cavalli, F. (1993) Detection of bcl-2/JH rearrangement in follicular and diffuse lymphoma: concordant results of peripheral blood and bone marrow analysis at diagnosis. *Br. J. Cancer* **67,** 922–925.
42. Lambrechts, A. C., Hupkes, P. E., Dorssers, L. C. J., and van't Veer, M. B. (1994) Clinical significance of translocation t(14;18) positive cells in the circulation of patients with stage III or IV follicular non-Hodgkin's lymphoma during first remission. *J. Clin. Oncol.* **12,** 1541–1546.
43. Gribben, J. G., Freedman, A. S., Neuberg, D., Roy, D. C., Blake, K. W., Woo, S. D., et al. (1991) Immunologic purging of marrow assessed by PCR before autologous bone marrow transplantation for B-cell lymphoma. *N Engl J Med* **325,** 1525–1533.
44. Price, C. G. A., Meerabux, J., Murtagh, S., Cotter, F. E., Rohatiner, A. Z. S., Young, B. D., et al. (1991) The significance of circulating cells carrying t(14;18) in long remission from follicular lymphoma. *J. Clin. Oncol.* 9, 1527–1532.
45. Lopez-Guillermo, A., Cabanillas, F., McLaughlin, P., Smith, T., Hagemeister, F., Rodriguez, M. A., et al. (1998) The clinical significance of molecular response in indolent follicular lymphomas. *Blood* **91,** 2955–2960.
46. Ault, K. A. (1979) Detection of small numbers of monoclonal B lymphocytes in the blood of patients with B-cell lymphoma. *N. Engl. J. Med.* **300,** 1401–1405.
47. Horning, S. J., Galila, N., Cleary, M., and Sklar, J. (1990) Detection of non-Hodgkin's lymphoma in the peripheral blood by analysis of the antigen receptor gene rearrangements: results of a prospective trial. *Blood* **75,** 1139–1145.
48. Summers, K. E., Davies, A. J., Matthews, J., Jenner, M. J., Cornelius, V., Amess, J. A., et al. (2002) The relative role of peripheral blood and bone marrow for monitoring molecular evidence of disease in follicular lymphoma by quantitative real-time polymerase chain reaction. *Br. J. Haematol.* **118,** 563–566.
49. Gribben, J. G., Neuberg, D., Barber, M., Moore, J., Pesek, K. W., Freedman, A. S., et al. (1994) Detection of residual lymphoma cells by polymerase chain reaction in peripheral blood is significantly less predictive for relapse than detection in bone marrow. *Blood* **83,** 3800–3807.
50. Freedman, A. S., Neuberg, D., Mauch, P., Soiffer, R. J., Anderson, K. C., Fisher, D. C., et al. (1999) Long-term follow-up of autologous bone marrow transplantation in patients with relapsed follicular lymphoma. *Blood* **94,** 3325–3333.
51. Gribben, J. G., Neuberg, D., Freedman, A. S., Gimmi, C. D., Pesek, K. W., Barber, M., et al (1993) Detection by polymerase chain reaction of residual cells with the bcl-2 translocation is associated with increased risk of relapse after autologous bone marrow transplantation for B-cell lymphoma. *Blood* **81,** 3449–3457.

52. Corradini, P., Astolfi, M., Cherasco, C., Ladetto, M., Voena, C., Caracciolo, D., et al. (1997) Molecular monitoring of minimal residual disease in follicular and mantle cell non-Hodgkin's lymphomas treated with high dose chemotherapy and peripheral blood progenitor cell autografting. *Blood* **89,** 724–731.
53. Corradini, P., Ladetto, M., Pileri, A., and Tarella, C. (1999) Clinical relevance of minimal residual disease monitoring in non-Hodgkin's lymphomas: a critical reappraisal of molecular strategies. *Leukemia* **13,** 1691–1695.
54. Moos, M., Schulz, R., Martin, S., Benner, A., and Haas, R. (1998) The remission status before and the PCR status after high-dose therapy with peripheral blood stem cell support are prognostic factors for relapse-free survival in patients with follicular non-Hodgkin's lymphoma. *Leukemia* **12,** 1971–1976.
55. Apostolidis, J., Gupta, R. K., Grenzelias, D., Johnson, P. W., Pappa, V. I., Summers, K. E., et al. (2000) High-dose therapy with autologous bone marrow support as consolidation of remission in follicular lymphoma: long-term clinical and molecular follow-up. *J. Clin. Oncol.* **18,** 527–536.
56. Bendandi, M., Gocke, C. D., Kobrin, C. B., Benko, F. A., Sternas, L. A., Pennington, R., et al. (1999) Complete molecular remissions induced by patient-specific vaccination plus granulocyte-monocyte colony-stimulating factor against lymphoma. *Nat. Med.* **5,** 1171–1177.
57. Czuczman, M. S., Grillo-Lopez, A. J., White, C. A., Saleh, M., Gordon, L., LoBuglio, A. F., et al. (1999) Treatment of patients with low-grade B-cell lymphoma with the combination of chimeric anti-CD20 monoclonal antibody and CHOP chemotherapy. *J. Clin. Oncol.* **17,** 268–276.
58. Roberts, W. M., Estrov, Z., Ouspenskaia, M. V., Johnston, D. A., McClain, K. L., and Zipf, T. F. (1997) Measurement of residual leukemia during remission in childhood acute lymphoblastic leukemia [see comments]. *N. Engl. J. Med.* **336,** 317–323.
59. Nucifora, G., Larson, R. A., and Rowley, J. D. (1993) Persistence of the 8;21 translocation in patients with acute myeloid leukemia type M2 in long-term remission. *Blood* **82,** 712–715.
60. Dolken, L., Schuler, F., and Dolken, G. (1998) Quantitative detection of t(14;18)-positive cells by real-time quantitative PCR using fluorogenic probes. *Biotechniques* **25,** 1058–1064.
61. Ladetto, M., Donovan, J. W., Harig, S., Trojan, A., Poor, C., Schlossnan, R., et al. (2000) Real-time polymerase chain reaction of immunoglobulin rearrangements for quantitative evaluation of minimal residual disease in multiple myeloma. *Biol. Blood Marrow Transplant* **6,** 241–253.
62. Jenner, M. J., Summers, K. E., Norton, A. J., Amess, J. A., Arch, R. S., Young, B. D., et al. (2002) JH probe real-time quantitative polymerase chain reaction assay for Bcl-2/IgH rearrangements. *Br. J. Haematol.* **118,** 550–558.
63. Pongers-Willemse, M. J., Verhagen, O. J., Tibbe, G. J., Wijkhuijs, A. J., de Haas, V., Roovers, E., et al. (1998) Real-time quantitative PCR for the detection of minimal residual disease in acute lymphoblastic leukemia using junctional region specific TaqMan probes. *Leukemia* **12,** 2006–2014.

64. Donovan, J. W., Ladetto, M., Zou, G., Neuberg, D., Poor, C., Bowers, D., et al. (2000) Immunoglobulin heavy-chain consensus probes for real-time PCR quantification of residual disease in acute lymphoblastic leukemia. *Blood* **95,** 2651–2658.
65. Summers, K. E., Goff, L. K., Wilson, A. G., Gupta, R. K., Lister, T. A., Fitzgibbon, J. (2001) Frequency of the Bcl-2/IgH rearrangement in normal individuals: implications for the monitoring of disease in patients with follicular lymphoma. *J. Clinical Oncology* **19,** 420–424.
66. Overbergh, L., Giulietti, A., Valckx, D., Decallonne, R., Bouillon, R., Mathieu, C. (2003) The use of real-time reverse transcriptase PCR for the quantification of cytokine gene expression. *J. Biomolecular Techniques* **14,** 33–43.
67. Real-time PCR. http://dorakmt.tripod.com/genetics/realtime.html. Date accessed: January 1, 2005.
68. Estalilla, O. C., Medeiros, L. J., Manning, J. T., Jr., Luthra, R. (2000) 5'→3' exonuclease-based real-time PCR assays for detecting the t(14;18)(q32;21): a survey of 162 malignant lymphomas and reactive specimens. *Mod. Pathol.* **13,** 661–666.
69. Applied Biosystems. http://www.appliedbiosystems.com. Date accessed: January 1, 2005.

Index

G

Kolibri 360 GmbH
Ferdinand-Jühlke-Straße 7
99095 Erfurt, Deutschland
produktsicherheit@kolibri360.de